EPH-Gestosis

Diagnose und Resultate

3. Meeting der Organisation Gestose, 23.–25. Oktober 1970, Paris
4. Meeting der Organisation Gestose, 8.–10. Oktober 1971, Florenz

Herausgegeben von
E. T. Rippmann und *Ch. Rippert*
O.G., Organisation Gestose, Aarau/Schweiz

Mit 200 Abbildungen und
100 Tabellen

1972

Walter de Gruyter · Berlin · New York

ISBN 3 11 004022 0

Satz: IBM Composer Walter de Gruyter & Co., Berlin – Druck: Mercedes-Druck, Berlin 61 – Printed in Germany.

Umschlag: Thomas Bonnie, Hamburg

Vorwort

Die ORGANISATION GESTOSE (O.G.) legt ihren 1. Kongreßband vor. Er umfaßt die Vorträge, Diskussionsbeiträge, sowie die Berichte der Studiengruppen des 3. und 4. Meetings in Paris, 1970 und Florenz, 1971. Damit erfährt der 1970 erschienene Band „Die Spätgestose (EPH-Gestose)"* die erwartete Fortsetzung.

Die O.G. hat die sich anläßlich des 1969 in Basel abgehaltenen Symposiums über die EPH-Gestose gestellten Aufgaben in Angriff genommen. Je mehr die Arbeit voranschreitet, desto besser erkennen wir das große Ausmaß der Probleme, die auf uns warten. Die EPH-Gestose ist nicht länger ein isoliertes, klinik-intern zu behandelndes Krankheitsbild. Die Fragestellung nach Ursachen, kausaler Behandlung, Prophylaxe, nach immediater und später Folge muß mit Spezialisten der medizinischen und paramedizinischen Fachgebiete diskutiert werden. Wir benötigen ihre Kenntnisse, ihre diagnostischen und therapeutischen Möglichkeiten. Die Zusammenarbeit auf interdisziplinärem Gebiet im internationalen Rahmen hat in der Bildung der Studiengruppen über die Spezialgebiete der EPH-Gestose in Florenz ihren vielversprechenden Anfang genommen.

In Aarau soll im Jahre 1972 die Zusammenarbeit intensiviert werden. Damit sollen neue Impulse für weitere Ausbreitung der Forschung auf der Basis allgemein akzeptierter, grundlegender Parameter gesetzt werden.

Oktober 1972

O.G.
Organisation Gestose
E. T. Rippmann
Ch. Rippert

* Die Spätgestose (EPH-Gestose)
Internationales Symposium an der Universitäts-Frauenklinik Basel, April 1969. Herausgeber: Dr. *E. T. Rippmann* (Schwabe & Co. Basel, 1970).

Inhalt

Das Signet der Organisation Gestose (O. G.)

E. T. Rippmann

Die Vereinheitlichung der Parameter und Definitionen der EPH-Gestose ist die Grundlage für die Vergleichbarkeit von Forschungsresultaten.

Die Vereinheitlichung der Nomenklatur (a) und der Klassifikation (b) führt uns zur Definition der Cardinalsymptome E, P und H, sowie der Fälle von EPH-Gestose, die primär ohne Cardinalsymptome auftreten (c). Aus den Symptomen ergibt sich die Diagnose und die Beurteilung der Schwere der Erkrankung durch den Gestose Index (GI) (d). Eine fehlende Diagnostik, die daher ungenügende Therapie bedeuten eine große Gefahr für Mutter und Kind. Zunehmende Verfeinerung diagnostischer Maßnahmen ermöglicht eine causale Therapie und reduziert die perinatale mütterliche und kindliche Morbidität und Mortalität (e). Durch solche vorangetriebene Maßnahmen hoffen wir, Ursachen der EPH-Gestose abgrenzen zu können (f). Sechs Faktoren helfen uns in unseren Bemühungen um eine ungestörte Schwangerschaft (g):

1. Beratung vor der Heirat (premarital counceling).
2. Gesundenuntersuchungen in Hinblick auf eine zu erwartende Schwangerschaft.
3. Abklärung und Behandlung von vorbestehenden Krankheiten vor der Schwangerschaft oder im schwangerschaftsfreien Interval.
4. Frühe Erfassung der EPH-Gestose.
5. Gewissenhafte Führung durch die gefährdete Schwangerschaft.
6. Kausale Therapie.

Eine solche Prophylaxe, getragen von den erwähnten Maßnahmen, ist anzustreben (h). Die Organisation Gestose (O.G.) möchte alle Bemühungen auf dem Gebiete der EPH-Gestose koordinieren und fördern und damit zu Erfolg und Fortschritt führen.

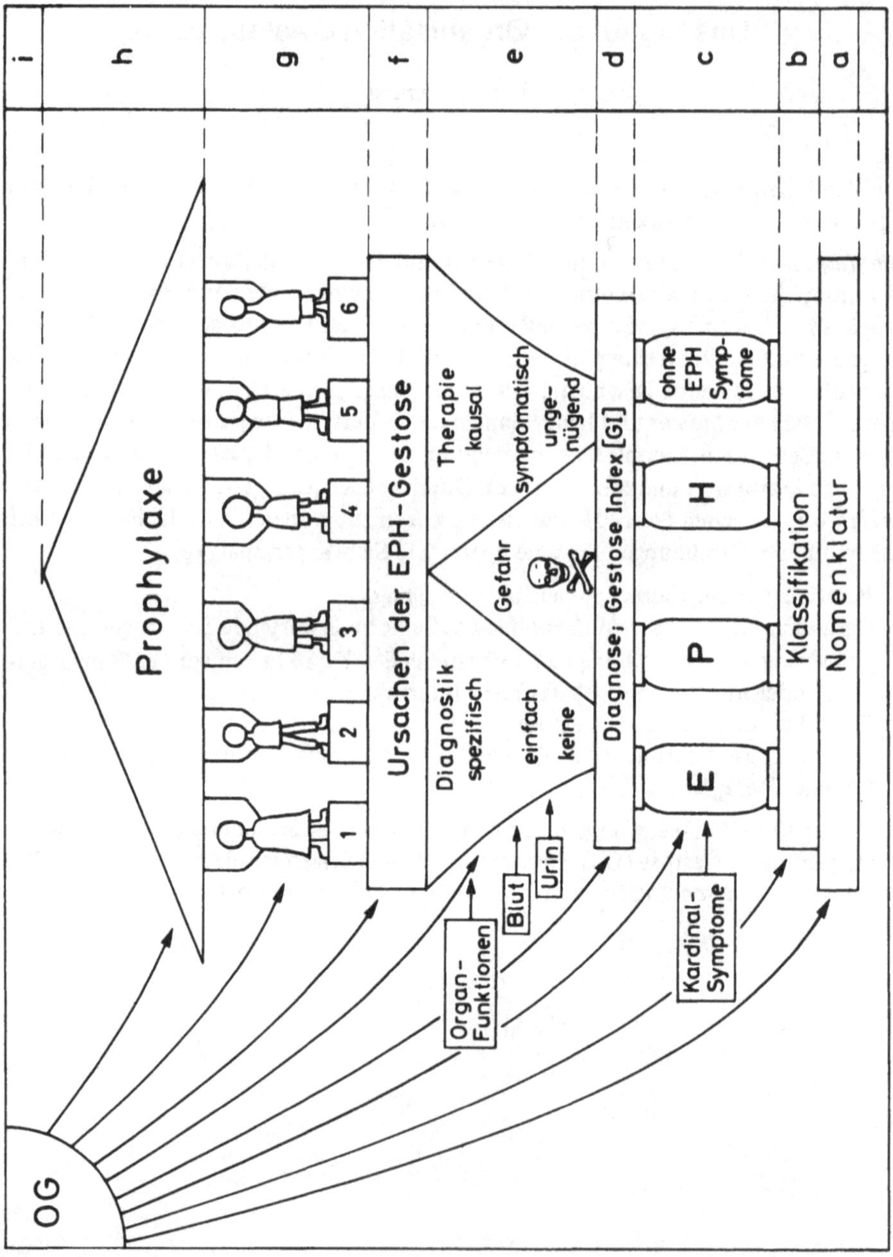
i
h
g
f
e
d
c
b
a
OG
Prophylaxe
1
2
3
4
5
6
Ursachen der EPH-Gestose
Diagnostik
spezifisch
einfach
keine
Gefahr
Therapie
kausal
symptomatisch
unge-
nügend
Diagnose; Gestose Index [GI]
E
P
H
ohne
EPH
Symp-
tome
Klassifikation
Nomenklatur
Organ-
Funktionen
Blut
Urin
Kardinal-
Symptome

Greetings to the Members of The Organisation Gestosis

G. W. Theobald

Hon. Research Fellow, U.C.H. Obstetric Hospital, London, W.C.1.,
Ex Assistant Master, The Rotunde Hospital, Dublin,
Late Consultant Obstetrician and Gynaecologist to St. Luke's Maternity Hospital and the Royal Infirmary, Bradford,
Formerly Professor of Obstetrics and Gynaecology, The Chulalongkorn University, Bangkok, Siam

I remember with very great pleasure my visit to Lausanne when I had the privilege of meeting so many members of the Organisation Gestosis. I only wish that such a Society had existed years ago and should like to wish the members the best of good fortune in their future research programmes. I would like, however, to suggest that in their search for new facts they do not neglect what has already been learned in the fight to save both mothers and babies. Obstetricians are not quite such fools as some think: they have recognized and obviated retrolental fibroplasia; they have virtually abolished puerperal sepsis; they have not only recognized the Rhesus factor but have learned to treat affected babies and may in time abolish the condition; they have reduced maternal mortality almost to zero and infant mortality from about 400 to about 30 per thousand; and they have learned to prevent both eclampsia and imminent eclampsia.

Many would agree that *all* the "pregnancy toxaemias" represent a breakdown in one or more of the maternal homeostatic mechanisms, and that in the majority of the cases occurring in Europe the woman starts pregnancy with pre-existing defects, such as renal disease, "essential" hypertension, or hypoplasia of the arterial tree. All that can be done is to improve the woman's nutrition and afford her rest in bed. Rest in bed is another form of nutrition for it makes possible the flow of a higher fraction of her blood through the placenta.

The abolition of all maternal mortality from "toxaemia" as well as of both eclampsia and imminent eclampsia, therefore, depends on persuading *all* general practitioners to send *all* patients who have a blood pressure of or exceeding 140/90 mm. Hg, proteinuria, severe oedema and *sudden* weight gain for observation and rest in hospital. These cases *must* be accepted. This may necessitate sending normal patients home 48 hours after the baby is born and thereby make it possible to increase antenatal beds at the expense of lying-in beds. Further, it is important to induce labour in all women with hypertension, with or without proteinuria, once they reach Term minus 14 days. This short communication no doubt appears dogmatic but this seemed the only way to keep it short. I verily believe that the implementation of these ideas could save many maternal and foetal lives without the necessity for a single hour's research.

E

Weight Gain/Watermetabolism

Weight Gain During Pregnancy

J. C. McClure Browne

Institute of Obstetrics and Gynecology, Hammersmith Hospital, London

In recent years, because of the extremely low figures for maternal mortality, it has been possible to direct more and more attention to perinatal mortality. From a pathological point of view the major causes of perinatal loss today are asphyxia and prematurity. In my own Department in 1969 there were 1916 deliveries with 60 perinatal deaths, a perinatal mortality rate of 31.8 per 1000. The commonest causes of perinatal death were asphyxia: 17 out of 60, and prematurity: 16 out of 60 deaths. The commonest clinical associations with asphyxial death were pre-eclamptic toxaemia (41%) and prolonged pregnancy (29.7%). The clinician knows well that in these cases the foetus may be small for dates with increased risk of respiratory distress syndrome and of handicap in later life, or it may become distressed in labour or may even die in utero before labour begins. In such cases there is a typical postmortem appearance, the foetus being small for dates, thin and undernourished with little body fat and the cord and membranes may be stained with meconium. The small for dates syndrome is seen in prolonged pregnancy, essential hypertension and what I call "the hypertensive diathesis". In pre-eclampsia the syndrome is seen only if there is underlying essential hypertension. It has been well documented that urinary oestriol excretion gives an indication of foetal wellbeing and that there is a close correlation between liquor volume and placental function. It is also possible to detect foetal growth failure by means of ultrasonic measurements. These methods however are sophisticated and are not widely available.

Although for many years it has been customary to associate water retention, excessive weight gain and pre-eclamptic toxaemia, little attention has been paid to poor weight gain or weight loss. Yet if there is intra-uterine death there is maternal loss of weight and it is clear that a pregnancy which is progressing well shows a steady maternal weight gain.

For a long time I have been convinced that failure to gain weight or even loss of weight is of ill omen and more recently other writers have agreed with me. In a controlled group studied from January 1966 to June 1968 we found that the overall incidence of small for dates was 10.4% of all deliveries. The small for dates group showed a smaller weight gain up to 34 weeks and from 34 weeks onwards this was more marked. The mean weight gain from 34 weeks until delivery in the small for dates groups was 0.18 kg per week compared with 0.31 kg per week in the control group.

In the small for dates group static or diminishing weight was three times as common as in the control group.

From 34 weeks onwards changes in maternal girth were also highly significant. Those women giving birth to small for dates babies showed a 77% incidence of static or decreasing girth, while in the control series only 48% showed such features. When static or decreasing weight and girth were examined there was a highly significant association between these features and the incidence of small for dates babies. Moreover in labour foetal distress occurred four times more often in the small for dates babies. The highest incidence of foetal distress occured (23%) in those women whose weight and girth tended to decrease in the last six weeks of pregnancy. This compared with 8% in controls. In hypertension static or diminishing weight and girth were highly indicative of small for dates babies. In a series of 54 cases of essential hypertension weight and girth were found to be increasing in 33 and no small for dates babies were born. In 21, however, weight and girth were static or diminishing and in this group 11 small for dates babies (51%) were born. The incidence of foetal distress in labour was also significantly increased in those cases where weight and girth were static or diminishing.

It is clear then that static or diminishing weight and girth are strongly suggestive of foetal malnutrition and of foetal distress in labour. It is interesting that oestriol excretion, weight and girth seem to correlate quite closely.

In cases of EPH-gestosis again static or diminishing weight appeared to be indicative of probable small for dates or dysmature babies. A gestosis index of more than 2.5 showed a doubled incidence of dysmaturity but this association was not nearly so strong as that of static or decreasing weight and girth with dysmaturity.

Definition of the Sign E, P and H

J. C. McClure Browne

Institute of Obstetrics and Gynecology, Hammersmith Hospital, London

E: Edema Discussion

The definition of edema should include only clinical pitting edema, the pitting being most apparent in the region of the heels, on the subcutancous surface of the tibia. It is also evidenced by swelling of the hands with tightness of the rings, and puffiness of the face, especially around the eyes. The earliest evidence of edema of the face is disappearance of the minute wrinkles which surround the eyes and give expression to the face. The disappearance of these wrinkles leaves the woman with the appearance of having applied too much cosmetic in order to mask these skin-changes.

Excess weight gain should not be automatically considered an indicator of edema. While excessive gain in weight *may* be due to edema it is most commonly due to over-eating. It may on the other hand be due to the presence of a multiple pregnancy or sometimes hydramnios. Nevertheless it may be in retrospect the first sign of the onset of pre-eclampsia which has later become clinically manifest.

In deciding whether weight gain is in fact excessive, it is important that the gain in weight during pregnancy be related to the weight before the pregnancy began. In the first trimester there is often some decrease in weight because of nausea or vomiting and when this passes off there may be an apparently very rapid gain in weight which is in fact only due to return of the body fluids to normal. In the third trimester (when gestosis commonly occurs) the average normal weight gain is 450g/week.

In my opinion it is unwise to specify that if the edema persists after only one night's bed rest (as suggested in the circulated definition), it is considered to be clinically significant of gestosis. In my experience the pregnant woman undergoes a diuresis lasting for the first 48 hours after she is put to bed and clinical estimates of edema before this time has elapsed may be misleading. It has been my practice for some years to record at the first antenatal visit the woman's statement about her weight before pregnancy. Most women today are very weight-conscious and can give fairly accurate figures about it.

A further point worthy of note is that as excessive weight gain in the pregnant woman has several causes it is useless to wait until it occurs and only then to advise dietary restriction, to see whether in fact the excessive gain has been due to over-eating. To find this out at this stage will take two vital weeks and the informative value that excessive weight gain may have as an early warning of EPH-gestosis will be lost. I think that every woman should be advised at her first antenatal visit as to the diet that she should take, the emphasis being on high protein with low carbohydrate and relatively low fat, and whenever she is seen at later visits she should be exhorted to follow this plan. In this way an excessive weight gain, if it is observed, is much more likely to be due to fluid retention and to give early warning of impending EPH-gestosis. Many of the most severe cases of edema, often occurring in a matter of hours in a woman heavily sedated because of impending eclampsia develop during a period when there is absolutely no fluid intake and when no increase in weight can occur. This must imply a transference of fluid from the intracellular to the extracellular compartment. Failure to gain weight, or loss of weight, in the absence of an overt cause such as gastro-intestinal disturbance, is of grave significance for the foetus, but seems to have but little direct significance for the mother.

Materne Gewichtszunahme, Kindliches Geburtsgewicht, Perinatale Prognose: Durch welche Faktoren beeinflußt?

L. Tervilä

Stadtkrankenhaus, Lathi, Finnland

Als durchschnittliche Gewichtszunahme der Mutter während der Schwangerschaft kann man im allgemeinen etwa 11% ihres gewöhnlichen Körpergewichts annehmen. Dieser Wert schwankt jedoch beträchtlich von Fall zu Fall. Je nach Größe der Frucht, Größe der Plazenta und Flüssigkeitsretention in den mütterlichen Geweben. Im folgenden wird der Einfluß gewisser Faktoren auf die Gewichtszunahme der Mutter, die Korrelation dieser Gewichtszunahme mit dem Geburtsgewicht des Kindes und weiter mit der kindlichen Prognose untersucht.

Das Material bilden 3249 aufeinanderfolgende Geburten im Hebammeninstitut von Helsinki. Um den Einfluß des Alters zu ermitteln, wurden die Gebärenden in unter und über 30-jährige eingeteilt (Tab. 1). Man sieht, daß keine Korrelation zwischen Alter und Gewichtszunahme besteht; die Gewichtsdifferenz ist statistisch nicht signifikant. Die durchschnittliche Gewichtszunahme der Mütter während der Gravidität war im ganzen Material 11998 g und das durchschnittliche Gewicht der Kinder 3504 g. Auch im Gewicht der Kinder besteht kein statistisch signifikanter Unterschied.

Tab. 1. Smoothed mean increase in maternal body weight during pregnancy, its difference from the total mean for the series, smoothed mean birthweight of the children, and its difference from the total mean, in relation to the age of the mother.

Age		-29 years			30- years				
No. of Cases	Maternal Weight Increase, gm	Difference from Mean, gm	Mean Birthweight, gm	Difference from Mean, gm	No. of Cases	Maternal Weight Increase, gm	Difference from Mean, gm	Mean Birthweight, gm	Difference from Mean, gm
2.479	12.036	+ 38	3.494	- 10	767	11.776	- 222	3.524	+ 20

Um den Einfluß der Parität zu klären, haben wir die Patientinnen in Erst- und Mehrgebärende eingeteilt (Tab. 2). Die Gewichtszunahme der Mütter wies auch bei dieser Gruppierung keine signifikante Differenz auf. Im Geburtsgewicht der Kinder dagegen stellte sich wieder die altbekannte Tatsache heraus, daß das Gewicht der Frucht mit zunehmender Geburtenzahl ansteigt.

Tab. 2. Smoothed mean increase in maternal body weight during pregnancy, its difference from the total mean for the series, smoothed mean birthweight of the children, and its difference from the total mean, in relation to the parity of the mother.

Parity	Primiparae				Multiparae				
No. of Cases	Maternal Weight Increase, gm	Difference from Mean, gm	Mean Birthweight, gm	Difference from Mean, gm	No. of Cases	Maternal Weight Increase, gm	Difference from Mean, gm	Mean Birthweight, gm	Difference from Mean, gm
1.574	12.321	+ 323	3.420	- 84	1.675	11.753	- 245	3.598	+ 94

Mit Hilfe der Varianzanalyse wurde eine sehr große Signifikanz bezüglich Einfluß der mütterlichen Konstitution auf diese Faktoren erhalten (Tab. 3). Die Gebärenden wurden in Gruppen mit unter und über 160 cm Körperlänge sowie mit 55, 56–65 und über 66 kg Körpergewicht eingeteilt. Ein signifikanter Unterschied läßt sich sowohl in der Gewichtszunahme der Mütter als auch im Geburtsgewicht der Kinder nachweisen. Bei langen Frauen ist die Gewichtszunahme größer als bei kleinen, und bei schlanken größer als bei korpulenten.

Tab. 3. Smoothed mean increase in maternal body weight during pregnancy, its difference from the total mean for the series, smoothed mean birthweight of the children, and its difference from the total mean, in relation to the height and weight of the mother.

Height	–159 cm					160– cm				
Pregravid Maternal Weight, kg	No. of Cases	Maternal Weight Increases, gm	Difference from Mean, gm	Mean Birthweight, gm	Difference from Mean, gm	No. of Weight, gm	Maternal Weight Increases, gm	Difference from Mean, gm	Mean Birthweight, gm	Difference from Mean, gm
–55	557	11.578	- 420	3.317	- 187	694	12.858	+ 860	3.462	- 42
56–65	293	10.898	- 1100	3.474	- 30	1.242	11.994	- 4	3.548	+ 44
66–	54	9.778	- 2200	3.627	+ 123	409	12.020	+ 22	3.680	+ 176

Die Geburtsgewichte der Kinder sind direkt proportional sowohl zur Körperlänge wie zum Körpergewicht der Mütter. Die Analyse läßt jedoch nicht erkennen, ob das Körpergewicht oder die Körperlänge der Mutter mit größerer Signifikanz mit dem Geburtsgewicht der Kinder korreliert.

Für die Untersuchung des Einflusses der Toxämie auf die Gewichtszunahme der Mütter wurden die Gebärenden den Teilfaktoren der Toxämie gemäß in Gruppen eingeteilt, wie aus Tab. 4 ersichtlich ist.

Tab. 4. Smoothed weight increase in maternal body weight in each toxaemia symptom and Symptom combination group and its difference from the total mean, and from the control group.

Symptom	No. of Parturients	Mean Body Weight Increase, gm	Difference from Mean, gm	Difference from Control Group, gm
1. Controls	1.435	10,990	- 1.008	0
2. Oedema	1.118	13,220	+ 1.222	+ 2.230
3. Proteinuria	145	10,680	- 1.318	- 0.096
4. Hypertension	77	12,000	+ 0.002	+ 1.010
5. Oedema + proteinuria	184	13,080	+ 1.082	+ 2.090
6. Oedema + hypertension	111	14,210	+ 2.212	+ 3.220
7. Proteinuria + hypertension	52	11,230	- 0.768	+ 0.240
8. Oedema + proteinuria + hypertension	98	14,980	+ 2.982	+ 3.990
Total	3.220[1]	Mean 11.998		

[1] Body weight increase of 21 parturients not known.

Man sieht, daß in all denjenigen Gruppen, in denen das Krankheitsbild mit Ödem einhergeht, die Mütter höheres Körpergewicht als durchschnittlich aufwiesen. In den anderen Gruppen war durchschnittliche oder geringere Gewichtszunahme zu vermerken.

Die Geburtsgewichte der Kinder in den verschiedenen Toxämiegruppen sind in Tab. 5 zusammengestellt, wo der früher festgestellte Einfluß der Geburtenzahl eliminiert ist.

Tab. 5. Mean birthweight of children in each toxaemia symptom and symptom combination group after elimination of effect of parity.

Symptom	No. of Parturients	Mean Birthweight, gm	Difference from Mean Birthweight of Total Series, gm
1. Controls	1.453	3.441	- 63
2. Oedema	1.130	3.578	+ 74
3. Proteinuria	144	3.511	+ 7
4. Hypertension	80	3.437	- 67
5. Oedema + proteinuria	173	3.578	+ 74
6. Oedema + hypertension	113	3.500	- 4
7. Proteinuria + hypertension	53	3.375	- 129
8. Oedema + proteinuria + hypertension	103	3.580	+ 76
Total	3.249	Mean 3.504 birthweight	

Statistisch signifikant schwerer sind die Kinder in den Gruppen ödematöser Frauen. Andererseits sind die Geburtsgewichte in den Gruppen mit Hypertonie ohne Ödem signifikant kleiner als durchschnittlich. Obwohl die Proteinurie an sich keinen Einfluß auf das Gewicht der Kinder zu haben schien, verminderte sie zusammen mit der Hypertonie deutlich das Geburtsgewicht.

Die obigen Resultate brachten uns auf den Gedanken, die Kinder der ödematösen Mütter könnten vielleicht eine erhöhte Flüssigkeitsretention haben. Aus diesem Grunde untersuchten wir 1127 nacheinander geborene Kinder bezüglich des Gewichtsverlustes und der Flüssigkeitsaufnahme in den fünf ersten Lebenstagen. Nicht berücksichtigt blieben alle Kinder, deren Mütter Proteinurie oder Hypertonie aufgewiesen hatten, alle Mehrlingsgeburten soeie die Kinder unter 2500 g Geburtsgewicht. Die Ödempatientinnen wurden außerdem noch aufgeteilt in eine Gruppe mit vorgängiger Diuretikabehandlung und ohne Behandlung.

Die Ergebnisse sind aus Tab. 6 ersichtlich. Weder bezüglich Gewichtsverlust noch Flüssigkeitsbedarf bestehen signifikante Unterschiede zwischen den verschiedenen Gruppen. Daraus läßt sich der Schluß ziehen, daß die Kinder der ödematösen Mütter tatsächlich schwerer sind und nicht etwa eine Flüssigkeitsretention in Frage kommt.

Tab. 6. Weight loss and fluid intake per gram of birthweight during 4–5 postnatal days of children of gravidas with untreated oedema or oedema treated with diuretics, compared with non-oedematous gravidas.

Birthweight, gm	Controls		Untreated Oedema		Treated with Diuretics	
	Weight Loss, gm	Fluid Intake, gm	Weight Loss, gm	Fluid Intake, gm	Weight Loss, gm	Fluid Intake, gm
2500–3000	0.19	0.13	0.21	0.14	0.19	0.13
3010–3500	0.17	0.12	0.18	0.11	0.17	0.11
3510–4000	0.16	0.10	0.16	0.10	0.16	0.10
4010–	0.16	0.09	0.15	0.09	0.16	0.10

Überprüft man schließlich die perinatale Mortalität in den verschiedenen Toxämiegruppen (Tab. 7), lassen sich mehrere Übereinstimmungen in den Beobachtungen über das Gewicht der Kinder feststellen. Die Mortalitätszahlen für Ödemgruppe und Kontrollgruppe sind genau gleich. Die Proteinurie erhöhte die Mortalität leicht; die deutlich höchste Sterblichkeit wurde in der Hypertoniegruppe verzeichnet. Auch waren bei polysymptomatischer Gestose mit Hypertoniebeteiligung die Mortalitätszahlen höher. Die Beteiligung von Ödem schien die Sterblichkeit zu vermindern.

Tab. 7. Distribution of cases into toxaemia groups according to single symptoms and symptom combinations, and number and incidence of perinatal deaths in each group.

Symptoms	Total No. of Cases	Total No. of Deaths	Perinatal Mortality Rate
Controls	1473	20	1.4
Oedema	1147	17	1.5
Proteinuria	151	7	4.6
Hypertension	88	8	9.1
Oedema + proteinuria	181	8	4.4
Oedema + hypertension	122	9	7.4
Proteinuria + hypertension	59	6	10.2
Oedema + hypertension + proteinuria	115	12	10.4
Total	3336	87	

Der Anteil der Frühgeburten scheint ganz ähnlich zu korrelieren (Tab. 8). Die Kontrollgruppe, die Ödemgruppe und die Proteinuriegruppe verhalten sich annähernd gleich. In der Hypertoniegruppe sind am meisten Frühgeburten zu beobachten; während die Beteiligung von Ödem diese Frequenz verminderte. Diese Tabelle ist deshalb bedeutsam, weil die Mortalität der Frühgeburten einen so großen und von Jahr zu Jahr relativ immer größer werdenden Teil von der Kindersterblichkeit im Laufe des ersten Lebensjahres ausmacht.

Tab. 8. Distribution of cases into toxaemia groups according to single symptoms and symptom combinations, and number and incidence of underweight children and their mortality in each group.

Symptoms	Notal No. of Cases	Birth Weight 650–2500 g			
		No. of Births	Incidence of Births	No. of Deaths	Incidence of Deaths
Controls	1473	85	5.8	16	1.1
Oedema	1147	37	3.2	10	0.9
Proteinuria	151	6	4.0	3	2.0
Hypertension	88	11	12.5	5	5.7
Oedema + proteinuria	181	7	3.9	1	0.6
Oedema + hypertension	122	8	6.5	6	4.9
Proteinuria + hypertension	59	8	13.6	5	8.5
Oedema + hypertension + proteinuria	115	18	15.7	10	8.9
Total	3336	680		56	

Es hat also den Anschein, daß starke Gewichtszunahme der Mutter während der Schwangerschaft und manifestes Ödem die kindliche Prognose verbessern. Vielleicht ist das Ödem das Erscheinungsbild einer Abwehrreaktion des Organismus gegen die schwerere Form der Toxämie, gegen die Hypertonie.

References

Tervilä, L. u. *E. Krokfors:* Do Age and Parity influence the Nature of Toxaemia? Ann. Chir. & Gyn. Fenn. 54 (1965) S. 355.

Krokfors, E. u. *L. Tervilä:* Correlation of the Standard of Living to the Nature of Toxaemia of late Pregnancy. Ann. Chir. & Gyn. Fenn. 55 (1966) S. 219–226.

Krokfors, E. u. *L. Tervilä:* Influence of the Maternal Constitution on the Nature of Toxaemia of late Pregnancy. Ann. Chir. & Gyn. Fenn. 55 (1966) S. 227–232.

Krokfors, E. u. *L. Tervilä:* Correlation of the Nature of Toxaemia of late Pregnancy to the Birthweight of the Child and to Maternal Weight Increase during Pregnancy. Ann. Chir. & Gyn. Fenn. 55 (1966) S. 289–295.

Tervilä, L. u. *E. Krokfors:* Correlation of Nature of Toxaemia of Pregnancy to Perinatal Mortality and Underweight of Newborn. Ann. Chir. & Gyn. Fenn. 55 (1966) S. 109–111.

Tervilä, L. u. *E. Krokfors:* Oedema Matris et Fetus. Ann. Chir. & Gyn. Fenn. 55 (1966) S. 69–71.

Weight Gain in Pregnancy

B. Vedra, E. Pavlikova

Institute for Care of Mother and Child, Prague–Podoli, CSSR

The weight gain in pregnancy can be estimated in two ways:

1. as the difference between the weight *actually measured* and the *unreliable figure of the prepregnant weight* given by the pregnant woman. The exactness of such an estimate depends on the reliability of the memory and on the knowledge of the patient. The weight gain is given in *kg since the beginning of pregnancy.*
2. as a difference of the weights actually measured at two occasions in pregnancy. The exactness of this figure depends only on the exactness of the measurements. It is not dependent on the memory of the patient. The difference of two actually measured weights divided by the number of days between the two occasions gives the daily nett weight gain.

Weight increase in kg since the begin of pregnancy

Table 1 gives the data of the weight increases in 5 weeks intervals in normal pregnancy

Tab. 1. Weight gain in pregnancy.

Week	n	$\bar{x}$	s	Range of weight gains $\bar{x} \pm 1$ s	$\bar{x} \pm 2$ s	$\bar{x} \pm 3$ s
10 ± 2	89	1.6	2.8	- 1.2 to 4.4	- 4.0 to 7.2	- 6.8 to 10.0
15 ± 2	194	2.6	2.5	0.0 to 5.1	- 2.5 to 7.6	- 5.0 to 10.2
20 ± 2	267	4.6	2.9	1.8 to 7.5	- 1.1 to 10.3	- 4.0 to 13.2
25 ± 2	334	7.2	3.3	3.9 to 10.6	+ 0.6 to 13.9	- 2.7 to 17.2
30 ± 2	400	9.6	3.6	6.0 to 13.2	+ 2.4 to 16.8	- 1.2 to 20.4
35 ± 2	529	11.8	4.0	7.8 to 15.9	+ 3.7 to 19.9	- 0.3 to 23.9
40 - 2	441	13.4	4.3	9.1 to 17.6	+ 4.9 to 21.9	+ 0.6 to 26.2

Table 2 – EPH-gestosis

Tab. 2. Weight gain in normal pregnancy.

Week	n	$\bar{x}$	s	Range of weight gains $\bar{x} \pm 1$ s	$\bar{x} \pm 2$ s	$\bar{x} \pm 3$ s
10 ± 2	39	0.9	3.6	- 2.7 to + 4,4	- 6.3 to + 8.0	- 9.9 to 11.6
15 ± 2	105	2.1	2.5	- 0.4 to + 4.6	- 3.0 to + 7.1	- 5.5 to 9.6
20 ± 2	132	3.9	2.3	+ 1.5 to + 6.2	- 0.8 to + 8.6	- 3.2 to 10.9
25 ± 2	151	6.3	2.8	+ 3.5 to + 9.0	+ 0.7 to + 11.8	- 2.0 to 14.5
30 ± 2	162	7.9	2.8	+ 5.1 to + 10.8	+ 2.3 to + 13.6	- 0.5 to 16.4
35 ± 2	220	10.6	3.7	+ 7.0 to + 14.3	+ 3.3 to + 17.9	- 0.3 to 21.6
40 ± 2	209	11.9	3.7	+ 8.2 to + 15.7	+ 4.4 to + 19.4	+ 0.7 to 23.1

Table 3 – weight increases regardless whether the pregnant remained healthy or became gestotic.

Tab. 3. Weight gain in EPH-gestosis.

Week	n	$\bar{x}$	s	Range of weight gains $\bar{x} \pm 1$ s	$\bar{x} \pm 2$ s	$\bar{x} \pm 3$ s
10 ± 2	50	2.2	1.9	+ 0,3 to 4.1	- 1.6 to 6.0	- 3.5 to 7.9
15 ± 2	89	3.4	2.4	+ 1.0 to 5.8	- 1.4 to 8.2	- 3.8 to 10.5
20 ± 2	135	5.6	3.2	+ 2.4 to 8.7	- 0.8 to 11.9	- 4.0 to 15.1
25 ± 2	183	7.8	3.1	+ 4.7 to 10.9	+ 1.5 to 14.1	- 1.6 to 17.2
30 ± 2	238	10.6	3.5	+ 7.1 to 14.1	+ 3.5 to 17.7	+ 0.0 to 21.2
35 ± 2	309	12.7	3.2	+ 9.5 to 15.9	+ 6.4 to 19.1	+ 3.2 to 22.2
40 ± 2	232	14.7	4.6	+ 10.1 to 19.2	+ 5.5 to 23.8	+ 0.9 to 28.4

The tables are expressed as diagramms in Fig. 1, 2 and 3 respectively.

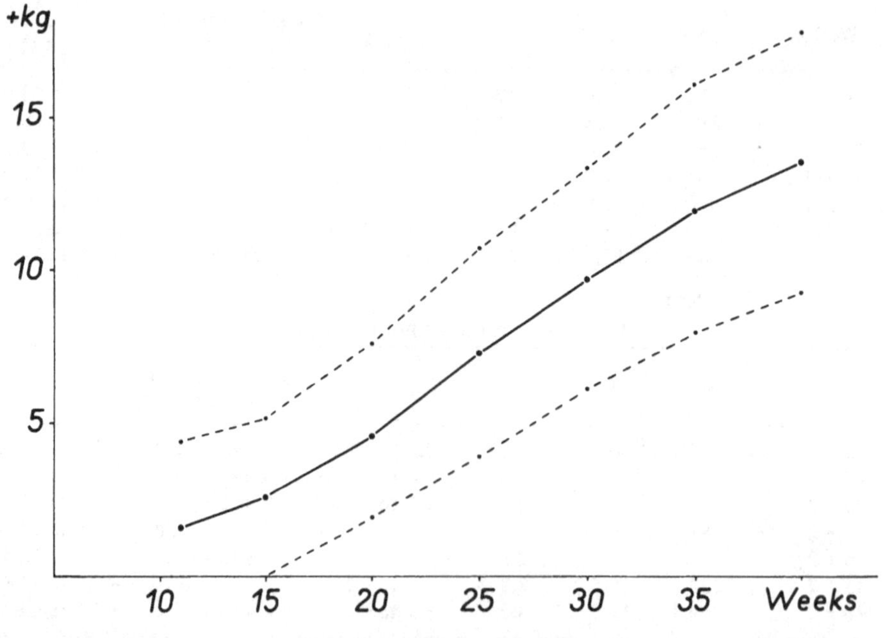

Fig. 1. Weight gain in pregnancy

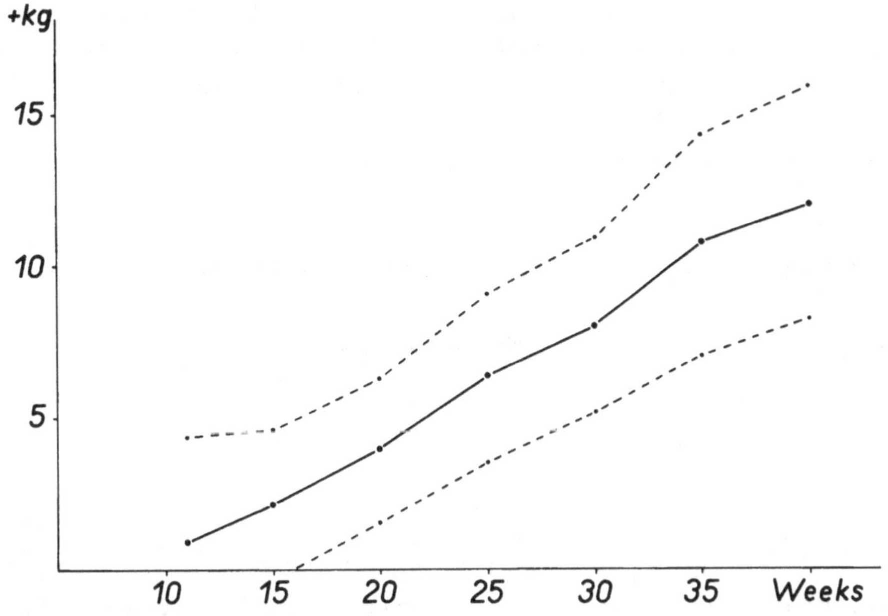

Fig. 2. Weight gain in normal pregnancy

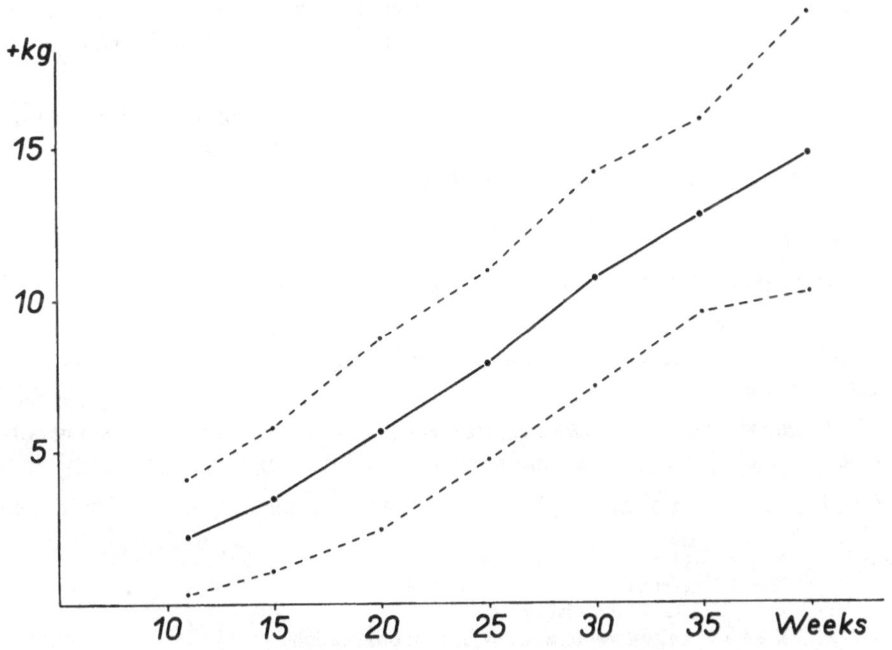

Fig. 3. Weight gain in EPH-gestosis

As can be seen from the tables, the range of weight gains both in normal and gestotic pregnancy is extremely broad and both groups cover themselves to a very great extent.

Statistically we can state that the greater the weight gain, the greater is the probability of the development of EPH-gestosis in the last months of pregnancy.

Individually, the value of this estimate is rather dubious.

The daily nett weight gain

The daily nett weight gains – average and range of individual observations – are given in Tab. 4.

Tab. 4. Daily weight gain g/24 hours.

	n = 463, s = 2.7		
$\bar{x}$	67,4		
$\bar{x} \pm 1$ s	45,7	–	89,1
$\bar{x} \pm 2$ s	24,0	–	110,8
$\bar{x} \pm 3$ s	2,3	–	132,5

It can be stated that the greater is the nett weight gain, the greater is the probability of the development of edema.

On Fig. No. 1, 2 and 3 we can see that the weight curves between the $10. \pm 2$ and $35. \pm 2$ week, or between the 13th and 37th week of pregnancy are almost linear. That means that the daily nett weight gain in this period of gestation is on the average constant.

The decline from the linearity at the 11th and 40th week is of minimal practical value and can be omitted. For practical purposes the beginning of the weight increase can be extrapolated approximately to the 10th week.

Remarks for the praxis

1. The measurement must be made exactly and under standard conditions.
2. The weight gain between the 10th and 24th week (calculated either as daily or weekly increase) should be the same as between the 24th week and any next occasion.
3. *The acceleration of the weight increase after the 24th week signalises some abnormality,* usually pathologic accumulation of interstitial fluid.
4. Graphical recording of the weight changes is recommended. A weight diagramme is

Remarks:
n	number of estimations
$\bar{x}$	average
s	standard deviation
$\bar{x} \pm 1$ s	enclose approximately 66% of observations
$\bar{x} \pm 2$ s	enclose approximately 95% of observations
$\bar{x} \pm 3$ s	enclose approximately 99% of observations

of pracitcal value if it is made precisely. A normal millimetre-paper should be used. At the horizontal line the time is recorded, 1 millimeter equal to 1 day. The first day of the horizontal line is the first day of the last menstruation. At the vertical line measured weights are plotted against the time, 1 millimeter equal to 0.10 kg. Zero is equal to the weight given by the patient.

The linearity of the weight curve after the 13th week (practically after the 10th) excludes pathologic retention of fluids.

Reference

Vedra, B., E. Pavlíková: J. Obstet. Gynaec. Brit. Cwlth. 76 (1969) S. 873.

Preclinical Detection of EPH-Gestosis

Maher Mahran, F.R.C.S., Ph.D. (Edin.) M.R.C.O.G.

Department of Obstetrics and Gynecology, Ain Shams University, Cairo, UAR

This work is the extension at Ain Shams University Cairo of an original work from Edinburgh University in collaboration with Department of Obstetrics and Medical Physics Unit.

There are two aspects of water metabolism: a static and a dynamic one. The static aspect deals with measurement of total body water. This was evaluated in one hundred pregnant women using tritiated water. The average total body water % body weight for 34 normal pregnant women during the first half of pregnancy was 56.2%, and for 32 normal pregnant women during the second half of pregnancy it was 57.5%. The average total body water in 26 preeclamptic patients was 61.8% of body weight with significant rise (*Mahran,* 1964). But we have to realize that measurement of total body water represents a static momentary aspect of water equilibrium in the body.

The dynamic aspect could be assessed in terms of 'Turnover Time' of water in the body. This is the average time a molecule of water remains in the body. This also may be expressed as the percentage of total body water changed each day. A turnover rate of 7.7% of total body water/day was found for normal women (*Shloerb* et al, 1950; *Haley* and *Woodburg,* 1952). In 1953 Hutchison et al. suggested that the turnover rate is decreased in EPH and in women suffering of essential hypertension.

Material

One hundred and thirty two pregnant women. 87 normal of whom 40 were during the first half of pregnancy, 32 were during the second half of pregnancy, 10 were in the first 10 days after delivery and 50 patients suffering of EPH constitute the material of this work. All preeclamptic patients had a B.P. of 150/90 or more with edema and/or proteinuria. None of the patients received either hypotensive or diuretic therapy.

Method

The technique for determination of water turnover rate is a simple one. The patient drinks a glass of milk containing, 5 millicurie of tritiated water after completely evacuating the bladder. She is asked to collect early morning specimens of urine for 5 days. Urine samples are distilled and one milliliter is counted in liquid scintillation counter. The results of activity of the consecutive (5days) are plotted on a semilogarithmic scale. The following equation is used to determine the disappearance constant or the fraction of total body water which is replaced during unit of time (t)

$$(THO)t = (THO)O \times e^{-\lambda t}$$

λ = disappearance constant or fraction of total body water which is replaced during unit time (t)
(THO)O = concentration of tritiated water at the beginning of the period (t)
(THO)+ = concentration of tritiated water at the end of the period (t)

Results

The detailed results of turnover rate in normal pregnancy and early puerperium are shown in Tab. 1. It is clear that there is no significant difference between the turnover rate of water during normal pregnancy comparing the first and second half. There is a striking increase in water turnover rate during the puerperium. The disappearance constant is nearly doubled.

Tab. 1. Water Turnover Rate in Normal Pregnant Women.

Type	Number	Disappearance constant		Statistical Control		
		Mean	S.D.	t	P.	Sig.
Normal Preg. (1st)	40	.091	.011	.17	.8	–
Normal Preg. (2nd)	32	.093	.034	.05	.9	–
Early Postpartum	10	.177	.038	7	.001	++
Total	82					

It is clear from Tab. 2 comparing the turnover rate in normal pregnant women during the second half and in women suffering of EPH-gestosis that there is a significant reduction in water turnover in preeclamptic patients, the disappearance constant in normal women is .093 ± .034 while in preeclamptic patients it is .059 ± .031.

Tab. 2. Water turnover rate in normal pregnancy and in women with EPH-Gestosis.

Type	Number	Disappearance Constant				
		mean	S.D.	*	P	Sig.
Normal	32	.093	.034	3	.01	*
EPH	50	.059	.031			
Total	82					

It was logic to extrapolate our thinking to the possibility that such rigidity in water turnover might start sometime before there is a clinically detectable water retention either by abnormal weight gain or by flank edema.

To answer this question we estimated the turnover rate of water in 36 pregnant women between 12 and 20 weeks pregnancy-chosen at random with no previous history of preeclampsia. Among these 36 patients 6 had a disappearance constant less than .06 which we considered the lowest limit for normality. (Tab. 2) They had a disappearance constant .043, .045, .046, .055, .055, .058. These six patients were followed up until delivery. Four patients developed frank signs of EPH and were admitted to antenatal wards. One patient developed abnormal weight gain at 28 weeks and responded well to conservative measures as an outpatient. One patient did not show any abnormality clinically later on.

Tab. 3.

Number	Name	Age	Parity		Fate
1	S.A	22	P	.043	EPH-gestosis
2	M.N	25	M	.045	EPH-gestosis
3	S.M	26	M	.046	Abn. Wt. gain
4	F.A	19	M	.055	EPH-gestosis
5	A.M	18	P	.066	–
6	M.O	20	M	.058	EPH-gestosis

Discussion

While we are waiting for the exploration of the etiology of preeclampsia the two important therapeutic measures which succeeded in marked reduction of fetal loss and maternal mortality are early detection of the disease when apparently it can be easily arrested and termination of pregnancy in cases which fail to respond to treatment.

It is unfortunate that preeclampsia is an asymptomatic disease and the only symptom which the patient might notice, that is edema, is considered by many whether patients or doctor as a normal associate of pregnancy. In developing countries many women do not attend ante-natal care regularly or even at all and so they miss the only chance of early detection. That is why there is a striking difference between the incidence and the complications of the private patients and patients attending casually antenatal clinics (*Mahran,* 1970). Early detection is either by discovering cases showing early signs of the disease or by the proper record of weight gain and any abnormal increase. In our antenatal clinic any abnormal increase in weight is considered a warning sign and we advise immediately our patients to limit salt, water and high caloric diet. Egyptian women are usually overweight and particularly those in free hospital class.

Eight out of ten women would prefere salty food during pregnancy. Drinking too much water and soft drinks is customary especially during summer, which lasts for about 5 months.

If the patient does not respond to the simple dietary measures, a diuretic is prescribed. Abnormal weight gain could be due to water retention or deposition of fat. Differentiation between both depends on the rate of weight gain which is faster in water retention and also on the response to diuretic drugs. In a previous statistical analysis of 24079 records it was indicated that women who gain weight relatively rapidly between the twelfth and twentieth week of pregnancy are more liable to become edematous than those who gain weight slowly. The work also indicated that women who develop edema later in pregnancy show an appreciably higher rate of weight gain than normal women long before edema appears.

The measurement of water turnover rate is an even earlier method of preclinical detection of preeclampsia. It is also a method which could be used to differentiate between water retention and fat deposition in cases of abnormal weight gain. Clinically the method is easy and in most of our cases it was done as an outpatient procedure. However we cannot recommend its use except in research work. Nevertheless there is a possibility that during the incubation period of the disease certain biological changes might be detected by simple clinical tests not entailing the use of radioisotopes. From our findings it seems possible that diminished water turnover is a reversible process and there could be many abortive cases of preeclampsia which disappear before they are born in full picture.

In conclusion I would like to say that diminished water turnover rate and abnormal weight gain are two preclinical stages which take place during the first half of pregnancy and lead to the appearance of the full clinical picture including edema in the late months of pregnancy.

Acknowledgements

I whish to acknowledge the help of the staff of the Atomic Energy Commission for their help in counting the radioactive samples of urine.

References

Haley, H. B. and *J. W. Woodbury:* J. Clin. Invest 31 (1952) S. 635.

Hutchison, D. L., A. A. Pleutl and *H. C. Taylor Jr.:* J. Clin. Invest. 32 (1953) S. 235.

Mahran, Maher: J. Obstet. Gynaec. Brit. Cwlth 51 (1964) S. 218.

Schloerb, P. R., Priis-B. J. Handsen, I. S. Edelmann, A. K. Soloman and *F. D. Moore:* J. Clin. Invest 29 (1950) S. 1296.

Thomson, A. M., F. E. Hytten, W. Z. Billewicz: J. Obstet. Gynaec. Brit. Cwlth 51 (1967) S. 218.

Some Aspects of Water Metabolism in EPH-Gestosis

Maher Mahran, F.R.C.S., Ph.D. (Edin.) *M.R.C.O.G.*

Department of Obstetrics and Gynecology, Ain Shams University, Cairo, UAR

We diagnose EPH by the classic triad of signs: hypertension, edema and proteinuria. Edema is the clinical manifestation of disturbance of water metabolism in EPH. The clinical association between edema and eclampsia was noted back in 1797 by Demoret (Nordenstrahl, 1952). In the early years of this century Zangenmeister introduced the concept of water as the 'toxin of pre-eclampsia'.

The aim of this work is to study edema in EPH and to try a re-evaluation of its significance in relation to fetal prognosis and maternal pathology in Egyptian women. This is stimulated by a personal feeling that the significance of water disturbance in EPH has been underestimated before being properly evaluated.

From 1965 through 1969 we admitted in our department 1080 patients diagnosed as pre-eclampsia. Of these there were 606 patients with edema of different grades (56%).

We classified edema into 3 grades:

Grade I when edema does not extend beyond the lower limbs (81%).

Grade II When edema extends to the anterior abdominal wall or to other parts in a minimal way (15%).

Grade III When edema was generalized and marked (4%).

So it is clear that edema in EPH mainly presents as edema of the lower limbs (81%) and it is generalized in only 19% of cases.

The average age in grade I is 27.3 years, in grade II 27 years and in grade III 30.4 years. There is a tendency for edema to be generalized in older patients (Tab. 1 and Fig. 1).

Tab. 1. Distribution of Age Among Edematous Patients (606 patients with EPH-gestosis).

	15–19 years	20–24 years	25–29 years	30–34 years	35–39 years	40 or more years
Edema I	53	128	114	77	89	31
Edema II	13	29	11	15	15	9
Edema III	1	4	4	4	5	4

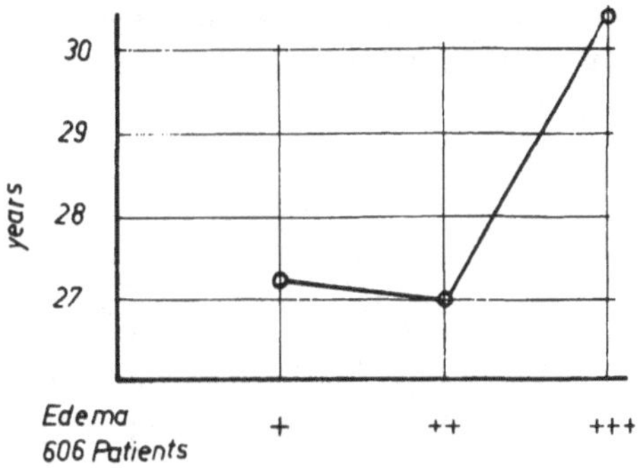

Fig. 1. Average Age

The average parity is 3.35, 3 and 4.77 for the 3 successive grades (Tab. 2). Again there is a tendency for edema to acquire a generalized form with increasing parity (Fig. 2).

Tab. 2. Distribution of Parity Among Edematous Patients (606 patients with EPH-gestosis).

Parity	Edema I	Edema II	Edema III	Whole group
Primipara	207 (42%)	47 (51.1%)	9 (41%)	263 (43.4%)
Multipara	143 (29%)	20 (21.7%)	4 (18%)	167 (27.6%)
Grand Multipara	142 (29%)	25 (27.2%)	9 (41%)	176 (29%)
Total	292 100%	92 100%	22 100%	606 100%

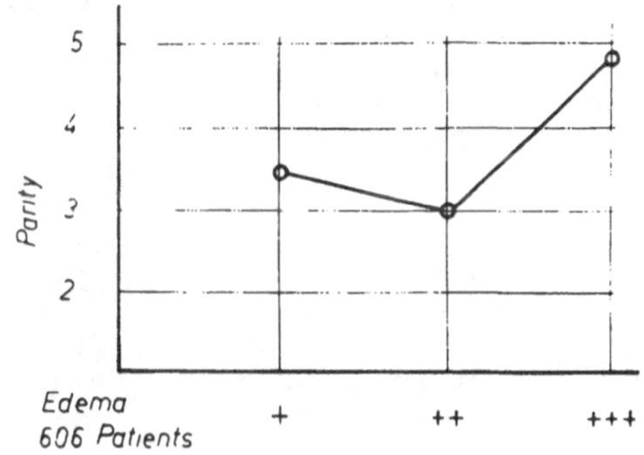

Fig. 2. Average Parity

The average systolic pressure in grade I is 151.1 mm/Hg in grade II 162 mm/Hg and in grade III 172.5 mm/Hg. In patients belonging to grade I-group 89.4 mm/Hg is the average diastolic pressure, for grade II it is 102.7 mm/Hg and in grade III it is

107.3 mm/Hg. A linear relation exists between the extent of edema and the rise of blood pressure. The relation is more linear with the systolic blood pressure (Fig. 3 and Fig. 4).

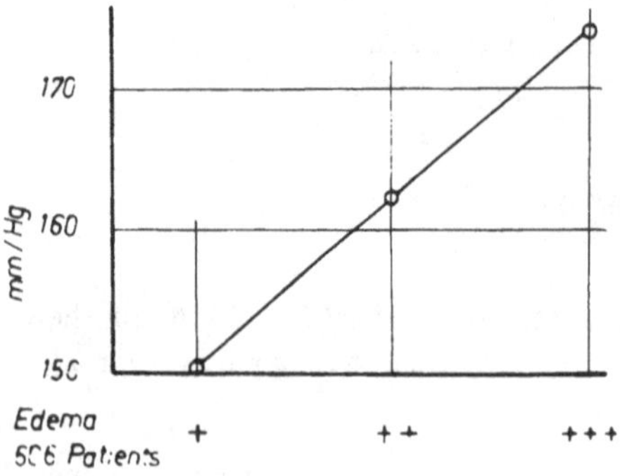

Fig. 3. Average Systolic B. P.

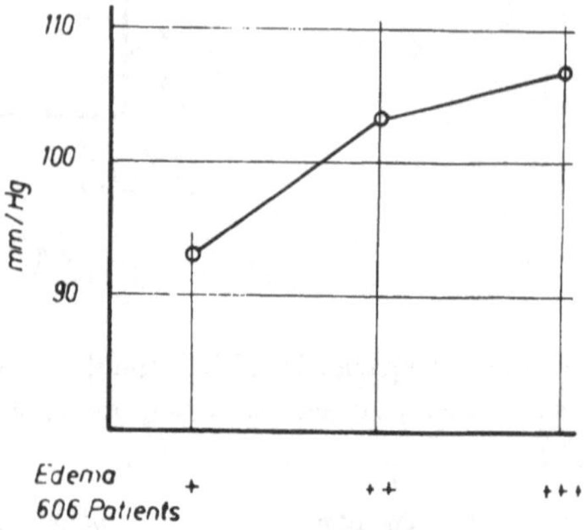

Fig. 4. Average Diastolic B. P.

The relation between edema and proteinuria was investigated (Tab. 3). In grade I 58% of the patients had proteinfree urine in grade II 31.5% had proteinfree urine but with

Tab. 3. Distribution of Proteinuria in Edematous Patients (606 Patients with EPH-gestosis).

	P 0	P I	P II	P III
Edema I	286 58%	91 18.5%	97 19.7%	18 3.8%
Edema II	29 31.5%	24 26.1%	25 27.2%	14 15.2%
Edema III	5 22.7%	4 18.2%	11 50%	2 9.1%

edema grade III only 22.7% had their urine free of protein. So it is clear that the greater the extent of edema the higher is the incidence of proteinuria; but our figures did not show a parallel relation between the extent of edema and the degree of proteinuria. This could possibly be due to the relative small number of patients in group III and II (Fig. 5).

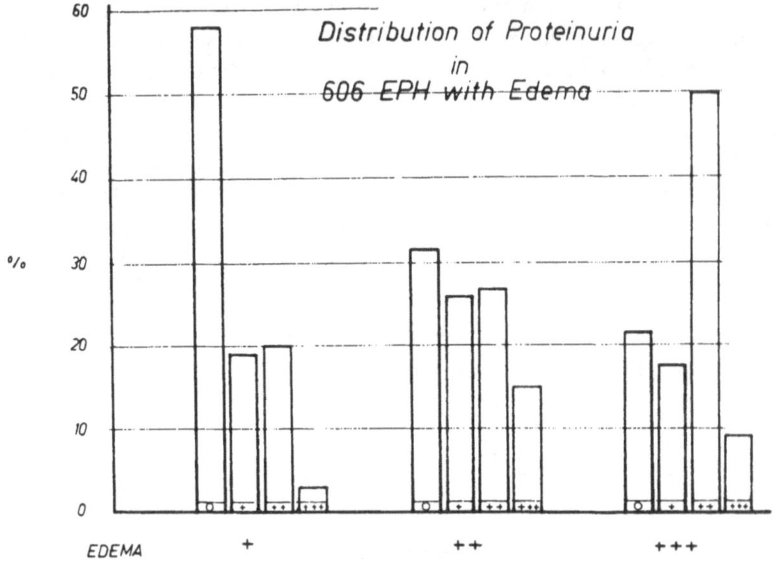

Fig. 5. Distribution of Proteinuria in 606 EPH with Edema

The fetal prognosis was studied in relation to the incidence of prematurity, small for dates (SFD) and stillbirth (S.B.). It is very clear that edema causes a rise in fetal complications. There is no significant difference when edema was localized to the lower limbs or extending to the lower abdominal wall but when edema is massive and generalized there is a sharp rise in fetal complications particularly in S.B. incidence (Fig. 6).

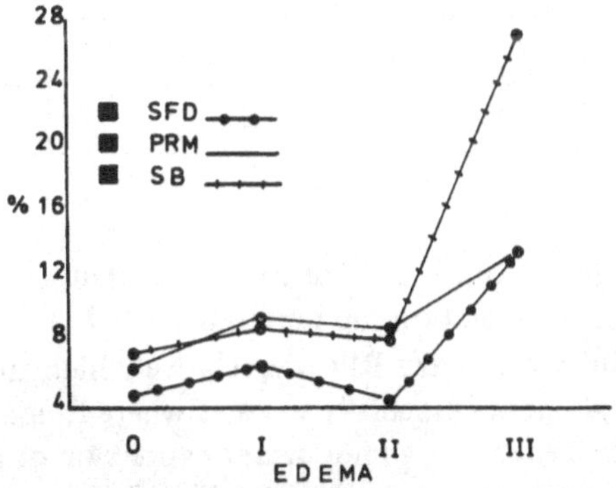

Fig. 6. Fetal Prognosis and Edema (606 EPH with Edema)

It is difficult to dissociate the study of water metabolism from renal pathology. Among a group of 30 successful renal biopsies in EPH patients I have chosen only 6 cases who had generalized edema and relatively mild or moderate proteinuria. The renal pathology proved in all cases to be the characteristic glomerular capillary endotheliosis (*Altchek,* 1961; *Dieckmann* et al., 1958; *Pirani* et al., 1960; *Pollak* and *Nettles,* 1960). Each biopsy was graded by a simple system which we designed for EPH cases where the lesion is mainly glomerular (Fig. 7). The detailed results are shown in Tab. 4. The B.P. varied between 140/80–150/90 mm/Hg. The proteinuria

Glomerular Lesion in EPH

Normal	0
Doubful	1
Mild	2
Moderate	3
Severe	4

$$RPI = \frac{\text{sum } (G_1 + G_2 \ldots)}{\text{Total number of G}}$$

Fig. 7. **Renal pathological grading**

Tab. 4. RPI in EPH with Generalized Edema.

No	Age	Par	S	D	P	F	G.I.	G	RPI
1	22	P	140	90	3.0	S.E	6	10/10	2.6
2	32	M	140	80	0.5	S	3	4/6	2.5
3	22	M	140	80	1.0	N	4	5/5	2.5
4	25	M	150	90	1.5	S	5	4/7	2.9
5	19	P	140	80	2.0	S.E	4	12/12	1.9
6	25	P	150	90	2.5	S	6	8/10	2.9

between .5–3 g/L. There was one mild case and 5 moderate cases according to the G.I. Although there was a parallel relationship between the G.I. and the renal pathological index (RPI) – except in case 4 –, the RPI was relatively high and the glomerular lesion was advanced in many glomeruli especially in cases where fundal changes were present. This points to generalized edema as an important expression of renal pathology not less significant than hypertension or proteinuria. This finding would be more convincing if edema was the only sign, and this is what we are trying to investigate at the moment.

Edema is an abnormal increase in the amount of extracellular water. There is a very important question to be answered: Is edema normal or abnormal? Is it physiological or pathological? or both? When a man has edema this is abnormal, but when the patient is a pregnant woman some consider this normal, while others consider it abnormal. However there is a rather general agreement that if edema is associated with hypertension or proteinuria it is pathological. Although most obstetricians probably accept that edema per se in pregnancy is not necessarily pathological, yet they regard it with suspicion (*Lancet,* 1967). If edema is massive, even when only localized to the lower limbs, or if it is generalized we always treat it with rest and diuretics, naturally assuming that it is abnormal. Still, the important question is: does physiological edema exist? Should I consider any edema, even massive in absence of hypertension or proteinuria, a normal finding?

Edema of the leg is considered physiological. The explanation is not difficult. The combination of increased intravenous pressure due to the pressure of the enlarged uterus and the diminished colloid osmotic pressure due to hydraemia could account for increased filtration through the capillaries of the lower limbs. But why does edema occur only in about one third of cases? Why does edema not occur in cases of supine hypotensive syndrome where a definite obstruction of the inferior vena cava occurs? The fact that some insist that leg edema which disappears after recumbency within 48 hours should be considered physiological is to be taken with caution. Because we know that other forms of edema due to general causes appear at first in the lower limbs and diminish or disappear from the legs by recumbency and are associated with nocturnal polyuria. Further studies are needed to exclude any associated ultrastructural changes in the kidney before the term physiological is postulated.

If physiological edema exists a line of demarcation is necessary between it and pathological edema. If there is associated hypertension and or proteinuria there is no problem. If edema is generalized, even with normal B.P. and proteinfree urine, it should be considered abnormal. However still leg edema alone could be pathological.

If edema is generalized it is very important to study its distribution. There are many factors which take part in the distribution of edema in different parts of the body like gravity and localized pressure. Estrogen might play a role. It is known that the ground-substance in some areas of the body such as the sex skin of monkeys and the cock's comb is influenced by sex hormones. A chemical change brought about by estrogen makes the ground substance more hygroscopic. This softening of the ground substance is clear in normal pregnancy in certain areas like the cervix, pelvic joints and nipples. Such a phenomenon might occasionally explain why edema affects selectively certain areas to a greater extent, like for instance edema of the vulva, where tissues are steroid sensitive (*Gersh* and *Catchpole,* 1960; *Zachariae,* 1959).

One of the difficulties of proper assessment of edema is the lack of a grading system. I believe there are at least two important factors to be noticed in any grading. The first is the extent of the affected part of the body. The second is the extent of edema itself in any part affected. Because of the lack of a satisfactory grading system, *Nelson,* (1955) and *Macgillivray* (1961) avoided mentioning edema in the definition of grading of pre-eclampsia. *Thomson* et al., in their extensive epidemiological study of edema, classified edema into two groups; localized and generalized. The third group was the no-edema-group (*Thomson* et al., 1967).

When we classified edema into 3 groups severe edema was isolated as a separate group and the information of this group was not diluted by other groups. In restudying the fetal prognosis in our patients we found that the distinction of generalized edema into two groups revealed the deletarious effect of edema grade III where prematurity is 13.6% compared to 8.7% in grade II; the percentage of small for dates is 13.6 compared to 4.3% in grade II and S.B. % is 27.2% compared to 8.7% for grade II i.e. more than three times higher. The figures of S.B. % is more significant as the babies of edematous patients are usually overweight and this reduces relatively the incidence of prematurity and small for dates. If we add the results of grade II and III the deletarious effect of grade III edema will disappear because of the better prognosis of the much bigger number of grade II.

The fact that abnormal weight gain preceedes symptoms of EPH and the appearance of edema and proteinuria is not a new observation. It has been studied and confirmed by many workers (*Davey* et al., 1961; *Fiser* and *Dvorak*, 1960; *Huter* et al., 1965).

It was demonstrated that women who develop edema later in pregnancy show an appreciably higher rate of weight gain long before edema appears. The records indicate that women who gain weight relatively rapidly between the 13th and 20th week are more liable to become edematous than those who gain weight slowly (*Hytten* et al., 1966; *Thomson* et al., 1967).

It was also demonstrated that abnormal weight gain between the 20th and 30th weeks preceedes the appearance of proteinuria (*Hamlin*, 1952; *Thomson* and *Billewicz*, 1957; *MacGillivray*, 1961).

Another aspect of water metabolism disturbance is the decreased water turnover rate which preceedes abnormal weight gain and edema. This is probably the earliest disturbance in water metabolism in EPH (*Mahran*, 1964).

It is important to remember that edema or expansion of the extracellular water compartment is not the only abnormality in EPH. At a later stage there will be an increase in the intracellular water content as has been demonstrated by combined estimation of total body water using tritrium and extracellular water using ^{24}Na (*Mahran*, 1970). The intracellular space expansion might be responsible for serious cellular damage and many of the serious signs and symptoms of pre-eclampsia (*Lancet*, 1967).

Finaly I would like to mention that edema might not be associated with water retention but could be due to shift of water from the intracellular space to the extracellular space so that disappearance of edema in some cases of eclampsia might be due to movement of water in the opposite direction and signify bad prognosis.

In conclusion I stress the importance and the need of more prospective studies in water metabolism in pregnancy particularly its kinetic aspect.

References

Altchek, A.: J. Amer. Med. Ass. 175 (1961) S. 791.

Davey, D. A., W. J. O'Sullivan and *J. C. Mc Clure Browne:* Lancet 1 (1961) S. 519.

Dieckmann, W. J., C. P. McCartney and *J. P. Jr. Harrod:* Amer. J. Obstetr. Gynec. 75 (1958) S. 634.

Editorial: Lancet 2 (1967) S. 197.

Fiser, M. and *Z. Dvorak:* Cs. Cynek 25 (1960) S. 604.

Gersh, I. and *H. R. Catchpole:* Perspect. Biol. Med. 3 (1960) S. 282.

Hamlin, R. H. J.: Lancet 1 (1952) S. 64.

Hüter, K. A., F. Ehlers and *B. Schelte:* Geburtsh. u. Frauenheilk. 25 (1965) S. 385.

Hytten, F. E., A. M. Thomson and *N. R. Taggart:* J. Obst. Gynaec. Brit. CWlth 73 (1966) S. 553.

Mac Gillivray, I.: J. Obstet. Gynaec. Brit. CWlth 68 (1961) S. 557.

Mahran, M.: J. Obstet. Gynaec. Brit. CWlth 51 (1964) S. 218.

Mahran, M.: Under Publication (1970).

Nelson, R. R.: J. Obstet. Gynaec. Brit. Emp. 62 (1955) S. 48.

Pirani, C. L., R. Pollak, J. B. Lennigan, J. B. Nettles, P. Stein: Path et microbiol. 24 (1961) S. 586.

Pollak, V. E. and *R. M. Mark:* Amer. J. Med. 30 (1961) S. 181.

Pollak, V. E. and *J. B. Nettles:* Amer. J. Obstetr. Gynaec. 79 (1960) S. 866.

Thomson, A. M. and *W. Z. Billewicz:* Brit. Med. 5, 1 (1957) S. 243.

Thomson, A. M., F. E. Hytten and *W. Z. Billewicz:* J. Obstet. Gynaec. Brit. Cwlth. 74 (1967) S. 1.

Zachariae, F.: Acid mucopolysaccharides in the genital system and their role in the mechanism of ovulation. Periodica, Copenhagen (1959).

How to Measure Proteinuria

The Investigation of Proteinuria in Pregnancy

H. P. McEwan

The Royal Maternity Hospital, Glasgow, U.K.

Two main problems exist in regard to proteinuria of pregnancy. The first relates to diagnosis and this rests mainly on the fact that our criteria for the diagnosis of pre-eclampsia are so vague. The second problem is in relation to prognosis. Many attempts have been made to relate the degree and severity of proteinuria to the outcome of pregnancy, but this shows only a very general relationship and in many cases one is disappointed by the results.

We have investigated proteinuria in detail by means of immuno-electrophoresis and we have today chosen to describe the results in several groups of patients. First of all normal patients, secondly those with essential hypertension, thirdly pre-eclampsia and fourthly nephritic conditions which may be lumped under the general heading of nephrosis.

Owing to the small amount of protein even when the proteinuria is gross, the urine requires to be concentrated. This can be done by several methods and a concentration of between 50 and 100 times the volume can readily be achieved. This is a diagram of immuno-electrophoresis. The concentrated specimen of urine is placed in a well, indicated here, and an electric current passed along the agar gel. This results in separation of the protein and subsequently an antiserum is placed in troughs which diffuse in towards the line of travel of the protein at right angles to it and gives rise to precipitation arcs which can be *recognised* when the plate is ready for inspection.

Next slide. This slide indicates the results which can be seen in cases of essential hypertension. These do not vary very much from the findings in normal patients. There is a distinct arc of precipitation related to albumin and almost nothing else, sometimes a faint precipitin arc can be seen with some other proteins, but by and large albumin is the only protein seen.

Fig. 1. Urinary Protein Pattern Hypertension

Second slide. In pre-eclampsia the number of proteins appearing in urine is greatly increased. We have albumin, transferrin, gamma G globulin but also alpha$_1$-glycoprotein, haemopexin, ceruloplasmin and as the condition increases in severity so do the number of protein arcs.

Next slide. A noticeable feature was the appearance of large molecule proteins. One protein which particularly interested us was alpha$_2$-macroglobulin which can be seen in this position.

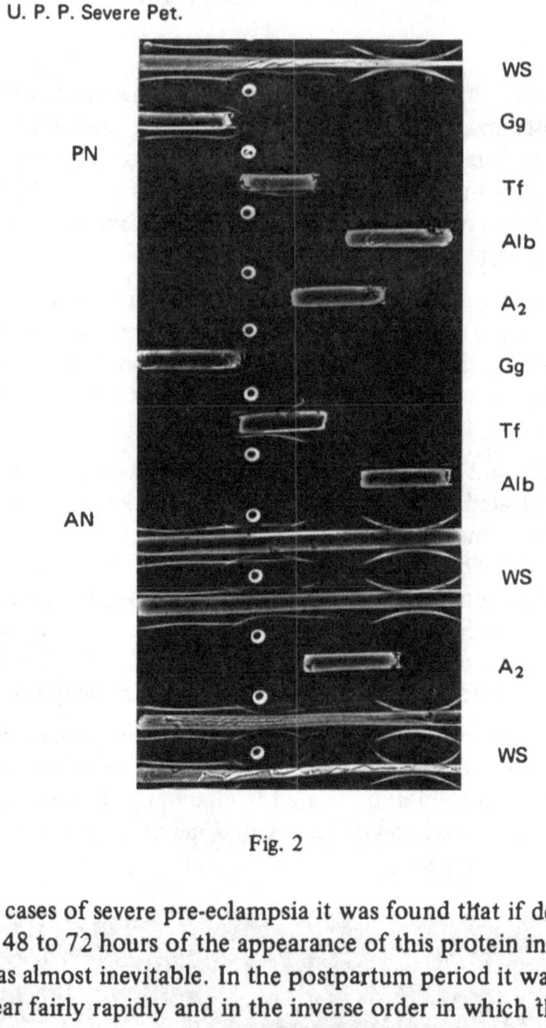

Fig. 2

Following these cases of severe pre-eclampsia it was found that if delivery was not achieved within 48 to 72 hours of the appearance of this protein in the urine, intrauterine death was almost inevitable. In the postpartum period it was noted that these proteins disappear fairly rapidly and in the inverse order in which they appeared in the antenatal period, i.e., large molecule proteins disappeared first and last the smaller molecular proteins.

The next slide shows the pattern found in nephritic conditions. It will be noted that the number of protein arcs is greater than that found in severe pre-eclampsia and was unrelated to the degree of proteinuria. Alpha$_2$-macroglobulin was present in the nephritic cases throughout pregnancy and was unrelated to the degree of proteinuria. Furthermore it persisted in the postpartum period with no tendency to disappear. It was found, on following these cases, that the prognosis as far as the outcome of pregnancy was not affected. Whereas in severe pre-eclampsia where the appearance of alpha$_2$-macroglobulin heralded the onset of intra-uterine death, there was no significance found in relation to this protein, in the cases with nephrosis.

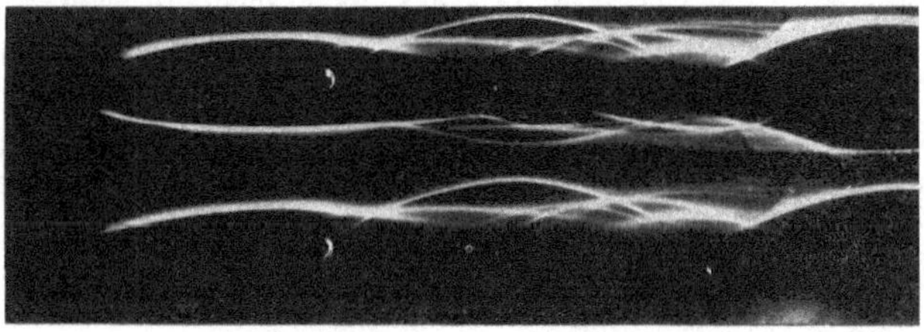

Fig. 3. Urinary Protein Pattern Nephrosis

I would now like to present two cases, one of pre-eclampsia and one of nephrosis complicating pregnancy, to illustrate how immuno-electrophoresis can be of value in differentiating between pre-eclampsia and kidney disease.

Case I is of Mrs. A. aged 26 Para (2 + 0) a known case of nephrosis. Proteinuria had been present *throughout* and between the two previous pregnancies both of which were uneventful. She was first seen in this pregnancy when twelve weeks pregnant. Blood pressure was normal. A protein level of 0.7 g per cent. was present. On immuno-electrophoresis, wide spectrum antiserum and with antiserum to albumin, transferrin, gamma G globulin and alpha$_2$-macroglobulin precipitin arcs were demonstrated.

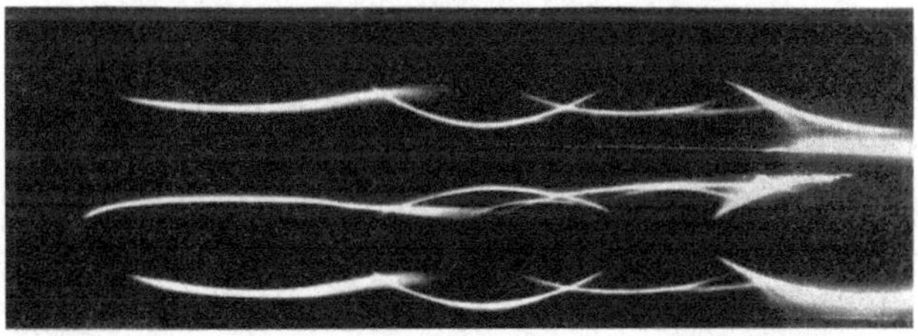

Fig. 4. Urinary Protein Pattern Severe Pre-Eclampsia

This pattern continued throughout pregnancy and was still seen six months after delivery. Labour was induced at term with delivery of a live female child weighing 3.6 kg. Urine protein level ranged from 0.4 to 0.9 g per cent. Renal biopsy permormed four months after delivery showed changes typical of membranous glomerulo-nephritis.

Next slide. This is a section of a glomerulus in this case. *Next slide.* At the right hand and left hand side the urine has been subjected to wide spectrum antiserum and in the centre the individual antisera, albumin, transferrin gamma G globulin and alpha$_2$-macroglobulin. There is no change in the protein pattern and alpha$_2$-macroglobulin can be detected both antenatally and postnatally.

Case II is of an unmarried primigravida aged 22. She had no previous illness. When first seen at the thirtieth week of pregnancy her blood pressure was normal and there was no proteinuria. One week later, blood pressure had risen to 140/105 mm/Hg and 0.2 per cent protein was present in the urine. Immuno-electrophoresis revealed definite reaction to albumin, transferrin and gamma G globulin but none to alpha$_2$-macroglobulin. The patient was admitted. Despite sedation and diuretics blood pressure rose to 160/115 mm/Hg and on the immuno-electrophoresis picture alpha$_2$-macroglobulin was demonstrated. At 33 weeks surgical induction was performed with delivery of a live female child weighing 2 kg. By the fourth postnatal day, urinary protein level was 0.05 g percent. Blood pressure was normal and immuno-electrophoresis revealed traces of albumin, transferrin, gamma G globulin but no alpha$_2$-macroglobulin.

Next slide. This illustrates the protein patterns found antenatally and postnatally. After delivery there is a decrease in the number of proteins and disappearance of alpha$_2$-macroglobulin.

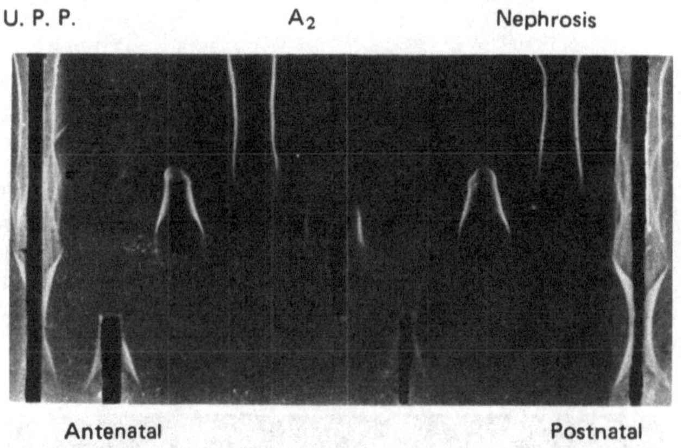

Fig. 5

In conclusion we find that this is a *useful* method of analysing proteinuria in pregnancy. It provides a method of differentiating between nephrotic conditions and pre-eclampsia. In nephrosis irrespective of the degree of proteinuria, large molecule proteins are always found. In the case of pre-eclampsia large molecule proteins only appear when the disease becomes very severe and the presence of alpha$_2$-macroglobulin is of dire prognostic significance heralding the onset of intra-uterine death.

What Methods should be given in the Definition of Proteinuria besides the Esbach and Paper-Sticks Method?

A. Cretti

II. Frauenklinik der Medizinischen Akademie, Bialystok, Polen

In the definition of proteinuria proposed by Organisation Gestosis the level of proteinuria is given as estimated by the method of *Esbach* and the paper-sticks method. But there are countries where *Esbach* is not used at all, and the paper-sticks method not employed in hospitals. In the effort to make our definitions more widely acceptable it seems justified to add also the cut-off-points for other procedures, besides Esbach and the paper-sticks method.

As far as I know the most widely used methods (besides *Esbach* and paper-sticks) are the procedure of heating the urine with acetic acid and the procedure with nitric acid. Both methods were developed from the qualitative tests to the quantitative ones by means of using variously diluted urine. Knowing how much the urine was diluted, it is quite simple to calculate the concentration of protein.

I have no experience with the method of heating with acetic acid – as far as I know it is used in France. We use nitric acid alcording to *Brahberg, Roberts* and *Stolnikow.* It was developed from the qualitative method of *Heller.* We found it reliable and relatively simple.

So the proposal is to add to the definition of proteinuria and in the Gestosis Index also the value of proteinuria as estimated by the test with nitric acid, and, if we can consider the test of heating with the acetic acid reliable, to add the cut-off-point for this test too.

What are the levels from these tests which would correspond to given levels of proteinuria estimated by the method of *Esbach*? To answer this question, comparative studies of these methods would be needed. We have not performed such studies, but we have done numerous estimations of proteinuria by the method with nitric acid. We found that in healthy pregnant women, even during such physical strain as labour, proteinuria estimated by method with nitric acid never exceeded 0.1%. So we considered the values of above 0.1% as abnormal and consequently we have put this level as cut-off-point for proteinuria in our own definition of proteinuria as a sign of gestosis.

But it was not a comparative study with the method of *Esbach* or paper-sticks method. So the question remains open: What are the levels of proteinuria estimated with other methods corresponding with the given levels resulting from method of *Esbach* and paper-sticks method?

Measurement of Urinary Protein

J. Studd

Birmingham Maternity Hospital, Queen Elizabeth Medical Center, Birmingham, G.B.

It is proposed by the Organisation Gestosis that the daily urinary protein loss should be one of the three parameters of the Gestosis Index.

We would all agree that the quantity of proteinuria is a very valuable guide to the severity of the disease whether the EPH-gestosis is due to glomerulonephritis or to the condition that we usually call pre-eclampsia. It is vital, therefore, that we choose an accurate method of urinary protein estimation; if not, any conclusions that we may make based upon the Gestosis Index will have little scientific or critical validity.

In the United Kingdom we employ two simple methods of urinary protein estimation.

1. Albustix.
2. *Esbach*'s albuminometer.

These are convenient methods for use in the ward or clinic and can be performed by the nurse.

I have compared the accuracy of these two methods with the accepted biochemical method for measuring both serum and urinary protein. This is the Biuret technique which is accurate and described in all standard textbooks of clinical biochemistry.

1. *Albustix.* Readings were taken from 651 consecutive four-hour urinary collections. The columns were read against the colour chart provided reading from nil to + + + protein.

The first slide shows the mean values and the standard error of the 651 observations with varying degrees of proteinuria.

The second slide shows the distribution of urinary protein concentration as measured by the Biuret method for each Albustix gradation. Only six false positives were obtained in this series.

These observations indicate that the Albustix strips provide a satisfactory semi-quantitative measure of proteinuria particularly at low levels but the wide scatter of the concentrations of protein in the cases recorded as three-plus or four-plus indicate the difficulty of reading these higher concentrations with accuracy by this method and suggest that the colour range provided is possibly too wide for useful practice. It is clear, therefore, that some other method must be used if one wishes to measure accurately large amounts of protein in the urine and the Organisation Gestosis has suggested that *Esbach*'s method is satisfactory for this.

2. *Esbach's albuminometer.* The *Esbach* result were obtained from 145 24-hour collections from 11 obstetric patients with proteinuria. Eight of these patients had severe pre-eclampsia and three had pregnancies complicated by the nephrotic syndrome. As before, the *Esbach* result was compared to the result obtained by the Biuret estimation. This slide (No. 3) demonstrates that *Esbach*'s method is inaccurate for all degrees of proteinuria. Moreover, at low levels the errors are magnified and at higher levels and at higher concentrations it reads approximately one-third or one-half of the true proteinuria.

Although it is accepted that *Esbach*'s is only a semi-quantitative method of protein estimation, its use continues in most hospitals in the United Kingdom and the continent of Europe in the belief that it is a useful, quick, convenient ward technique that may be performed by the nursing staff. Both the *Esbach*'s technique and the Biuret method require a 24 hour urine collection but the former has to stand for a further 24 hours before reading whereas the Biuret method is one of the simplest of laboratory assays permitting large numbers of specimens to be examined in less than one hour and is a standard biochemical service offered by most laboratories.

Perhaps in time a use may be found for the hundreds of *Esbach*'s tubes that we have in our hospitals. I have used them to make elegant pipe racks and am currently attempting to make a set of Papageno's magic pipes for a University production of Mozart's Die Zauberflöte, but I am convinced that it has no place in the measurement of urinary protein in the year 1970.

Proteinuria in Single Specimens

A. Cretti

II. Frauenklinik der Medizinischen Akademie, Bialystok, Polen

In the definition of proteinuria and in the Gestosis Index, proposed by the Organization Gestosis, the cut-off-points are given as relating to 24 h urine.

Rippmann in the Bulletin of the Büro für Geburtshilfe und Gynäkologie, p. 1735, draws our attention to the fact, that the cut-off-points for proteinuria in single specimens of urine are not yet estimated in our classification. Of course the estimation of proteinuria in 24 hours collection of urine is the most reliable method and it should remain in our definition. But is is obvious that the collection of 24 hours urine is not easy to perform, everywhere, especially not in the out-patients practice. Our proposed criteria for diagnosis and classification should be easily accessible not only in hospitals but also for the general practitioner or even midwife in a small village.
In my opinion there is still another reason for considering the single-specimen-value in the definition of proteinuria. Let us take a patient with severe gestosis who was just admitted to the hospital. Shall we wait full 24 hours for the result of proteinuria estimation? I think this would not be the best way. We should immediately know how far advanced the renal lesions are because this has important implications for the management. Therefore in such a case we estimate the proteinuria in a single specimen, besides the evaluation of proteinuria in 24 h urine.

The reasons mentioned above are sufficiently important to give in our definition also the cut-off-points for single specimens, besides the cut-off-point for 24 hours urine.

If now we agree with such proposal, we come to quite difficult a point, namely, what level of proteinuria in single specimen could be considered as corresponding to a given level of proteinuria in a 24 hours urine? This question is very complicated, because the amount of excreted urine depends on many various factors, such as orthostatic factor, water intake, diuresis, drugs, changes in the process of gestosis involving the kidneys. All these factors can change in few hours. According to our experience the differences between the levels of single-specimen-proteinuria and 24-hours-proteinuria are not very great in severe proteinuria of for instance 5‰ and above. But in the milder cases the differences are sometimes considerable.

It has already been proposed to define proteinuria as the level of proteins in 24 hours urine and in single specimens. I don't know whether these proposals are based on many comparisons of single-specimen-proteinuria with the 24-hours-proteinuria in the same patients.

So I would like to put the following questions for the discussion:

1. Shall we wait for the results of large scale studies, based on sufficiently numerous simultaneous estimations of proteinuria in 24-hours-urine and proteinuria in single specimens? (Can we anticipate any binding conclusions from these studies?)

2. Or shall we a priori determine the cut-off-point for single specimen proteinuria? For example, the cut-of-point for the first morning portion voided midstream? As the conditions of the first morning specimen would be similar for all patients, and after bed-rest the orthostatic factor would play not a great role.

The Radial Immunodiffusion Method for Quantitative Estimation of Proteinuria

V. Wagner, I. Klofacova, B. Vedra, J. Hampl

Institute for the Care of Mother and Child, Prague – Podoli

The radial immunodiffusion method is valuable especially for determination of very small concentrations of protein in the urine. The minimal concentration of protein which can still be detected is 1 mg%, which answers approximately to the losses of 10–15 mg per 24 hours (calculated for urine volumes 1000 ml, resp. 1500 ml per 24 hours).

Material

1. ***Buffer solution.*** Barbital buffer ph 8.6, ionic strength 0.1, diluted by the same volume of distilled water before use.
2. ***Glass.*** Slides 8.5 × 8.5 cm, washed in detergent, rinsed in tap water and distilled water, sterilised.
3. ***Antisera.*** Horse-anti-human serum (HaHu) produced by SEVAC Prague.
4. ***Agar.*** Ionagar No. 2 (Oxoid London) dissolved in concentration of 1.5% buffer solution (see above). To prevent bacterial contamination Sodium azid 1:1000 was added. The plates can be stored for 7–10 days at 4° C in moist chamber.
5. ***Preparation of plates.*** To 11.2 ml of 1.5% agar dissolved at 100° C in autoclave, cooled down to 50° C 2.5 ml diluted Horse-anti-human serum is added (must be also preheated to 50° C). This mixture (13.7 ml) is poured on the surface of preheated slide which must be placed in equilibrial position until cooling.
6. ***Standards.*** Normal human serum standard (NHS) is prepared by pooling several samples of serum obtained from healthy population, the concentration of total protein is determined by use of gradient cylinder method (*Lowry* and *Hunter*, J. Biol. Chem. 159 (1945) S. 465). The dilutions of standards are prepared between 0 to 70 mg% or some standardized preparation (e.g. Behringwerke: Standard-Humanserum) can be used.

Procedure

By the use of a needle (diameter 2.4 mm) 35 holes are cut on the agar layer on the plate (seven rows, in each 5 holes in distances of 15 mm).

The first and last row are used for filling with the standard solutions, the other holes are used for filling with urine samples in duplicates or triplicates. Into each hole approximately 0.004 ml of urine can be poured by use of a Pasteur pipette with long and sharp tip. The reflexion of surface disappears when the level of liquid reaches the surface of agar layer.

The plates are placed for 48 hours at room temperature in a moist chamber.

In direct light and black background the diameters of immuno-precipitation rings are read by help of a magnifying eye piece (8 ×) with micrometer built in.

Evaluation

Mean values of duplicates or triplicates of standard solutions are used for preparation of a calibration curve in semilog scale, which is used for calculation of actual concentrations of protein in samples.

The method of radial immunodiffusion detects the minimal concentrations of 1–3 mg%, which answers to calculated losses of proteins on the border fo physiology. Therefore the method can be recommended for the research projects dealing with the pathophysiology of proteinuria.

Criteria of Hypertension

Measurement of the Diastolic Blood Pressure

A. Cretti

II. Frauenklinik der Medizinischen Akademie, Bialystok, Polen

What is the reason of talking about such a simple routine method as the measurement of blood pressure? One of the main aims of Organisation Gestosis is to unify the criteria for diagnosis and classification of gestosis. Only in this way it is possible to make the material from various centers comparable. What is the present situation from this point of view, concerning the measurement of diastolic blood pressure?

Even if various centers agree that the cut-off-point level of diastolic blood pressure in gestosis is (for example) 90 millimeters of mercury, and that all cases with a diastolic blood pressure above this value should be regarded as gestotic, at present time the material from various centers is not comparable.

This is because some centers register the diastolic pressure value at the moment when the sounds begin to be muffled (beginning of the Phase IV of *Korotkoff*'s sounds), but others at the moment when the sounds disappear completely (beginning of the Phase V). The difference between the level of the first diastolic pressure and the level of the second diastolic pressure is usually about 10 millimetres of mercury, but sometimes may be even 20 millimeters. The center, where the first diastolic pressure is registered will have of course a higher rate of gestosis cases and these cases would be less severe than in the center where the second diastolic pressure is measured. Therefore the material from these two centers is incomparable, especially in mild cases. But also the groups of patients with more severe forms of gestosis would differ.

The best solution would be to unify the method of measurement. There were already some trials to be more accurate, or to estimate both diastolic pressures and to take both of them into consideration. Some authors also advised to measure both diastolic pressures and to calculate the mean value. These two methods may be valuable but one can doubt if they are not to laborious for an average busy obstetrician in out-patient department or for a general practitioner. Moreover we ought to remember that our classification is foreseen not only for hospitals but for general use too.

So it seems that two solutions remain:

1. to accept first diastolic pressure, or
2. to accept second diastolic pressure.

In considering this dilemma one can start from various points of view.

I. Which value is nearer to the real diastolic pressure, measured directly by cannulation of an artery?

Such comparison was made by *Roberts* et al. (1953). There appeared to be no constant differences between the diastolic pressure recorded directly and the diastolic pressure recorded indirectly regardless of whether the first reading or the second reading is used. But such simultaneous observations were much to few to establish the magnitude and constancy of this error. At present we do not know whether the true diastolic pressure is more closely related to the first diastolic pressure or to the second diastolic pressure.

II. Which method is easier and simpler and therefore offers a smaller possibility of errors, even when done by an unexperienced person?

To recognize a change in the character of sounds, to estimate accurately the moment at which the *Korotkoff*'s sounds become muffled is certainly more difficult than to determine the moment of their complete dissapearance. Therefore it seems that estimation of the second diastolic pressure is simpler and fewer errors may be expected.

III. What implications for diagnosis, classification, statistics and for management can be anticipated when we choose the first diastolic pressure and what implications if we choose the second diastolic pressure?

If the first diastolic pressure will be chosen, more patients will be diagnosed as gestotic and more gestotic patients will be regarded and treated as patients with severe gestosis. Concerning the statistics of results, the rate of mortality and rate of complications will be lower, because there will be more mild cases. If we decide to accept the first diastolic pressure, the treatment will begin earlier; this can have important effect on the result of therapy.

Closing my remarks on the measurement of the diastolic pressure I hope that the points mentioned above will be useful for the discussion which is now to follow. In my personal opinion, the relation between each diastolic pressures and the true diastolic pressure is not known exactly until now. Thus it is not so very important to decide which diastolic pressure would be chosen. But it is important to choose one of them and accept it all over the world, as to make the material from various centers more comparable.

Die Technik der Blutdruckmessung

R. F. Vollman

National Institutes of Health, Bethesda, Maryland, USA

Die Diagnose der EPH-Gestose stützt sich primär auf die Symptomatik. Die Häufigkeit dieser Schwangerschaftskomplikation hängt somit einerseits von der Definition der pathologischen Zustände: Ödem (E), Proteinurie (P) und Hypertonie (H) ab, andererseits von der Meßtechnik der einzelnen Parameter. Während für die Bestimmung von Ödemen und den Nachweis der Proteinurie keine Übereinstimmung erzielt werden konnte, ist die Grenze zwischen normalem Blutdruck (135/85) und der Hypertonie (140/90) weitgehend akzeptiert, wenn auch nicht unbestritten.

Die Methodik der Blutdruckmessung beeinflußt jedoch das Ergebnis, läßt Hypertonien diagnostizieren, wo keine sind, respektive normale Werte bei Hypertonie erheben.

Die Section on Obstetrics des Perinatal Research Branch der National Institutes of Health, Bethesda, Maryland, USA, haben deshalb bei 12 großen Kliniken der Vereinigten Staaten eine Umfrage über die Technik der Blutdruckbestimmung durchgeführt. Dabei wurde gefragt nach dem Zeitpunkt in der Konsultation, der Position der Patientin, nach der Seite, auf welcher die Blutdruckmessung ausgeführt wurde. Man bat um die Spezifizierung des Blutdruckapparates, der Breite der Manchette, der Genauigkeit beim Ablesen des systolischen und diastolischen Wertes. Sodann fragten die Autoren, ob eine schriftliche Anleitung zur Verfügung stand.

Das Resultat* zeigt eine breite Streuung der Antworten in allen Richtungen. Somit ist die Vergleichbarkeit der Untersuchungsergebnisse sehr fraglich. Die Anwendung einer einheitlichen und allgemein akzeptierten Definition eines Symptomes ist ungenügend. Eine wichtige Voraussetzung stellt die Standardisierung der Meßtechnik dar.

* Genaue Angaben siehe:
E. Friedmann, Ist International Task Force on Toxemia, National Institutes of Health, Perinatal Research Branch, Section on Obstetrics, Bethesda, Maryland, USA, 6.–8. Dezember 1971.

Schriftliche Stellungnahme zur Diskussion über die Blutdruckmessung

Prof. Dr. L. C. Chesley

State University of New York. Downstate Medical Center, Department of Obstetrics and Gynecology

The American Heart Association recommends taking the change of sound (phase 4) as the diastolic pressure. That was their original recommendation, in force for many years. About 15 years ago, they changed to disappearance of sound (phase 5), but recently they have reverted to their original standard.

I have always used phase 4, because when we started our follow-up study of eclamptic women more than 35 years ago that was the standard.

Prof. Dr. V. Friedberg

Universitätskliniken Mainz, Frauenklinik

Sie fragen mich an zu welchem Zeitpunkt wir den diastolischen Wert bei einer Blutdruckmessung bestimmen. Ich glaube, es gibt bei den Internisten eine enorme Literatur darüber, inwieweit der „abklingende Ton" den effektiven diastolischen Wert widergibt. Darüber besteht selbst bei den Internisten keine Einigkeit – wie mir gerade hier Herr Professor Schölmerich versichert hat, der wohl in Deutschland zu den führenden Kreislaufspezialisten gehört. Bei meiner Anfrage bei meinen Assistenten mußte ich die verschiedensten Auffassungen erleben, wobei es überwiegt, daß der diastolische Wert mit dem „leiserwerden des Tones" angegeben wird. Ich möchte aber nicht glauben, daß für unsere bisherige Toxikosestatistik der gemessene diastolische Wert als sicher anzusehen ist und ich habe daher auch meist bei meinen früheren Arbeiten – in Kenntnis der unklaren Situation der Messung des diastolischen Druckes – meistens den systolischen Druck herangezogen, obwohl ich mir bewußt bin, daß gerade bei der Toxikose der diastolische Wert für die Prognose wichtiger ist als der systolische Wert.

E P H

Applying the Symptomatic Classification

Symptomatic Classification

J. C. McClure Browne

Institute of Obstetrics and Gynecology, Hammersmith Hospital, London, G.B.

I have attempted to assess the significance of edema, proteinuria and hypertension as symptoms in regard to prognosis. In the years 1961–1967 at Hammersmith Hospital there were 16 174 deliveries. EPH-gestosis, defined as a blood pressure greater than 150/100 on one occasion, with or without edema and proteinuria, occurred 2957 times (an incidence of 18.4%). In these cases there was no maternal death and no eclamptic. Our only yardstick then was perinatal mortality and the incidence of perinatal mortality in these EPH-gestosis cases was 38 per 1000. When proteinuria was absent the perinatal mortality was 19 per 1000. When proteinuria was present it was 93 per 1000. The serious significance of proteinuria is therefore clear. Moreover the perinatal mortality varies with the degree of proteinuria, the greater the amount of protein in the urine the higher the perinatal mortality.

The degree of hypertension also has serious implications. In a series of over 6000 cases we recorded the initial reading of diastolic blood pressure at the first visit before 16 weeks gestation. The higher the initial reading of diastolic pressure, the greater the perinatal mortality, and a sharp change occurred when the initial diastolic pressure was above 80. The same was true of the initial systolic blood pressure, any reading above 140 giving a greatly increased perinatal mortality. I believe it is important that at the first antenatal visit the blood pressure reading which should be recorded is that obtained first of all. Any subsequent drop at a later reading, perhaps 20 minutes later after resting, should be ignored. It is the response of the woman to the stress of her first antenatal visit which is important. The woman with a hypertensive tendency will almost invariably show an initial rise of blood pressure. It is worthy of note that the perinatal mortality is considerably increased when the maximum diastolic blood pressure recorded at any time during pregnancy is above 110.

Edema, though well recognised as part of the EPH-gestosis syndrome, is of less significance. 36% of our 2957 cases had edema, but in only 15% – less than half of the cases with edema – was it more than slight and in no case was it severe. In none of the perinatal deaths was edema the only feature and it was never marked.

It seems therefore that hypertension and proteinuria are by far the most important signs of EPH-gestosis and the occurrence of proteinuria must always be regarded as of most serious prognostic significance.

Zur Anwendung der symptomatischen Klassifikation der Spätgestosen

C. Goecke

Universitäts-Frauenklinik, Würzburg, BRD

Erhebliche Abweichungen in den regionalen und internationalen Gestosestatistiken haben deutlich gemacht, daß die bisherige unterschiedliche Einteilung der Spätgestosen unbefriedigend ist und eine Neuordnung der Gestosenomenklatur wünschenswert erscheint. Die „Organisation Gestose" schlug daher eine neue und für alle praktikable Einteilung vor.

Da die Pathogenese der Spätgestose noch ungeklärt ist, will sich diese Einteilung zunächst auf die nachweisbaren klinischen Symptome beschränken. Dem entspricht die Einteilung in

- monosymptomatische Gestosen
  - Ödeme
  - Proteinurie
  - Hypertonie
- polysymptomatische Gestosen
- drohende Eklampsie
  - subjektive und objektive Zeichen nachweisbar:
  - motorische Unruhe, Hyperreflexie, Sehstörungen, Oligurie, Anurie
- Eklampsie

Eine solche symptomatische Einteilung kann jedoch nur einheitlich durchgeführt werden, wenn Einigung über die Definition der Hauptsymptome erzielt wurde.

Man sollte von pathologischen Ödemen sprechen, wenn Beinödeme nach Bettruhe noch nachweisbar sind, wenn Ödeme an den Händen oder im Gesicht oder generalisierte Ödeme bestehen, und ferner, wenn die Gewichtszunahme der Schwangeren über 350 g/Woche vor dem 6. Schwangerschaftsmonat oder über 500 g/Woche nach dem 6. Monat beträgt.

Man sollte von einer pathologischen Proteinurie sprechen, wenn die Eiweißausscheidung 0,4 g/l Harn übersteigt. Obwohl die Eiweißbestimmung nach *Esbach* ungenau ist, wurde diese Methode wegen ihrer Einfachheit weiterhin empfohlen. Eine Eiweißausscheidung von 0,4 g‰ und weniger sollte jedoch ebenfalls, im besonderen im Hinblick auf eine Harnweginfektion, abgeklärt werden. Eine Hypertonie liegt vor, wenn der systolische Blutdruck 140 mm/Hg oder mehr beträgt und ein diastolischer Blutdruck von 90 mm/Hg oder mehr gemessen werden kann.

Diese vorgeschlagene symptomatische Klassifikation wurde retrospektiv bei nahezu 2500 Schwangeren und Gebärenden mit Zeichen einer Gestose angewandt (Universitäts-Frauenklinik Würzburg; 1950–1969). – Die Häufigkeit der EPH-Gestose betrug 7,5% (Tab. 1). Der Anteil polysymptomatischer Gestosen lag über 80%. Die Eklampsiehäufigkeit betrug im Durchschnitt 3,9%; sie ist in den vergangenen Jahren deutlich geringer geworden. – Die perinatale kindliche Mortalität und Untergewichtigkeit (unter 2500 g) steigt deutlich mit der Schwere der Erkrankung (Tab. 2). Bei monosymptomatischer Gestose ist die Komplikationshäufigkeit nur gering (Tab. 3). Besteht nur eine Proteinurie, so ist die Untergewichtigkeit bei Neugeborenen deutlich, liegt nur eine Hyptertonie vor, so ist die perinatale kindliche Mortalität gesteigert. Ödeme als alleiniges Symptom scheint die Komplikationsrate nicht zu beeinflussen.

Tab. 1. Häufigkeit der Gestoseformen bezogen auf die Zahl der mit Zeichen einer EPH-Gestose hospitalisierten Schwangeren und Gebärenden und bezogen auf die Gesamtzahl der entbundenen Mütter.

	% der EPH-Gestosen (n = 2417)		% der Entbindungen (n = 32 232)	
monosymptomatische EPH-Gestose	7,1		0,5	
Ödeme		6,3		0,48
Proteinurie		0,5		0,03
Hypertonie		0,3		0,02
polysymptomatische EPH-Gestose	80,1		6,0	
drohende Eklampsie	8,9		0,7	
Eklampsie	3,9		0,3	
insgesamt	100,0		7,5	

Tab. 2. Perinatale kindliche Mortalität und Untergewichtigkeit (< 2500 g) bei verschiedenen Gestoseformen (n = 2417).

	perinatale Mortalität %	Geburtsgewicht unter 2500 g
Monosymptomatische EPH-Gestose	7	12
Polysymptomatische EPH-Gestose	11	14
Drohende Eklampsie (n = 215)	24	37
Eklampsie (n = 94)	38	47

Tab. 3. Perinatale kindliche Mortalität und Untergewichtigkeit (< 2500 g) bei monosymptomatischer EPH-Gestose.

	perinatale Mortalität %	Geburtsgewicht unter 2500 g
Ödeme	5,0	11,8
Proteinurie	5,2	21,0
Hypertonie	9,3	11,6

The Signs of EPH-Gestosis. Correlation to Different Obstetrical Parameters

L. Tervilä

Municipal Hospital, Lathi, Finnland

For this meeting we have in Helsinki repeated an old statistical observation published in 1965–66 about the correlation between the symptoms of gestosis and perinatal mortality and different other parameters. The material of 2000 gestosis-cases was divided into groups according to the symptoms or combinations of symptoms as we can see in Tab. 1.

Tab. 1. Wirkung der verschiedenen Symptome der EPH-Gestose.

	Gesamtzahl	Gewicht	< 2500 g %	Apgar 0–6 %	Perinat. mort. %
Kontrolle	2001	3425	5,35	5,70	2,40
E	565	3585	2,30	6,90	0,88
P	40	3420	7,50	7,50	0,00
E + P	47	3638	0,00	14,89	2,13
H	313	3293	7,35	10,86	1,92
H + E	718	3543	3,62	9,19	1,53
H + P	93	3057	19,35	20,43	6,45
H + P + E	163	3199	17,18	14,11	3.07

In all the groups where oedema occurs, the weights of the newborns are significantly high. On the other hand in the groups with hypertension without oedema the children are smaller than average. Although proteinuria does not alone have a very marked effect, together with the hypertension it clearly diminishes the birthweight.

If we study the perinatal mortality and the Apgar-scores in the different groups, we see that the highest Apgar-indices occur in the groups with oedema and the lowest in groups with hypertension. The number of the underweight newborns seems to correlate in the same manner. The groups with proteinuria have, however, a few more small children than might have been expected.

I would like to make these facts still more clear with the following tables, where the symptoms are divided into even smaller groups.

First the hypertension in Tab. 2. In all four criteria, there is a worsening if the blood-pressure is higher. It is not so easy to say whether the systolic or the diastolic blood-pressure would correlate better. Maybe we have not chosen the limits correctly.

Tab. 2. Wirkung der Hypertonie auf die Neugeborenen.

	Gesamtzahl	Gewicht	< 2500 g %	Apgar 0–6 %	Perinat. mort. %
Kontrolle	2001	3425	5,35	5,70	2,40
Blutdruck Syst. –144	1212	3561	3,30	8,00	0,74
Blutdruck Syst. 145–	790	3310	10,55	12,30	3,18
Blutdruck Diast. –89	767	3557	3,18	3,13	0,91
Blutdruck Diast. 90–	1235	3404	8,05	7,42	2,20

Similarily for proteinuria (Tab. 3) the groups show a very good correlation with the criteria.

Tab. 3. Wirkung der Proteinurie auf die Neugeborenen.

	Gesamtzahl	Gewicht	< 2500 g %	Apgar 0–6 %	Perinat. mort. %
Kontrolle	2001	3425	5,35	5,70	2,40
Proteinurie –0,3‰	1659	3506	4,20	8,62	1,33
Proteinurie 0,4–1,0‰	213	3384	9,86	14,08	1,88
Proteinurie 1,1– %	130	3021	24,62	16,92	6,15

Finally if we divide the gestotic pregnant women into three groups with oedema (Tab. 4) we see that the correlations are now quite the opposite. The worse the oedemas, the better the babies.

Tab. 4. Wirkung des Ödems auf die Neugeborenen.

	Gesamtzahl	Gewicht	< 2500 g %	Apgar 0–6 %	Perinat. mort. %
Kontrolle	2001	3425	5,35	5,70	2,40
Keine Ödeme	509	3278	10,41	11,79	2,36
Wenig Ödeme	342	3410	6,43	11,11	2,34
Reichlich Ödeme	1151	3559	4,25	8,43	1,22

My conclusion is that it is possible that oedema is related to the defence mechanism of the body against gestosis and to take it as a positive point of the gestosis-index is, perhaps, wrong.

Influence de l'EPH Gestose sur le nouveau-né

Cl. Amiel, A. Thomine

Maternité de Port-Royal, Centre des Prématurés, Paris, France

Les gestoses ont été analysées à la Maternité de Port-Royal, dans le Service du Professeur *Varangot,* selon les critères proposés à la deuxième session de Janvier 1970. Cette analyse est rétrospective et a porté sur le nombre total des grossesses en 1969. Les chiffres recueillis permettent d'apprécier la fréquence, le retentissement sur la croissance intra-utérine, la mortalité. – Les résultats de la Maternité de Port-Royal sont dans l'ensemble très comparables à ceux obtenus par le Docteur *Welti* à la Maternité Universitaire de Lausanne.

Materiel et methodes

Au cours de l'année 1969 à la Maternité de Port-Royal, 1812 grossesses ont été enregistrées; le nombre total des naissances est de 1852. Le nombre total des nouveaux-nés d'un poids inférieur à 2500 gr est de 187, soit 10% des naissances. Parmi ces enfants, 35 sont des hypotrophiques, c'est à dire d'un poids de naissance trop petit pour leur âge gestationnel. La plupart d'entre eux ne sont pas prématurés et ont un âge gestationnel supérieur à 38 semaines. 6 d'entre eux sont à la fois hypotrophiques et prématurés (Tab.1).

Tab. 1. Materiel d'étude – Maternité Port Royal – 1969.

	Nombre	%
Total des grossesses	1812	
Total des naissances	1852	
Nouveau-nés d'un p inférieur à 2500 g	187	10% des naissances
Hypotrophiques	35	1,8
Prématures	152	8,2
Toxémie gravidique	161	8,8% des grossesses

L'age gestationnel est calculé en semaines complètes après le premier jour des dernières règles. Lorsque cette date est imprécise ou aberrante, il est apprécié sur des critères cliniques de maturation actuellement considérés comme satisfaisants: *critères morphologiques* d'une part mais surtout *neurologiques.* En effet la maturation cérébrale se poursuivant parallèlement à la durée de gestation, l'état du tonus et des reflexes primaires permet de retrouver cet âge gestationnel. Les conditions d'équipement n'ont pas permis, sauf dans quelques cas particuliers, d'utiliser les critères bio-électriques comme élément de confirmation.

La définition de l'hypotrophie choisie pour ce travail repose sur la situation du poids de naissance par rapport à l'âge conceptionnel sur la courbe dite de croissance intra-utérine de Lubschenco Tout nouveau-né situé au dessous du 10e *percentile* est hypotrophique, quelque soit son âge conceptionnel.

La définition de la pathologie maternelle la classification adoptée ici est celle proposée par le comité de nomenclature de l'Organisation Gestosis. La classification symptomatique inclut tous les cas où l'un ou plusieurs des symptômes suivants étaient présents:

1. *l'albuminurie* inclut arbitrairement les protéinuries supérieures à 0,5 g/L.
2. *L'oedème* trop difficile à apprécier est défini par une prise de poids excessive, fixée à 2 kg par mois, 13 kg pendant la totalité de la grossesse.
3. *l'hypertension* commence à 14/9 Cm/Hg.

Resultats et commentaires

Le diagnostic d'EPH-gestose a été porté 161 fois sur 1812 grossesses, soit dans 8,8% des cas.

La distribution des 161 cas d'EPH-gestosis selon les symptômes présents est représentée Tab. 2. On peut noter que parmi les formes monosymptomatiques la protéinurie isolée est rare, 11 cas. Les formes oedémateuses pures, hypertensives pures, ou polysymptomatiques se partagent la presque totalité des cas. Ces chiffres sont extrêmement voisins de ceux constatés à Lausanne. La Fréquence globale est également très proche (8,7% à Lausanne).

Tab. 2. Classification symptomatique dans 161 grossesses avec toxémie.

Toxémie	Nombre de cas	Nombre de toxémies au début du travail	Nombre de toxémies transitoires au cours de la grossesse
Monosymptomatique			
Oedème (E)	50	32	18
Protéinurie (P)	11	11	0
Hypertension (H)	42	36	6
Polysymptomatique	53	50	3
Pre-éclampsie	4	3	1
Eclampsie	1	1	0
Total	161	133	28

La distribution selon l'étiologie (Tab. 3) donne des résultats également très proches de ceux de Lausanne. On doit cependant faire uns réserve sur le groupe des formes transitoires – les bilans rénaux faits dans les mois qui ont succédé à l'accouchement ne figurent souvent pas dans nos archives il est donc possible qu'un certain nombre de ces cas soit en fait surajouté à une maladie chronique.

Tab. 3. Répartition selon l'age gestationel des nouveau-nés dans 161 cas de toxémie gravidique.

Toxémie	Terme non connu	Prématurité 24–38 sem.	Nouveau-né a terme 38–42 sem.	Post-maturité 42–46 sem.
Monosymptomatique Oedeme	3	12	31	4
Protéinurie	0	6	4	1
Hypertension	1	13	22	6
Polysymptomatique	3	13	35	2
Pre-éclampsie	0	2	2	0
Eclampsie	0	0	1	0
Total	7	46	95	13

Distribution selon la maturité – la répartition selon l'âge conceptionnel est représentée au tab. 4. On peut noter que 46 enfants sont nés avant 38 semaines, soit dans 28% des cas. Cette fréquence est très supérieure à celle notée à Lausanne, (13 sur 237). Elle est 3 fois supérieure à celle retrouvée dans la population globale de la maternité.

Tab. 4. Classification étiologique de 161 grossesses avec toxémie gravidique.

Toxémie	Monosymptomatique E	P	H	Polysymp.	Pre-éclampsie	Eclampsie
Toxémie transitoire	50	8	39	45		
Toxémie surajoutée à une lésion chronique du rein		3		1		
Hypertension arterielle permanente			2	2	1	
Non classée			1	5	3	1
Total	50	11	42	53	4	1

Notons que sur ces 46 prématurés, 2 seulement sont nés après déclenchement.

Distribution selon la croissance intra-utérine. Celle-ci est représenté au tab. 5. Il apparait que 17 nouveaux-nés seulement sur 169 ont un poids de naissance inférieur au 10e

Tab. 5. Croissance intra-uterine chez 169 nouveau-nés apres toxémie gravidique.

Toxemie	Hypotrophie foetale	Croissance normale	Terme non connu
Monosymptomatique Oedeme	1	47	3
Protéinurie	3	10	0
Hypertension	2	40	1
Polysymptomatique	8	46	3
Pre-éclampsie	2	2	0
Eclampsie	1	0	0
Total	17	145	7

percentile sur la courbe de Lubchenco, soit 10% alors que 145 ont eu une croissance considérée comme normale – Cette proportion est légèrement supérieure à celle de Lausanne, (17 sur 269).

Par ailleurs on peut remarquer que parmi les nouveaux-nés hypotrophiques, au nombre de 35 à Port-Royal en 1969, l'EPH-gestosis est retrouvée dans 50% des cas (Tab. 6), des étiologies variées dans 25% des cas, pas d'étiologie décelable dans 25% des cas.

Tab. 6. Circonstances gestationelles observées chez 35 nouveau-nés hypotrophiques.

Grossesse	Nombre
Toxémie	17
Gemellité	3
Post maturité	1
Placenta praevia	2
Malformations foetales	2
	25
Pas d'anomalies	7
Non suivie	3
Total	35

Lorsque l'on considère (Fig. 1) la répartition de ces 35 nouveaux-nés selon leur poids, taille, et perimètree céphalique en relation avec l'âge gestationnel, on peut noter que les enfants nés après EPH-gestosis ne semblent pas différents des autres, et on peut retrouver chez tous la notion bien classique de l'atteinte prédominante du poids, moindre de la taille et du périmètre céphalique.

Mortalité périnatale

Elle est remarquablement basse (Tab. 7) puisque 4 norts-nés avant tout début de travail la résument, soit 2,4%. Elle est donc nettement inférieure aux chiffres de Lausanne

Tab. 7. Mortalité perinatale dans 161 grossesses avec toxémie.

Toxémie	Decès		
	Ante partum	Sub partum	Post partum
Monosymptomatique			
Oedemes			
Protéinurie	3		
Hypertension			
Polysymptomatique	1		
Pre-éclampsie			
Eclampsie			
Total	4		

(17/269). On peut remarquer également que l'EPH-gestosis représente ainsi une faible part de la mortalité périnatale à Port-Royal, (Tab. 8).

Tab. 8. Mortalité perinatale – Maternité Port Royal – 1969.

	Nombre	%o
Total des grossesses	1812	
Total des naissances	1852	
Morts-nés	34	18
Decès néonataux	26	14
Decès périnataux	60	32

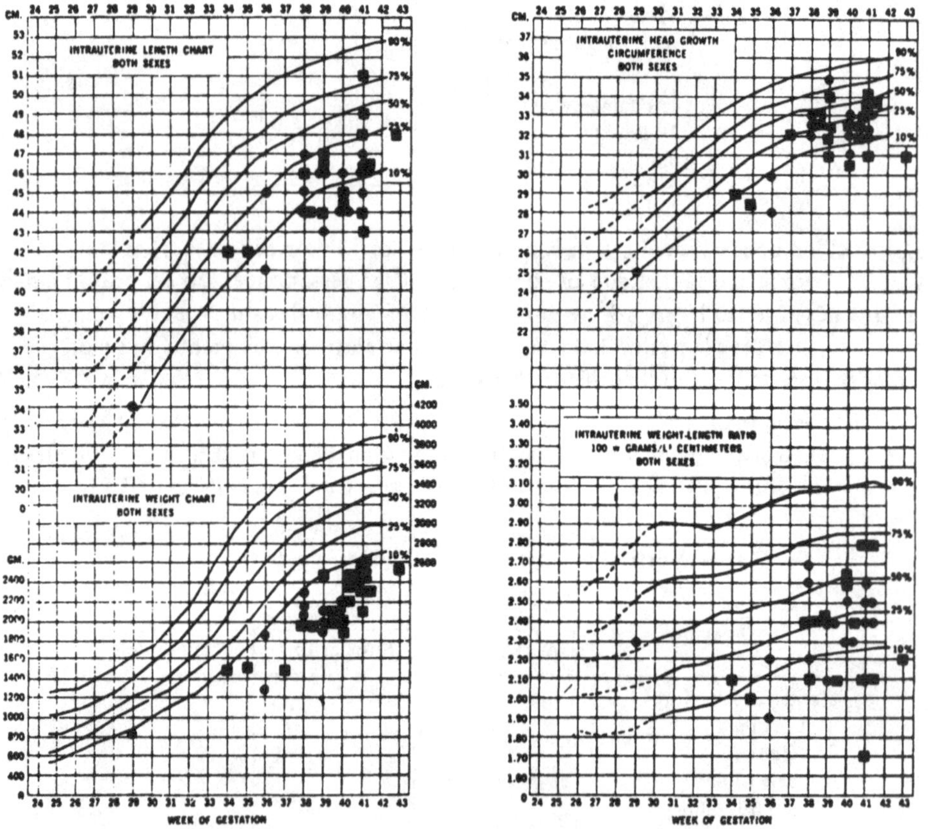

From Lubchenco, L.O., et al.: Pediatrics 37:403, 1966.
Additional copies available from Ross Laboratories, Columbus, Ohio 43216

● EPH GESTOSES
■ OTHER ETIOLOGIES

Fig. 1. Intra-uterine growth – gestational age distribution of 35 small-for-dates

Conclusion

Le faible pourcentage d'hypotrophie foetale a été une des surprises de cette analyse, en effet la majorité de ces enfants a eu une croissance intra-utérine peu ou pas perturbée, du moins d'après nos critères morphologiques grossiers.

Le taux très bas de mortalité représente un progrès remarquable sur les statistiques remontant à moins de 10 ans. D'une part une meilleure vigilance dans la surveillance des grossesses a entraîné cette baisse très sensible du taux des morts-nés. D'autre part une meilleure connaissance des problèmes néonataux particuliers à ce groupe d'enfants a rendu la mortalité infime dans les premiers jours de la vie.

Cependant, il reste dans quelques cas très sévères d'hypotrophie foetale de difficiles décisions thérapeutiques à prendre, louvoyant entre les risques de mort in utero et ceux d'une prématurité excessive. Il semble que selon chaque cas particulier, une décision de déclenchement puisse être discutée avec l'aide des examens biologiques, lorsque l'âge gestationnel a atteint environ 35 semaines et que la souffrance du foetus parait extrême.

Further Methods of Investigation

Serum- und Harnproteine bei EPH-Gestose

C. Goecke

Universitäts-Frauenklinik, Würzburg, BRD

Durch papierelektrophoretische Analysen der Proteine im Serum und Harn wurde versucht, diagnostische Hinweise bei EPH-Gestosen zu erhalten.

Im Vergleich mit den Werten gesunder Schwangerer (n = 65) zeigte sich bei etwa 100 Frauen mit meist schwerer Spätgestose (Tab. 1 a) eine deutliche Abnahme der Albumine und eine deutliche Zunahme der α- und β-Globuline. Die γ-Globuline zeigten keine Veränderungen. Zwischen leichter und schwerer Gestose ließen sich keine signifikanten Unterschiede feststellen. Hinweise auf eine im Vordergrund stehende Leber- oder Nierenbeteiligung ließen sich aus einem einzelnen Proteinogramm nicht ableiten.

Tab. 1a. Serum- und Harnproteine bei Nichtschwangeren, gesunden Schwangeren und bei EPH-Gestose.

	n	g‰ Esb.	Albumin (%)	Globulin (%)			
				α_1	α_2	β	γ
Präeklampsie Eklampsie	20	10,2	63,1	8,8	2,7	15,2	10,2

Auch am Ende der normal verlaufenden Schwangerschaft ist die Albuminfraktion im Vergleich zu Werten aus der Frühschwangerschaft oder zu Werten von nicht schwangeren Frauen vermindert. Infolge der Plasmavolumenzunahme und der Steigerung des Eiweißansatzes auf Kosten der Albumine kann jedoch eine Verminderung der Albuminsynthese nicht angenommen werden. Für die Globuline läßt sich unter Berücksichtigung einer Zunahme des Plasmavolumens um 30% eine ca. 70%ige Steigerung der Synthese errechnen. Die Hypalbuminämie und die meist fehlende Zunahme der γ-Globuline bei Gestose sind weniger Folge einer Synthesestörung als vielmehr Folge der Proteinurie.

Bei den im Harn ausgeschiedenen Proteinen (Tab. 1b) überwiegen die Albumine. In etwa der Hälfte der Fälle werden aus noch ungeklärter Ursache keine α_2-Globuline ausgeschieden. Mit den entsprechenden Serumdiagrammen zeigen die Harndiagramme weder eine Ähnlichkeit noch ein spiegelbildliches Verhalten.

Tab. 1b. Serumproteine.

	n	Gesamt EW (g %)	Albumin (%)	Globulin (%)			
				α_1	α_2	β	γ
Nichtschwangere	35	6,5 ± 0,1	61,0 ± 0,7	3,7 ± 0,5	7,7 ± 0,7	10,2 ± 0,8	17,4 ± 0,5
Schwangere m. III–VII	20	6,7 ± 0,3	56,2 ± 0,8	5,5 ± 0,5	10,2 ± 1,0	13,4 ± 0,9	16,7 ± 0,9
Schwangere m. VIII–X	45	5,9 ± 0,2	51,1 ± 0,6	6,0 ± 0,7	10,9 ± 0,9	16,0 ± 0,7	16,2 ± 0,6
leichte Prä-eklampsie (< 5)	21	5,5 ± 0,1	43,6 ± 1,6	7,5 ± 0,5	13,0 ± 0,9	18,4 ± 1,0	17,1 ± 0,6
schwere Prä-eklampsie (> 5)	53	5,7 ± 0,2	41,8 ± 1,0	8,7 ± 0,6	15,2 ± 0,9	18,6 ± 0,8	16,0 ± 0,5
Eklampsie	23	5,6 ± 0,1	46,5 ± 0,5	7,4 ± 0,7	12,1 ± 0,6	17,7 ± 0,8	16,1 ± 1,1

The Estimation of Serum Proteins in Gestosis

A. Cretti

II. Frauenklinik der Medizinischen Akademie, Bialystok, Polen

It is known that in gestosis there are changes in serumproteins, namely hypoproteinemia and dysproteinemia. Dysproteinemia shows as decreased level of albumins and increased level of alpha-1-globulins, alpha-2-globulins and beta-globulins. There is disagreement about the level of gamma-globulins. There are differences between the studies about the percentage of cases in which these changes occur and about their intensity. For such differences different diagnostic criteria of gestosis might be responsible, namely which cases are included in the groups studied.

The detection of serum protein changes can play a role in diagnosis. If we have a patient suspected of gestosis and we find the changes mentioned above – this helps us to recognize this case as one prone for developing a gestosis with full symptoms.

In the differential diagnosis, when we separate the gestosis from glomerulonephritis combined with nephrotic syndrom, the estimation of serum proteins can be also helpful. In gestosis we do not observe the so-called "crossed" uroplasmatic profile, which is usually met in nephrosis. In this phenomenon we see high urinary values of albumins, which are diminished in the serum, and low levels of alpha-globulins and beta-globulins, which are augmented in the serum. This too may sometimes help in differentiating the transitory gestosis from the superimposed one.

The changes in serum proteins play also a role in the evaluation of the severity of a case: the more advanced the changes, the more severe the case.

Moreover the estimation of serum protein changes is important from the therapeutical point of view. As we know a level of whole serum proteins below 5.5 g % or an albumine-level below 2.5 g % is sufficient "per se" to be the cause of oedema through changes in oncotic pressure. In our department we consider a level under 6.3 g % as hypoproteinemia. All our patients receive high-protein diet. But if a patient with a serum protein level below 6.3 g % has oedema we additionaly give infusions of human albumins, as the hypoproteinemia in these cases is usually associated with diminution of albumins. With such treatment we observe better results than with the administration of saluretics only. But if the level is below 5.6 g % we give human albumins even if there is no visible oedema or excessive weight gain.

According to our program we shall talk to-day about the standardizing of methods, which can be easily reproduced by the average personel taking care of pregnant women.

For determining whole serum proteins we have such a simple procedure as the method of *Philips* and *Van Slyke* at our disposal. Here no photocolorimeter is needed but only various solutions of copper sulfate. Unfortunately, this method can have an inaccurateness up to 10% or even 15%. However, the error can be diminished considerably if all the estimations are done by the same person and from time to time the results are confronted with a more accurate method, for example with the biuret method. And, of course, if the copper sulfate solutions are sufficiently often changed.

The estimation of whole serum protein by *Biuret* method is sufficiently accurate. Here the photocolorimeter is needed. This not very expensive apparatus is useful in laboratory for many various analyses and one is entitled to hope that in a not very far away future it would be available everywhere.

Where there is no possibility to employ the more accurate biuret method and if the method of Philips and Van Slyke is used, one should be aware of the possible error range of this last procedure and of the above described means to reduce the inaccurateness.

There is also a difficulty in interpreting the results of whole serum protein estimations, difficulty independent of the method used. This difficulty depends on variability of changes in blood volume. The volume of whole blood is usually diminished in gestosis when comparing it with healthy pregnant women, but it may vary from case to case. So the concentration of protein, which is estimated, depends on the blood volume in each single case. This may be one of the causes why the results of serum proteins are sometimes variable. However, determinations of blood volume are not simple and could not be as yet regarded as standardized routine methods.

The albumins can be determined not only by the paper electrophoresis but also by the precipitation-method which is easier and besides no apparatus for electrophoresis is then needed. Knowing the level of albumins we can abstract this figure from the value of whole serum protein and thus evaluate the level of globulins and thereby estimate the albumins to globulins quotient.

The paper electrophoresis, giving the more detailed information of the level of albumins, alpha-1-globulins, alpha-2-globulins, beta-globulins and gamma-globulins is nowadays quite widely used. Some authors represent the opinion that especially the increase of beta-globulins can be interpreted as a bad prognostic sign.

The method of immunoelectrophoresis is not very expensive. It is a semiquantitative method, giving information about more fractions than paper electrophoresis. We can judge from the precipitation lines if a protein fraction is present, or absent and if the level of a fraction is increased or decreased. However, one must have a great experience to evaluate properly the picture of immunoelectrophoresis.

The electrophoresis on polyacryloamid gel, the so called "disc electrophoresis" is in phase of introduction. It is certainly very valuable but it is to early to talk about the standardization of this procedure.

Serum Proteins in Pregnancy and EPH-Gestosis

J. Studd

Birmingham Maternity Hospital, Queen Elisabeth Medical Center, Birmingham, G.B.

During the last 15 years many workers have studied serum proteins in pregnancy and pre-eclampsia by paper electrophoresis with agreement that in normal pregnancy there is a fall in serum albumin and elevation of the beta-globulin fraction; an elevation of $alpha_1$-globulin and $alpha_2$-globulin and a fall in the gamma-globulin fraction has not been confirmed by all workers.

In EPH-gestosis there is a further fall in serum albumin and a probable rise in $alpha_2$-globulin and beta-globulin. There is not more information to be gained by work with paper electrophoresis because the proteins are only poorly separated into heterogenous bands whose only similarity is that of electrophoretic mobility. Further study must therefore be directed towards the changes occurring in individual proteins and I have studied this by using the method of immunoelectrophoresis as described by *Laurell.* This is not as yet a standard technique but all the proteins to be discussed can be easily estimated by the simple technique of immunodiffusion which is available to us all.

I have measured various serum proteins in 10 normal pregnancies and also in 10 patients with EPH-gestosis of considerable severity, all patients having a blood pressure of 160/110 or more and all patients having a proteinuria of more than 6 g per day. I have compared the patient's serum proteins in late pregnancy with the levels in the same patient's postpartum serum taken at three months. The results for changes in concentration of individual proteins are expressed as percentage of the patient's postpartum or non-pregnant level.

In normal pregnancy the serum albumin falls from 4.43 g % to 3.53 g % which represents a depression of 23%. However, in severe EPH-gestosis the fall in albumin is greater to 2.96 g % representing a fall of 34%. There is no significant change in total globulins in pregnancy or pre-eclampsia although there does appear to be a slight elevation in total serum globulins in EPH-syndrome.

Thyroxine binding prealbumin also demonstrates a considerable fall in normal pregnancy. The other proteins on this slide have all increased concentrations by the end of pregnancy and I would like to draw your attention to the elevation of transferrin, $alpha_2$-macroglobulin and beta-lipoprotein because these undergo further changes in concentration if the pregnancy is complicated by hypertension and proteinuria.

We see in the next slide the changes that occur in the serum proteins in the presence of severe pre-eclampsia. As already stated there is a fall in albumin and a fall in the two globulins of similar molecular weight that is, haemopexin and transferrin. It is probable that a fall in these proteins is a result of the loss of these three proteins in the urine which has been shown to be the case invariably when proteinuria complicates pregnancy, by *Helen McEwan.* Alpha$_2$-macroglobin and beta-lipoprotein show significant increases in the presence of proteinuria. I should point out that the changes in these five proteins, albumin, haemopexin, transferrin and also alpha$_2$-macroglobulin and beta-lipoprotein creates a serum protein pattern identical with that found in the nephrotic syndrome. In that situation it is believed that the depression of the serum proteins of intermediate molecular weight is a result of heavy loss of these proteins in the urine. The hypoproteinaemia then stimulates an increased liver synthesis of proteins which is unselective producing proteins of all sizes and molecular weights. The small ones are again lost to the defective glomerular basement membrane and the large macromolecules are retained, being too large to pass through the permeable kidney basement membrane. Serial studies have shown that the depression of albumin haemopexin and transferrin is directly related to the quantity and duration of the loss and that the elevation of beta-lipoprotein is similarly related to the duration of the proteinuria.

Zur Östrogen-Ausscheidung bei EPH-Gestose

C. Goecke

Universitäts-Frauenklinik, Würzburg, BRD

Bei ungestörter Schwangerschaft steigt die tägliche Östrogen-Ausscheidung im Harn kontinuierlich an und erreicht am Entbindungstermin eine Höhe von 30–50 mg Östrogene/24 Std. Ist die fetoplazentare Einheit durch Plazentainsuffizienz, Einschränkung der fetalen Zirkulation oder verminderte Bereitstellung der Östrogenvorstufen durch die fetalen Nebennieren gestört, so kann eine Abnahme der täglichen Östrogen-Ausscheidung diagnostische Hinweise geben.

Verschiedene Faktoren können jedoch den Wert der Harn-Östrogen-Bestimmung einschränken. Es konnte gezeigt werden [2, 3], daß

1. die Östrogen-Ausscheidung eng korreliert ist mit dem mütterlichen extrazellulären Raum im besonderen dem Plasmavolumen. – Bei extrazellulärer Wasserretention, vor allem bei Ödembildung können Östrogene im mütterlichen Organismus vermehrt retiniert werden.
2. die absolute Östrogen-Ausscheidung korreliert ist mit der Höhe der Diurese. – Wird vermehrt Harn ausgeschieden, so steigt die Östrogen-Ausscheidung an. Die natürliche und medikamentöse Diurese-Steigerung läßt somit auch die Östrogen-Ausscheidung zunehmen. Eine verminderte Östrogen-Ausscheidung kann daher bei behandelter Gestose gelegentlich nicht erkennbar sein.
3. eine gestörte Tubulus-Funktion der Nieren die Östrogen-Ausscheidung beeinträchtigt. – Bei Pfropfgestose mit renalem Grundleiden oder Pyelonephritis der Schwangeren kann eine verminderte Östrogen-Ausscheidung durch mangelhafte Tubulus-Funktion vorgetäuscht sein.
4. an die Schwangere verabreichte Medikamente sowohl die Östrogen-Bestimmung selbst als auch die Freisetzung der Östrogen-Vorstufen in den kindlichen Nebennieren beeinflussen [1].
5. Tag-zu-Tag-Schwankungen in der Östrogen-Ausscheidung über 50% des Ausgangswertes betragen können.
6. ein signifikanter Abfall der Östrogen-Ausscheidung erst 3–6 Stunden nach Ausfall der gesamten Plazenta zu erwarten ist. – Selbst 48 Stunden nach intrauterinem Fruchttod konnte in etwa 20% der Fälle noch eine Östrogen-Ausscheidung an der unteren Grenze des angegebenen Normbereiches gefunden werden.

Diese Faktoren gilt es bei der Beurteilung der Östrogen-Ausscheidung in durch EPH-Gestose gestörter Schwangerschaft zu berücksichtigen. Es besteht ferner eine enge Korrelation (r = 0,42) zwischen Östriol-Ausscheidung und der errechneten funktionstüchtigen Plazentaoberfläche. Durch genauere Direktbestimmungen der Plazentaoberfläche mit dem Integrationsverfahren wird z. Zt. versucht, einen verläßlichen Östrogen-Plazenta-Faktor zu errechnen.

Literatur

[1] *Däßler, C.-G.:* Acta endocr. (Kbh.) 53 (1966) S. 401.

[2] *Goecke, C.:* Wiener Med. Wschr. 119 (1969) S. 805.

[3] *Goecke, C., S. Timonen:* Arch. Gynäk. 203 (1966) S. 118.

Plasma Renin Activity

B. Vedra

Research Institute for the Care of Mother and Child, Prague-Podoli

The homeostasis of body fluids and the regulation of circulation and of blood pressure are closely connected. The integration of the salt metabolism, body fluid volumes and circulation is mediated through the system renin-angiotensin-aldosterone (RAA). Aldosterone is the most powerfull sodium retaining corticoid, angiotensin is the most effective stimulus for the secretion of aldosterone and at the same time a very powerfull pressoric agent.

Therefore, if we should better understand the pathophysiology of EPH-gestosis, we need more studies of the RAA-system.

Renin is an enzyme produced in the juxtaglomerular cells of the kidneys. By its enzymatic effect the renin substrate, i.e. alfa-2-globulins of the plasma, are depolymerized to the dekapeptide angiotensin I and by further enzymatic action to the oktapeptide angiotensin II. Under normal conditions in the body angiotensin II is quickly destructed by angiotensinase.

For the purpose of research projects regarding the RAA-system, the method of *Boucher* can be recommended. This method measures the plasma renin activity as the amount of angiotensin II produced in a given volume of plasma in 3 hours. The amount is given in nanogram %.

The technical details of the method can be found in the literature (see references to this paper).

The method consists of incubation of plasma with Dowex-resin at 37°C for 3 hours with vigorous shaking. The further steps are washing of the incubate, elution of angiotensin from the Dowex resin and purification of the eluate by repeated evaporation and sublimation of the solvents in a vacuum. The last step is bioassay in the nephrectomized rat.

References

Boucher, R. et al.: Canad. Med. Ass. J. 90 (1964) p. 194.

Vedra, B., A. Slaby: Sborník lék. 70 (1968) p. 335.

Screening of Proteinuria in EPH-Gestosis

B. Vedra, J. Hampl

Research Institute for the Care of Mother and Child, Prague-Podoli

By the help of very sensitive methods a certain small amount of protein in urine can be found also in healthy subjects. The quantity of excreted proteins almost never exceeds 50 mg/24 hours. The loss of 50 mg/24 hours corresponds, according to the volume of urine, to the concentrations of 3–5 mg %. Every proteinuria exceeding these figures should therefore be regarded as abnormality or pathology.

The screening methods which are used in pregnancy are based on the determination of protein concentration in a sample of urine. The most sensitive screening methods detect reliably the concentrations about 10 mg % which means that every proteinuria detected by some of the screening methods highly exceeds the borders of physiology.

From the variety of methods determining proteins in urine the following two methods can be recommended for screening:

1. *Paper strip method,* which detects concentrations around 10 mg %.
2. *Sulfosalicylic acid test.*

To approximately 5 ml of urine 1–2 drops of 30% acetic acid are added. Then 3–5 drops of sulfosalicylic acid are added consecutively. White clouds observed against black background mean usually protein. The lowest sensitivity is 8–10 mg %. When correctly performed the method has no falsely negative results.

If by help of a screening method protein in urine is detected, in every such case the quantitative estimation of protein lost in 24 hours should be made. For this purpose the concentration of protein in a mixed sample of the total 24 hour volume of urine is determinded. The concentration given in mg % multiplicated by the total 24 hour-volume of urine in ml and divided by 100 gives the quantity of proteins in mg lost in 24 hours.

A Technique for the Study of the Renal Pathology in EPH-Gestosis by the Electron Microscope

Maher Mahran, F.R.C.S., M.R.C.O.G., Ph.D. (Ed.), F.I.C.S.
Hossam E. Fadel, D.G.O., D.S., M.Ch. (Cairo), *A. Nassar* Ph.D. (London)

Departments of Obstetrics and Gynecology, and Anatomy, Faculty of Medicine,
Ain Shame University, Cairo, UAR

Interest in kidney pathology in gestosis had begun more than a century ago. Only post-mortem examination of the kidney was available at that time. The material consisted mainly of eclamptic women, and the attempts at specification of the renal lesion were not successful.

It was correctly realized that study of the renal pathology during life must give more accurate results. Needle biopsy of the kidney was attempted for the first time by *Alwall* (1952). However, the method has gained popularity only after the demonstration of its safety by *Iversen* and *Brun* (1951).

The use of percutaneous renal biopsy during pregnancy was delayed for some time because of the technical difficulties encountered due to the presence of the pregnant uterus, and for fear of unexpected complications. Modifications of the technique allowed the procedure to be undertaken during pregnancy, and since then the method was practiced in many centers for the study of the renal pathology in Gestosis (*Dieckmann* et al., 1957; *Spargo* et al., 1959 and *Pollak* and *Nettles,* 1960).

Since 1965 we have been using this technique. Over 100 pregnant and recently delivered women were subjected to percutaneous renal biopsy. Many of them have been subjected more than once.

The success of renal biopsy depends to a large extent on the understanding and cooperation of the patient. A nervous, irritable or uncooperative patient, is not a suitable candidate for this procedure. History of bleeding tendencies or abnormal bleeding or clotting time are considered contra-indications to the technique.

Radiographic localization of the kidney prior to the biopsy is advised by many authors (*Morris* et al., 1964 and *Smythe* et al., 1964). However, we thought that this might be hazardous to the foetus and we avoided this practice.

When a patient was selected for biopsy, a pint of cross-matched blood was prepared. An injection of pethidine 100 mg. I.M. was given $^1/_2$ h. before the determined time. She was then transferred to the delivery room.

Recently delivered women can be made to assume the usual prone position on a sandbag (*Kark* and *Muehrcke*, 1954). However, those pregnant patients specially near term cannot maintain this position, and so they are asked to sit on the edge of the delivery table.

After thorough sterilization of the skin (tincture iodine and alcohol), the landmarks are identified i.e. the lower border of the last rib, and the outer border of the quadratus lumborum muscle (on the right side). The point of entry of the needle is selected about 1 cm below and lateral to the renal angle thus delineated. This is assumed to mark the lateral part of the inferior pole of the right kidney.

Anaesthesia is achieved by local infiltration at this point with 8 ml of Xylocaine 0.5%. A thin lumbar puncture needle is then used to explore the site of the kidney. It is pushed in gently ± perpendicular to the skin surface and is felt to pass through the lumbodorsal fascia. The patient is then instructed to take a deep inspiration and then to hold her breath, while the needle is pushed further to pierce the renal capsule and penetrate for a short distance into the kidney substance.

N.B.: If the biopsy is attempted in the upright position an assistant exerts manual pressure backwards and upwards under the right costal margin. This is meant to stabilise the kidney effectively in the anteroposterior plane permitting nicer control of the needle as it is introduced into the kidney.

The patient is then allowed to breathe quietly. If the needle moves freely to and fro with respiration in a wide arc this means that it is really in the kidney substance. If the needle moves only a little or only through a narrow arc, it is usually in the perinephric fat or just hits the surface of the kidney. After ensuring that the exploratory needle had entered the kidney substance, it is removed, and the depth of the kidney estimated.

The biopsy needle we use in the *Franklin*'s modification of *Vim-Silvermann* needle. The trocar and canula are introduced in the same point and pushed inwards in the same direction and to the same depth taking care that the final push through the kidney capsule must be done while the patient holds her breath in deep inspiration.

The trocar is then removed, and the cutting prongs of the *Silvermann* needle are introduced within the canula. The cutting prongs are then pushed inwards for further 2 cm while the patient holds her breath in deep inspiration, and the canula is then pushed for these 2 cm to ensheath the piece of renal tissue thus severed, and then the canula with the cutting knife are removed rapidly together. The cutting knife is inspected for the presence of a core of renal tissue. If not, the attempt can be repeated once or twice before it is announced a failure.

A sterile dressing is applied to the puncture area and a tight abdominal bandage is applied for 24 hours, and the patient transferred back to her bed. She is instructed to lie quiet for the next 24 hours.

The pulse, temperature, and blood pressure are observed hourly and recorded. Urine passed from the patient is collected at 2–4 hours intervals and inspected for the presence of hematuria during the next 24 hours. Analgesics are prescribed if pain is complained of. Success of the biopsy is obtaining renal tissue. The success rate in our hands was 77.8% (*Fadel* et al., 1968). In most reported series in non-pregnant subjects, the success rate varied from 80–90%, the highest recorded success rate being 96% (*Kark* et al., 1958). During pregnancy, *Pollak* and *Nettles* (1960) reported a success rate of 84.7%. Our lower success rate is to be attributed to the adoption of the sitting position, to the avoidance of radiographic localization, and may be to the tendency of our patients to obesity which makes identification of the landmarks specially the outer border of the quadratus lumborum muscle more difficult.

Sometimes only medullary tissue is obtained. This makes the biopsy inadequate. Five glomeruli and their adjacent tubules are the minimum required for the biopsy to be considered adequate for pathologic evaluation (*Pollak* and *Nettles,* 1960).

Inadvertent puncture of other organs e.g. spleen, liver, or duodenum during attempts at renal biopsy has been reported (*Kerr,* 1960). In our series suprarenal tissue was sometimes obtained (*Attia* et al., 1970).

The complications of renal biopsy in our hands were fortunately, of minor importance. About 8% complained of flank pain, and 3.5% had gross hematuria which abated spontaneously within 36 hours and none required blood transfusion or intervention. *Dieckmann* et al. (1957) reported that only 1 patient required blood transfusion in their series of 122 patients. *Altchek* (1961) stated that many cases hat flank tenderness and hematuria. *Smythe* et al. (1964) reported the occurrence of perirenal hematoma once in a series of 91 patients. *McCartney* (1964) reported that blood transfusion was needed in 3 patients and nephrectomy done once in the course of 400 biopsies. *Schewitz* et al. (1965) on the other hand, reported a frightening incidence of complications of renal biopsy during pregnancy. Of 90 patients, 15 had gross hematuria, 4 had renal colic and 2 patients hat sugical intervention. One patient had rupture of the renal pelvis and the other died during the induction of anaesthesia for evacuating a perirenal hematoma. They compared their results with 450 biopsies in non-pregnant subjects and came to the conclusion that the use of renal biopsy in pregnant patients should be recommended with great caution.

Although this frightening experience was not confirmed by subsequent investigators, still it had resulted in the recommendation that biopsies are not to be attempted during pregnancy but better deferred till the early puerperium (*Fisher* et al., 1969).

Processing of the renal tissue

Renal tissue obtained at biopsy can be useful in many ways. In addition to the usual pathologic study by light and electron microscopes, it can be cultured bacteriologically to help in the diagnosis of asymptomatic pyelonephritis (*Hutt,* 1961). Renal biopsy specimens have been subjected to immunofluorescent studies (*Morris* et al., 1964 and *Fadel* et al., 1969). Also renal biopsy may be utilized in histochemical studies. In this communication we will describe in more detail our technique of processing renal tissue obtained at biopsy for ultrastructural studies.

The tissue obtained is cut into small pieces (1 × 1 mm) each which are then immediately fixed in 4% phosphate buffered glutaraldehyde (ph 7.4) for periods ranging from

3 days to one month and then stored in 0.2 M sucrose in phosphate buffer. Trimming to the proper size is done under the dissecting microscope and the tissue is then post fixed in 1% buffered $Os\ O_4$ for 3 hours.

Dehydration is ascending grades of ethanol as follows:
1. 70% ethanol (2 changes 15 minutes each).
2. 80% ethanol (2 changes 15 minutes each).
3. 96% ethanol (2 changes 15 minutes each).
4. Absolute ethanol (2 changes 30 minutes each).

Embedding is done in Epon 812 using the following mixtures:

Mixture A.	(Stable for many months at 4° C).	
	Epon 812	62 ml
	DDSA (Dodecynyl succinic anhydride)	100 ml
Mixture B.	(Stable for many months at 4° C).	
	Epon 812	100 ml
	MNA (Methyl nadic anhydride)	89 ml
Mixture C.		
	Mixture A	4 volumes
	Mixture B	6 volumes

To this mixture is added 2–2½% of the accelerator DMP (2, 4′, 6 tri dimethyl-amino phenol).

The resultant mixture has to be mixed thoroughly for at least 10 min. It is preferable to prepare it just before use but, it can be kept only for few days in deep freeze at - 20° C.

After absolute ethanol the tissue is put in equal volumes of propylene oxide and mixture C for 1 hour at room temperature.

Then it is put in another mixture of propylene oxide and mixture C 1:3 for 3 hours at room temp. Then every piece of tissue is embedded in a gelatin capsule (already dried in the oven at 60° C for 1 hour) in a fresh pure mixture C at 60° C for 2 days.

Sections about 600 Å thick are then cut using the *"Porter Blum"* microtome. The sections are stained on the grids using 5% aqueous solution of Uranyl acetate followed by lead citrate (*Reynolds*, 1963). The grids are then examined with AEI electron microscope at 80 KV using the double condenser system.

In conclusion, we can say that percutaneous renal biopsy is a safe procedure. It has served many purposes in the study of EPH-Gestosis.

The delineation of the specific glomerular lesion became possible (*Spargo* et al., 1959; *Pirani* et al., 1963; *Altchek* et al., 1968 and *Fadel* et al., 1970).

Many cases clinically diagnosed as EPH-Gestosis were shown by renal biopsy to be suffering from primary renal disease or essential hypertension (*McCartney* et al., 1964 and *Fadel* et al., 1970).

The fact that renal biopsy could be obtained repeatedly and safely from the same patient enabled us for the first time to study the natural history of the renal lesion in EPH-Gestosis. The lesion was founded by many authors to be completely reversible

(*Hopper* et al., 1961; *Dennis* et al., 1963 and *Fadel* et al., 1969). While others have shown that it is only partially reversible (*Pirani* et al., 1963 and *Fiaschi* and *Naccarato*, 1968).

Renal biopsy has also served to correlate renal function with renal pathology during life (*McCartney* and *Spargo*, 1961).

Renal biopsy has also been useful in the study of the pathogenesis of the kidney lesion. The demonstration of fibrin aggregates along the basement membrane of the glomeruli supports the presence of a process of disseminated intravascular thrombosis. While the absence of gamma-globulins and complement in the glomerular lesion speaks against an immunologic basis for the renal lesion (*Morris* et al., 1964 and *Fisher* et al., 1969).

The reported hypertrophy of the juxta glomerular cells suggests a role for the renin-angiotensin-aldosterone system in the pathogenesis of EPH-Gestosis (*Altchek* et al., 1968 and *Fisher*, 1969).

References

Altchek, A.: J.A.M.A. 175 (1961) p. 791.

Altchek, A., N. L. Albright and *S. C. Sommers:* Obstet. Gynec. 31 (1968) p. 595.

Alwall, N.: Acta Med. Scandinav. 143 (1952) p. 430.

Attia, O., H. E. Fadel, M. Mahran, M. S. Sabour and *M. N. El-Mahallawi:* Amer. J. Obstet. Gynec. 107 (1970) p. 889.

Dennis, E. J., C. M. Smythe, F. A. McIver and *H. G. Howe:* Amer. J. Obstet. Gynec. 87 (1963) p. 364.

Dieckmann, W. J., E. L. Potter and *C. P. McCartney:* Amer. J. Obstet. Gynec. 73 (1957) p. 1.

Fadel, H. E., M. S. Sabour, M. Mahran, D. Seif Eldin and *M. N. El-Mahallawi:* J. Egypt. Med. A. 51 (1968) p. 1029.

Fadel, H. E., M. S. Sabour, M. Mahran, D. Seif Eldin and *M. N. El-Mahallawi:* Obstet. Gynec. 33 (1069) p. 528.

Fadel, H. E., M. S. Sabour, M. Mahran, D. Seif Eldin and *M. N. El-Mahallawi:* In „Die Spätgestose" Internationales Symposium an der Universitätsfrauenklinik, April 1969. Schwabe & Co., Basel (1970) p. 39.

Fadel, H. E., M. S. Sabour and *M. Mahran:* J. Int. Fed. Gynaec. Obstet. (in Press).

Fiaschi, E. and *R. Naccarato:* Virchows Arch. Abt. A. Path. Anat. 345 (1968) p. 299.

Fisher, E. R., V. Pardo, R. Paul and *T. T. Hayashi:* Amer. J. Path. 55 (1969) p. 109.

Hopper, J., M. G. Farquhar, H. Yamauchi, H. P. Moon and *E. W. Page:* Obstet. Gynec. 17 (1961) p. 271.

Hutt, M. S. R., J. A. Chalmers, J. S. MacDonald and *H. E. De Wardener:* Lancet 1 (1961) p. 351.

Iversen, P. and *C. Brun:* Amer. J. Med. 11 (1951) p. 324.

Kark, R. M. and *R. C. Muehrcke:* Lancet 1 (1954) p. 1047.

Kark, R. M., R. C. Muehrcke, V. E. Pollak, C. L. Pirani and *J. H. Kiefer:* Arch. Int. Med. 101 (1958) p. 439.

Kerr, D. N. S.: Lancet 2 (1960) p. 1370.

McCartney, C. P.: Circulation 30, Suppl. II (1964) p. 37.

McCartney, C. P. and *B. Spargo:* Med. Clin. Nor. Amer. 1 (1961) p. 141.

Morris, R. H., P. Vassalli, F. K. Beller and *R. T. McClusky:* Obstet. Gynec. 24 (1964) p. 32.

Pirani, C. L., V. E. Pollak, R. Lannigan and *G. Folli:* Amer. J. Obstet. Gynec. 87 (1963) p. 1047.

Pollak, V. E. and *J. B. Nettles:* Medicine (Balt.) 39 (1960) p. 469.

Reynolds, R. S.: J. Cell. Biol. 17 (1963) p. 208.

Schewitz, L. J., I. A. Friedman and *V. E. Pollak:* Obstet. Gynec. 26 (1965) p. 295.

Smythe, C. M., W. S. Bradham, E. J. Dennis, F. A. McIver and *H. G. Howe:* J. Lab. Clin. Med. 63 (1964) p. 562.

Spargo, B., C. P. McCartney and *R. Winemiller:* Arch. Path. 68 (1959) S. 593.

EPH-Gestose und Pyelonephritis

H. Kremling

Universitäts Frauenklinik, Würzburg, BRD

Die Pyelonephritis wird heute als häufigste Nierenkrankheit angesehen. Ihre Frequenz ist im Bereich einer Allgemeinpraxis mit etwa 3% angegeben, im klinischen Bereich mit mehr als 5% und in großen Sektionsstatistiken zwischen 5 und 10%. Bei etwa der Hälfte dieser Verstorbenen war die chronische Pyelonephritis eigentliche Todesursache. Folgt man den Mitteilungen von *Raaschou* [12], *Kleeman, Hewitt* und *Guze* [8], so konnten nur etwa 30% der chronischen Verlaufsformen klinisch diagnostiziert werden. Die chonische Pyelonephritis befällt nach den Untersuchungen von *Sarre* [14] und *Brod* [2, 3] Frauen häufiger als Männer. Von 228 Patienten mit chronischer Pyelonephritis der Freiburger Medizinischen Poliklinik der Universität waren 66,5% Frauen; in dem von *Brod* [3] untersuchten Kollektiv mit 421 Patienten betrug ihr ihr Anteil sogar 71%. Der Häufigkeitsgipfel lag bei den Frauen zwischen dem 20. und 25. Lebensjahr (*Sarre,* [14]). Die chronische Pyelonephritis kann sich nach *Berning* und *Thiele* [1] direkt aus der akuten entwickeln, aber auch das Resultat wiederholter Rezidive sein. Ist die chronische Form weiter fortgeschritten, manifestiert sie sich durch Nierenversagen oder Kreislaufkomplikationen [1].

Unter den prädisponierenden Faktoren der Gestose wird die chronische Pyelonephritis als Grundleiden oft genannt. *Hochuli* und *Käser* [7] fanden bei 104 Patientinnen mit Spätgestose in 16,3% eine chronische Pyelonephritis, bei weiteren 9,6% mußte die chronische Pyelonephritis als Grundleiden als wahrscheinlich angesehen werden. *Friedberg* [5] hat diese Frage in einem eingehenden Referat kürzlich kritisch gewürdigt. In einem weiteren Kollektiv von 113 Frauen mit Spätgestose sah *Hochuli* [6] bei 22 eine chronische Pyelonephritis, bei 5 Nierenmißbildungen mit Pyelonephritis (insgesamt 23,1%); bei weiteren 18 eine wahrscheinlich chronische Pyelonephritis, ferner eine Patientin mit chronischer interstitieller Nephritis (insgesamt 40,7% der untersuchten Frauen). Bei eigenen, gemeinsam mit *Goecke* und *Heidland* [9] durchgeführten Nachuntersuchungen hatten von 113 Frauen mit Spätgestose 27 (23,9%) eine chronische Pyelonephritis. Die Ergebnisse dieser Untersuchung sowie die klinischen Befunde während und nach der Behandlung der Gestose wiesen bei weiteren 23 (20,3%) auf eine z. Zt. nicht aktive Pyelonephritis hin.

Die Diagnose „Pfropfgestose durch Pyelonephritis“, die meist erst nach der Entbindung gestellt wird, ist schon während der Gravidität vor allem aus therapeutischen Gründen anzustreben; denn neben den bei Gestose üblichen Maßnahmen muß die Pyelonephritis behandelt werden. Durch langfristige Therapie ist es möglich, nicht nur

die Spätfolgen bei der Mutter zu verringern, sondern auch die Prognose des Kindes zu bessern. Dies läßt sich zeigen am Beispiel von 128 Schwangeren mit chronischer Pyelonephritis, die von 132 Kindern entbunden wurden. 59 Schwangere mit chronischer Pyelonephritits wurden länger als 21 Tage behandelt. 57 Kinder (96,4%) hatten ein Geburtsgewicht über 3000 g, 2 unter 3000 g (3,6%). Fetus mortuus 0%.
30 Schwangere (31 Kinder) wurden weniger als 21 Tage behandelt: lediglich 9 Kinder (29,0%) wogen über 3000 g, 17 (54,8%) unter 3000 g. 5 Kinder (16,2%) waren intrauterin abgestorben. 39 Schwangere mit 42 Kindern blieben unbehandelt; nur 8 Kinder (19,0%) wogen über, 19 (45,3%) unter 3000 g, 15 Kinder (35,7%) waren intrauterin abgestorben. Die 8 Schwangeren, deren Kinder mehr als 3000 g wogen, hatten noch keine erheblich eingeschränkte Nierenfunktion [10].

Tab. 1. Chronische Pyelonephritis; 128 Schwangere, 132 Kinder.

	Therapie > 21 Tage	Therapie < 21 Tage	ohne Therapie	insgesamt
Geburtsgewicht > 3000 g	57	9	8 (1 × Gemini)	74
Geburtsgewicht > 3000 g	2	17 (1 × Gemini)	19 (1 × Gemini)	38
Fetus mortuus Gewicht > 3000 g	0	2	1	3
Getus mortuus Gewicht < 3000 g	0	3	14 (1 × Gemini)	17
Insgesamt	59	31	42	132

Bei der Diagnostik während der Schwangerschaft ist folgendes zu beachten: mit dem Befund Eiweiß im Harn sollte man sich grundsätzlich nicht begnügen. Wird eine Proteinurie festgestellt, sind weitere Harnuntersuchungen erforderlich, vor allem auf Bakterien, Leukozytenzylinder und Glitterzellen (Sternheimer-Malbin). Werden Leukozytenzylinder im Harnsediment gefunden, liegt eine aktive Pyelonephritis vor. Treten sie bei einer Glomerulonephritis auf, weisen sie auf eine komplizierende Pyelonephritis hin. Der Nachweis von Leukozytenzylindern gelingt meist nach Peroxydase-Färbung. Manchmal finden sie sich erst nach Provokation mit einem Eisensorbitolzitratkomplex (*Devi* und Mitarb. [4]). – Der diagnostische Wert der Glitterzellen (Sternheimer-Malbin) wird teils bezweifelt, teils anerkannt. Nach der lebhaften Diskussion um den diagnostischen Wert dieser Zellen ist *Reubi* [13], *v. Niederhäusern* und *Wildbolz* zuzustimmen, daß sie in größerer Zahl nur bei intrarenalen Entzündungen vorkommen. Begründeter Verdacht auf Pyelonephritis gravidarum oder Pfropfgestose durch Pyelonephritis besteht, wenn diese Zellen mehr als 25% aller Leukozyten betragen.

Hinweise auf die Diagnose „Pfropfgestose durch Pyelonephritis" geben:

1. Proteinurie und Bakteriurie.
2. Hypertonie und Bakteriurie.
3. Hämaturie und Bakteriurie.
4. Leukozytenzylinder und/oder Glitterzellen (Sternheimer-Malbin) sprechen eher für Pyelonephritis oder Pfropfgestose durch Pyelonephritis als für essentielle Gestose.
5. Der Konzentrationsversuch kann bei Pfropfgestose durch Pyelonephritis schon vor dem Anstieg des Serumkreatinin (oberer Grenzwert bei Schwangeren 0,8 mg %) eingeschränkt sein.
6. Die Provokation mit einem Eisensorbitolzitratkomplex (Jectofer) weist in 30–40% auf chronische Pyelonephritis oder Pfropfgestose durch Pyelonephritis hin. Nach Jectofer können die Leukozyten im Harn erheblich ansteigen (Ausscheidungsrate: 190 000 oder mehr).

Wesentlich sind die Kriterien der chronischen Pyelonephritis bei Schwangeren, die in Anlehnung an die von *Sarre* [14] und *Brod* [2, 3] genannten Befunde etwa folgende sind:

1. Entzündliche Erkrankungen der Harnorgane in der Anamnese.
2. Proteinurie unter 1,5‰ Esbach.
3. Im Harnsediment überwiegen die Leukozyten die Erythrozyten.
4. Nachweis von Leukozytenzylindern und/oder Glitterzellen.
5. Bakteriurie (negative Urinkulturen jedoch in 25–50%).
6. Vermehrtes Plasmakreatinin über 0,8 mg %.
7. Frühzeitig eingeschränkte Konzentrationsfähigkeit.
8. Hyponatriämie, Hypokaliämie.
9. Anämie.
10. Nichtheilende Zystitis trigoni, Zystitis zystica, Leukoplakie im Trigonum vesicae.
11. Wird eine Isotopennephrographie erwogen, gibt der reduzierte Aktivitätsanstieg in der Sekretionsphase, vor allem bei einseitigem Befund, Hinweise auf die chronische Pyelonephritis.

Bei Pfropfgestose durch Pyelonephritis sind die Kriterien wie folgt zu erweitern: die Proteinurie liegt meist über 1,5‰ Esbach. Der Blutdruck ist fast immer erhöht (über 135/85 mm/Hg). Für Diagnose und Prognose ist der diastolische Blutdruck entscheidender, da er als Gradmesser der funktionellen Arteriolenerkrankung gilt. Für den systolischen Blutdruck trifft dies nicht in gleichem Maße zu, da er auch von anderen Faktoren, wie Schlagvolumen, Windkesselelastizität abhängt. Ohne Zweifel finden sich bei Pfropfgestose durch Pyelonephritis sehr of Ödeme, die aber nicht sehr ausgeprägt sein müssen. Daß Ödeme auch bei chronischer Pyelonephritis ohne Gestose auftreten können (*Berning* [1]), darf nicht unerwähnt bleiben.

Durch sorgfältige Anamnese, eingehende klinische Untersuchung, Kenntnis der Kriterien der chronischen Pyelonephritis gravidarum und kritische Bewertung der Leitsymptome (Proteinurie, Bakteriurie, Hämaturie und Hypertonie) ist es möglich, Pfropfgestosen durch Pyelonephritis während der Gravidität wesentlich häufiger zu diagnostizieren, als dies bisher der Fall war.

Literatur

[1] *Berning, H., K. G. Thiele:* Pyelonephritis und chronische interstitielle Nephritis, in: Handbuch der inneren Medizin VIII/2. Teil. Springer, Berlin–Heidelberg–New York (1968).

[2] *Brod, J.:* Chronic pyelonephritis. Lancet I (1956) S. 973.

[3] *Brod, J.:* Infektionswege bei Pyelonephritis in: *Losse-Kienitz:* Pyelonephritis-Forschungsergebnisse 1966. Thieme, Stuttgart 57 (1967) S. 1.

[4] *Devi, P. K., V. D. Sutaria, P. Asolkar, M. Deshmukh:* Diagnosis of latent urinary tract infections in pregnancy. Amer. J. Obstet. Gynec. 97 (1967) S. 39.

[5] *Friedberg, V.:* Die Bedeutung der Pyelonephritis für den eklamptischen Symptomenkomplex und für andere Spätkomplikationen. 73. Tagung der Nordwestdeutschen Gesellschaft für Gynäkologie auf Helgoland 30./31. Mai 1970.

[6] *Hochuli, E.:* Bedeutung der Nachuntersuchungen in: Die Spätgestose (hrsg. von *E. T. Rippmann*). Schwabe u. Co., Basel–Stuttgart (1969) S. 292.

[7] *Hochuli, E., O. Käser:* Chronische Pyelonephritis und Präeklampsie. Geburtsh. u. Frauenheilk. 18 (1958) S. 1133.

[8] *Kleeman, Ch. R., W. L. Hewitt, L. B. Guze:* Pyelonephritis Medicine (Baltimore) 39 (1960) S. 3.

[9] *Kremling, H., C. Goecke, A. Heidland:* Nachuntersuchungen bei Spätgestose. Med. Welt 20 (N.F.) (1967) S. 1244.

[10] *Kremling, H., Th. Dimmling, K. Feltmann:* Prognose des Kindes bei Pyelonephritis gravidarum. Geburtsh. u. Frauenheilk. 29 (1969) S. 800.

[11] *Niederhäusern, W. v., E. Wildbolz:* Klinik der akuten und chronischen Pyelonephritis in: Handbuch der Urologie Bd. IX/1. Teil. Springer, Berlin–Göttingen–Heidelberg (1964).

[12] *Raaschou, F.:* Studies of chronic pyelonephritis, Kopenhagen: Munksgaard (1948).

[13] *Reubi, F.:* Nierenkrankheiten. H. Huber, Bern–Stuttgart–Wien (1970).

[14] *Sarre, H.:* Nierenkrankheiten. Thieme, Stuttgart (1967).

Diagnostik der Pfropfgestose in der Gravidität

H. Kremling

Universitäts Frauenklinik, Würzburg, BRD

Etwa 50% der Spätgestosen sind Pfropfgestosen. Die chronische Pyelonephritis ist als Grundleiden besonders häufig.

Hinweise auf die Diagnose Pfropfgestose durch Pyelonephritis geben:
1. Proteinurie *und* Bakteriurie.
2. Hypertonie *und* Bakteriurie.
3. Hämaturie *und* Bakteriurie.
4. Leukozytenzylinder *und/oder* Glitzerzellen (*Sternheimer-Malbin*) sprechen für Pyelonephritis oder Pfropfgestose durch Pyelonephritis und gegen essentielle Gestose.
5. Der Konzentrationsversuch kann bei Pfropfgestose durch Pyelonephritis schon vor dem Anstieg des Serum-Kreatinin (oberer Grenzwert bei Schwangeren 0,8 mg %) eingeschränkt sein.
6. Die Provokation mit einem Eisensorbitolzitratkomplex (*Jectofer*) weist in 30–40% auf Pfropfgestose durch Pyelonephritis oder Glomerulonephritis hin. Nach Jectofer können die Leukozyten im Harn erheblich ansteigen (Ausscheidungsrate: 190 000 oder mehr).

Methode

Spontane Entleerung der Harnblase. Nach 3 Stunden wird der Urin entweder durch Mittelstrahlmethode oder Katheterung in einem sterilen Gefäß aufgefangen. Intramuskuläre Injektion von 50 mg Jectofer. Nach weiteren drei Stunden erneute Harngewinnung.

Die Zahl der ausgeschiedenen Leukozyten wird in *beiden* Harnportionen auf folgende Weise ermittelt:
Aus jedem Gefäß werden 10 ml in je einem Reagenzglas 5 Minuten lang bei 2000 Umdrehungen zentrifugiert; von den 10 ml werden 9 ml abpipettiert und der Rest gut durchmischt. Auszählung der Leukozyten in der Neubauer-Zählkammer. Die Ausscheidungsrate pro Stunde (N) errechnet sich aus folgender Formel:

$$N = \frac{500 \times C \times V}{20 \times P}$$

V = ausgeschiedenes Harnvolumen in 3 Stunden
C = Anzahl der Leukozyten
P = Zeit in Stunden

7. Ob eine essentielle Gestose oder eine Pfropfgestose durch chronische Pyelonephritis vorliegt, läßt sich post partum durch Infusionsurographie definitiv klären. Kriterien der chronischen Pyelonephritis im Infusionsurogramm:

   a) Plumpe Kelche
   b) Stenose der Kelchhälse
   c) Erweiterung des Nierenbeckens
   d) Streifiges Nierenbeckenrelief
   e) Asymmetrie der Nierengröße und Konstrastmitteldichte
   f) Unregelmäßige Parenchymkonturen
   g) Hypotonie des Harnleiters

Technik der Infusionsurographie bei Wöchnerinnen

Am Tage vor der Untersuchung (ab 7. Tag post partum) ist das Serum-Kreatinin zu bestimmen; liegt der Wert über 5 mg %, sollte bei Wöchnerinnen die Infusionsurographie nicht durchgeführt werden.

Gezielte Allergie-Anamnese, jedoch keine Vortestung. Infusion des Kontrastmittels (z. B. Conray FL oder Urovison) innerhalb 5–10 Min. Nach der Übersichtsaufnahme wird die erste Aufnahme 10–15 Min. nach Infusionsbeginn angefertigt. Eine weitere Aufnahme erfolgt nach 30–60 Min. Am Arbeitsplatz sind bereitzustellen NNR-Steroide (in gelöster spritzfertiger Form) Plasmaexpander, Elektrolyt-Lösungen, Sauerstoff.

Ist die Vene punktiert, läßt man zunächst 1 ml des Kontrastmittels einlaufen. Erfolgt nach 3–5 Min. keine Reaktion, wird die Infusion fortgeführt. Die Nadel bleibt am Ende der Infusion noch etwa 10–15 Min. in der Vene, damit erforderliche Injektionen sogleich durchgeführt werden können.

Veränderungen am Augenhintergrund bei EPH-Komplex

G. Döderlein

München, BRD

Auf dem Deutschen Gynäkologenkongreß in Wien 1941 wurde nach Entwicklung der Grundlagen für eine „Systematische, ärztliche Vor- und Fürsorge in der Schwangerschaft" die Frage erörtert, ob man durch frühzeitige Diagnose und Behandlung der Prä-Eklampsie den Ausbruch einer Eklampsie verhüten könne. Die Aussichten, von mir bejaht, wurden damals skeptisch beurteilt. Inzwischen besteht internationale Einigkeit darüber, daß es auf Zahl und Abstände der im letzten Drittel der Schwangerschaft durchgeführten ärztlichen Untersuchungen ankommt, ob eine drohende Eklampsie erkannt, erfolgreich behandelt und somit verhütet werden kann.

Zu dem als klassische Trias der Prä-Eklampsie bekannten EPH-Komplex gesellt sich erneut die sorgfältige Beobachtung des Augenhintergrundes im letzten Trimenon der Schwangerschaft. Schon 1855 hat *A. von Graefe* die „Retinitis gravidarum" nach einem eklamptischen Anfall beschrieben. Damit war die Aufmerksamkeit auf typische Veränderungen an der Netzhaut und an ihren Gefäßen in der Schwangerschaft gelenkt. Wenn wir heute von „Retinopathia gravidarum" oder von „Retinopathia eklamptika" sprechen, so verstehen wir darunter zunächst funktionelle, zum Teil spastische Einengungen der Netzhautarterien. In ausgeprägten Fällen von schwerer „manifester" Prä-Eklampsie kommt es bei längerem Bestehen solcher Einengungen der Netzhautarterien zu ischämischen Trübungsherden im Netzhautparenchym, zum Papillenödem und schließlich zu Retinablutungen. *K. Mylius* hat diese Funktionellen Veränderungen am Gefäßsystem der Netzhaut in der Schwangerschaft zuerst gesehen (1929) und abgebildet.

Heute ist es möglich, mit dem Augenspiegel die Gefäßweite der Arterien und Venen in der Netzhaut objektiv zu messen. Zu solchen Messungen eignet sich ein Verfahren nach dem Heliometerprinzip. *Lobeck* hat die Methode 1934 an der Universitätsaugenklinik in Jena zusammen mit den Zeisswerken entwickelt.

Aus der Universitätsfrauenklinik in Jena wurden 1960 500 schwangere Frauen ab VII. Lunarmonat der Schwangerschaft in der dortigen Universitätsaugenklinik (*Fr. Hollwich*) ophthalmometrisch untersucht. Ergebnisse:

1. Schon in der normalen Schwangerschaft beobachtet man Engeinstellung der Netzhautgefäße: im VII. Monat 16%; im VIII. Monat 34%; im IX. Monat 37%; im X. Monat 38%.

2. Der Grad einer Engeinstellung der Netzhautarterien in der Schwangerschaft steht in direkter Proportion zur Höhe des Blutdruckes. Dieses Phänomen ist spezifisch für die Schwangerschaft, denn bei essentieller Hypertonie außerhalb der Schwangerschaft bleibt der Anstieg des Blutdruckes ohne Einfluß auf das Kaliber der Netzhautarterien. In unserem Jenaer Material (*Döderlein-Hollwich*) finden wir bei einem systolischen Blutdruck von 130 mm/Hg im Mittelwert eine Engeinstellung der Netzhautarterien in 27% der Fälle; bei über 130 mm/Hg in 37%; bei über 140 mm/Hg in 54%. *Mittelstraß-Wolfshagen* (Hamburg) haben in 327 Fällen von Präeklampsie und Eklampsie je nach Schwere der klinischen Symptome im EPH-Komplex in 45–85% der Fälle funktionelle und organische Netzhautveränderungen im Sinne von Gefäßspasmen und von Retinopathien gefunden.
3. Der Übergang von noch physiologischer Engeinstellung der Netzhautarterien in der Schwangerschaft zu pathologischen Werten ist fließend. Die tonische Engeinstellung der Netzhautarteriolen ist Vorstufe und Vorbedingung für den Arteriolenspasmus und schließlich für anatomische Veränderungen an der Netzhaut beim EPH-Komplex.
4. In Fällen von „latenter" oder „manifester" Prä-Eklampsie oder von Eklampsie erreichen normaler Weise nach der Entbindung Blutdruck und Kaliber der Netzhautarterien wieder normale Werte.

Der Ophthalmologe *Kyrieleis* (Marburg) konnte ophthalmoskopisch bei Fällen von EPH-Komplex die zunehmende Engeinstellung und das Auftreten von Gefäßspasmen an Arterien der Netzhaut direkt verfolgen. Sie entstehen in kürzester Zeit, lösen sich rasch und treten ebenso rasch an anderer Stelle wieder auf. Die Gefäßspasmen in der Netzhaut entstehen bei Schwangeren im III. Trimenon unter Umständen innerhalb weniger Stunden. Diese Beobachtung unterstreicht meine oftmals betonte Ansicht, daß die Eklampsie niemals als „Blitz aus heiterem Himmel" entsteht. Stets geht ihr das mehr oder minder ausgeprägte Stadium der Prä-Eklampsie voraus, auch wenn dies nur wenige Stunden dauert. Diese konzentriert und rasch ablaufenden Vorstadien einer Eklampsie sind klinisch äußerst schwierig zu erfassen. Der funktionelle Symptomkreis EPH-Prä-Eklampsie-Eklampsie kann wegen der fließenden Übergänge zu keinem Zeitpunkt als „leicht" oder als „schwer" bezeichnet werden. Das lehrt uns die Beobachtung der Netzhautarterien und ihrer rasch wechsenden Kaliber.

Deshalb wiederhole ich meinen Vorschlag, die Begriffe „leichte" oder „schwere" Form der Prä-Eklampsie durch „latente" und „manifeste" Prä-Eklampsie zu ersetzen.

Die retinale Gefäßkonstriktion ist beim EPH-Komplex als Frühsymptom regelmäßig nachzuweisen. Die klassische Symptomentrias: Ödeme, Proteinurie, Hypertonie, sollte durch das nie fehlende 4. Zeichen der Arteriolenspasmen in der Retina ergänzt werden (*F. Hollwich*).

Die Hoffnung von *Kyrieleis*, man könne vielleicht durch Messung des Druckes in den Netzhautarterien die diagnostischen und prognostischen Voraussagen beim EPH-Komplex noch verfeinern, hat sich bisher noch nicht erfüllt. Die Ophthalmodynamometrie mißt nur den Druck in der A.ophthalmica. Dieser ist direkt proportional zu den Druckverhältnissen im autonomen Bezirk der Gehirngefäße.

Literatur

Döderlein, G.: Zentralblatt f. Gynäkologie 65 (1941) S. 529.
Döderlein, G.: Arch. Gynäk.: 173 (1942) S. 175.
Döderlein, G.: Die Spätgestose (EPH-Gestose). Schwabe & Co., Basel–Stuttgart (1970) S. 388.
Döderlein, G. und *Hollwich:* Zentralblatt f. Gynäkologie 83 (1961) S. 413.
Kyrieleis, W.: Geburtshilfe & Frauenheilkunde 14 (1954) S. 869.
Mittelstraß, H. & O. Wolfhagen: Geburtshilfe und Frauenheilkunde 8 (1948) S. 671.
Mylius, K.: Abh. Augenheilk. Beihefte z. Ztschr. Augenheilkunde 10 (1929).

La place de la ponction biopsie rénale dans le cadre des toxémies gravidiques

G. Pontonnier

Maternité, Toulouse, France

Notre équipe a réalisé, depuis 1958, près de 150 P.B.R. soit pendant la grossesse, soit dans le post partum immédiat, soit dans le post partum éloigné chez des femmes ayant présenté un syndrome vasculo rénal de la gestation. L'étude de ces biopsies rénales en microscopie optique, électronique et en histochimie nous a permis de préciser un certain nombre de points concernant le syndrome „HTA-oedème-protéinurie", spécifique du troisième trimestre de la gestation, appelé toxémie gravidique pure, dysgravidie ou gestose.

Sur le plan nosologique

Contrairement au dogme classique, la dysgravidie n'est pas un syndrome purement fonctionnel mais est, au contraire, caractérisée par un substratum anatomo-pathologique spécifique.

En microscopie optique la lésion dysgravidique atteint d'une façon uniforme tous les glomérules des deux reins. Elle se caractérise par:

une turgescence du flocculus qui, venant au contact de la capsule de *Bowman,* efface la chambre de filtration,

une disparition des lumières capillaires qui supprime l'aspect aéré du glomérule normal, lequel apparait très ischémié.

L'examen optique est toutefois insuffisant car d'une part dans un certain nombre de cas les glomérules paraissent normaux, car d'autre part lorsque la lésion est présente sa nature véritable ne peut être déterminée. L'échelle d'observation glomérulaire est insuffisante, il convient d'étudier les corpuscules de Malpighi à l'échelle cellulaire.

En microscopie électronique les anses capillaires dysgravidiques apparaissent très ischémiques. La disparition de leur lumière est dûe à la conjonction de trois lésions:

hypertrophie endothéliale
hypertrophie mésangiale
dépôt fibrinoïde sous la membrane basale

Ces trois lésions ne sont jamais réunies avec une telle intensité dans les néphropathies d'autres origines.

Sur le plan diagnostique

La confrontation anatomo-clinique a mis en évidence les quatre points suivants:

1. Dans la majorité des cas les oedèmes constituent le premier signe, l'H.T.A. apparaît ensuite. La protéinurie est le symptôme le plus inconstant. La plupart des protéinuries découvertes au cours d'une dysgravidie sont dues à une infection urinaire. La protéinurie véritablement dysgravidique esr rare et de mauvais pronostic.
2. La dysgravidie surajoutée à une H.T.A.P. ou à une néphropathie chronique existe. Elle est la principale cause de l'apparente aggravation des affections vasculo-rénales chroniques pendant la grossesse.
3. Les H.T.A. gravidiques récidivantes sont en fait des dysgravidies surajoutées à des affections vasculo-rénales indépendantes de la grossesse et méconnues.
4. La dysgravidie peut se traduire par un syndrome néphrotique typique mais avec hypertension.

Sur le plan pronostique

Après corrélations anatomo-cliniques on peut considérer qu'il existe deux sortes de dysgravidies:

Dysgravidie cliniquement modérée se traduisant en microscopie optique par des glomérules normaux, et en microscopie électronique par des anses capillaires à lumières en partie conservées et où la lésion dominante est l'hypertrophie mésangiale.

Dysgravidie cliniquement sévère se traduisant par une ischémie glomérulaire nette en microscopie optique et par la coexistence du trépied lésionnel en microscopie électronique.

La pratique des biopsies sériées montre qu'en règle générale la lésion glomérulaire disparaît après l'accouchement.

Si les lésions constatées en microscopie électronique ont un caractère en principe réversible (hypertrophie endothéliale et mésangiale, dépôt fibrinoïde), dans un certain nombre de cas sévères on a pu constater l'existence de lésions dont la réversibilité est plus discutable:

épaississement de la membrane basale,
épaississement de la limitante élastique interne des artérioles rénales.

Sur le plan pathogénique

L'histochimie a démontré la présence dans les glomérules dysgravidiques de deux protéines anormales, l'une paraît proche de la fibrine l'autre du fibrinogène. Ces constatations sont à rapprocher de celles de *Vassali.* Cet auteur a mis en évidence, par immuno-fluorescence, un dépot de fibrine dans les glomérules de dysgravidie.

On peut donc considérer que les dysgravidies entrent dans le cadre des coagulopathies de consommation.

Conclusion

La P.B.R. a fait faire un bond en avant à nos connaissances sur les dysgravidies. Nous pensons cependant que si la pratique était justifiée pendant la grossesse pour effecteur un travail de recherche, elle ne se justifie plus actuellement. La P.B.R. n'a des indications que dans le post partum, en général éloigné, lorsque la persistence de signes pathologiques impose un bilan rénal complet, biologique, anatomique, radiologique, pour préciser la nature exacte de l'affection en cause.

To Assess Fetal Well-Being

Die Amnioskopie zur Überwachung des Föten bei EPH-Gestose der Mutter

J. W. Dudenhausen, E. Saling

Städtische Frauenklinik, Berlin-Neukölln, 1 Berlin 44

Die Amnioskopie ist ein Verfahren zum frühzeitigen Erkennen einer hypoxischen Gefährdung des Feten in der Spätschwangerschaft und zu Beginn der Geburt, solange die Blase steht.

Das Prinzip (Abb. 1) dieses Untersuchungsverfahrens besteht darin, daß man in den Zervikalkanal ein mit einer Beleuchtungsquelle versehenes, konisches Rohr einführt und das Fruchtwasser am unteren Eipol durch die intakten Eihäute betrachtet.

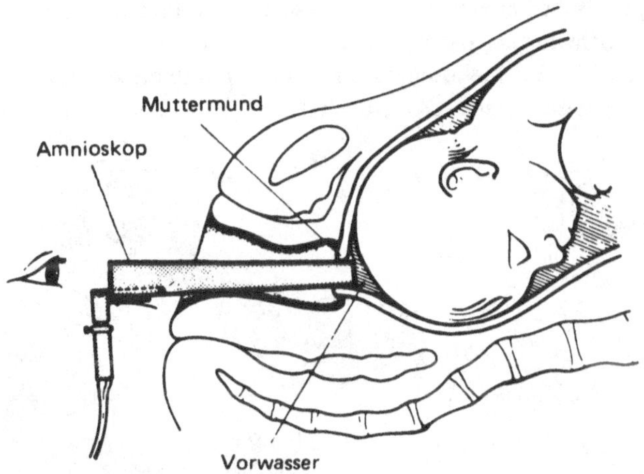

Abb. 1

Normalerweise ist das Fruchtwasser klar und enthält reichlich Vernixflocken. Auf eine erhöhte Gefährdung in utero weisen hingegen folgende amnioskopische Befunde hin und werden als positiv bezeichnet: Es liegt mekoniumhaltiges (= grünliches) Fruchtwasser vor, die Menge des Fruchtwassers ist stark reduziert oder es ist kein Fruchtwasser vorhanden. Wird ein solcher auf eine Plazentainsuffizienz und eine fetale Sauerstoffminderversorgung hinweisender Befund erhoben, so muß die Fruchtblase eröffnet

werden, damit der gegenwärtige Zustand des Feten durch Fetalblutanalysen genauer bestimmt werden kann.
Folgt man diesem Grundsatz, so findet man nur bei einem kleinen Teil der Feten, deren Mütter eine EPH-Gestose haben, eine Aziditätssteigerung. Wir haben (Abb. 2) bei 116, wegen einer EPH-Gestose amnioskopisch überwachten und positiv befundeten Feten kurz nach der amnioskopischen Diagnose mit Hilfe der Fetalblutanalysen die metabolische Azidität des Feten untersucht und fanden in nur 5 Fällen eine Präazidose, keinmal lag eine Azidose vor. 111mal war die Azidität des kindlichen Blutes im Normbereich.

pHqu4o	Zahl der Fälle
≤ 7, 19	0
7,20–7,24	5 (4,3%)
≥ 7, 25	111 (95,7%)
Insgesamt	116

Abb. 2. Fetale metabolische Azidität nach amnioskopisch festgestelltem grünem Fruchtwasser bei EPH-Gestose der Mutter

Wir wissen, daß die häufigste Gefährdung des Feten in der Spätschwangerschaft, die intrauterine chronische Sauerstoffminderversorgung infolge der Plazentainsuffizienz, in den letzten 6 Schwangerschaftswochen fast ausnahmslos zum Mekoniumabgang führt. Als Ursache für den Mekoniumabgang im Verlaufe dieser fetalen Sauerstoffminderversorgung wird die sog. O_2-Sparschaltung des fetalen Kreislaufes (Abb. 3)

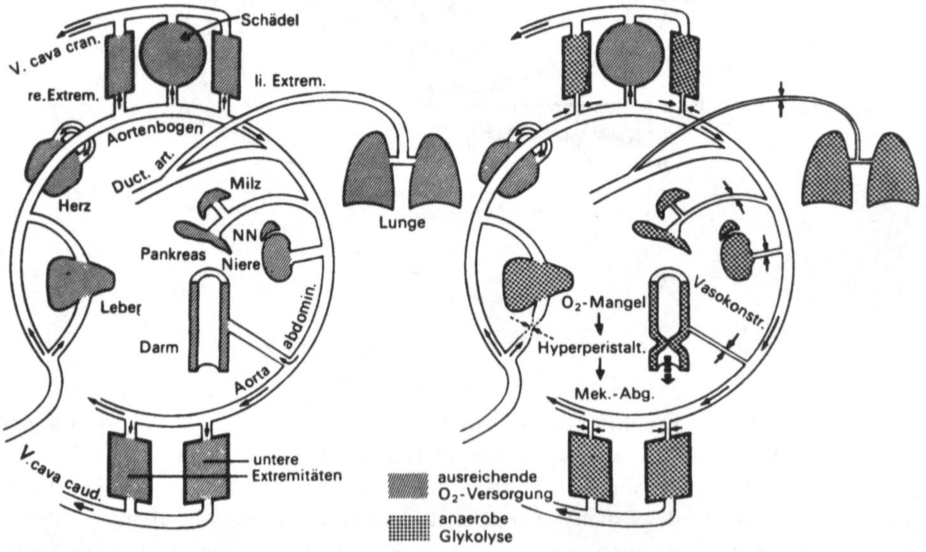

Abb. 3

angesehen. Darunter verstehen wir, daß in den für das intrauterine Leben nicht unbedingt lebensnotwendigen Organen, wie Lungen, Nieren, Muskulatur, Haut, Magen-Darm-Trakt, die Gefäße verengt und damit Durchblutung und Sauerstoffzufuhr vermindert werden. Am Darm z. B. ruft die lokale Hypoxie eine Hyperperistaltik hervor, und es kommt zum Mekoniumabgang. Die eingesparte O_2-Menge steht den lebensnotwendigen Organen (Gehirn, Herz, Plazenta) zur Verfügung.

Bei der Überwachung des durch eine EPH-Gestose der Mutter gefährdeten Feten halten wir die Amnioskopie je nach Schweregrad innerhalb der letzten 4 bis 6 Wochen und in Ausnahmefällen bis zu 8 Wochen vor dem Termin für indiziert. Die amnioskopische Überwachung erfolgt in 2tägigen Abständen. Auch nach einem medikamentös erzielten Rückgang der Gestosesymptome muß die amnioskopische Überwachung noch etwa eine Woche fortgesetzt werden.

Die EPH-Gestose ist zahlenmäßig die wichtigste Indikation zur Amnioskopie. Betrachtet man die Indikationen zur amnioskopischen Untersuchung (Abb. 4) bei den etwa 1200 amnioskopisch überwachten Frauen des Jahres 1969 an unserer Klinik, das sind etwa 48% aller Geburten an unserer Klinik, so erkennt man, daß über $^3/_4$ aller amnioskopisch überwachten Feten wegen einer EPH-Gestose der Mutter untersucht wurden.

	Häufigkeit
EPH-Gestose	78.5%
Terminüberschreitung	16.1%
Fragl. Blasensprung	7.2%
Rh-Unverträglichkeit	2.8%
Diabetes mellitus	1.1%
Alteration KHT	0.4%
Verdacht auf Inf. mortuus	0.1%
Verdacht auf Plac. praevia	0.2%
Andere Indikationen	3.4%

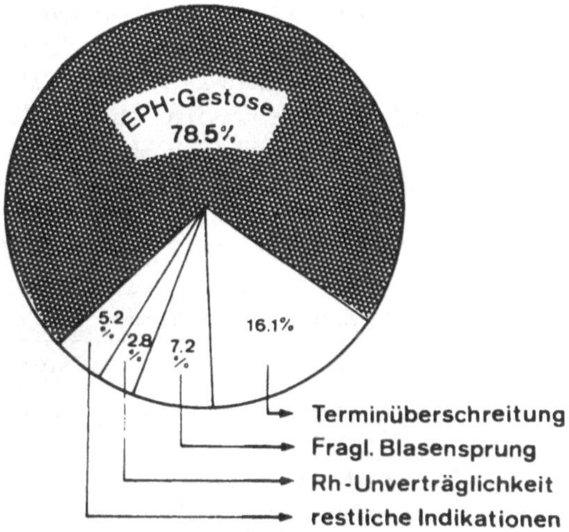

Abb. 4. Indikationen zur Amnioskopie (1969)

Reichwein hat bei einer Auswertung von über 1000 Fällen mit EPH-Gestose an unserer Klinik etwa 22% Fruchtwasserverfärbungen gefunden, die amnioskopisch oder sub partu festgestellt wurden. Betrachtet man bei diesen Frauen mit Fruchtwasserverfärbungen die Verteilung der Gestosesymptome (Abb. 5), so stellt sich heraus, daß 99% Blutdruckerhöhungen, 83% Ödeme und 38% eine Proteinurie hatten. Aus der Verteilung der Grade der Gestosesymptome ist ersichtlich, daß die höchsten Prozentsätze auf die leichten Gestosesymptome entfallen, das liegt natürlich daran, daß dieses Kollektiv auch das größte ist. Für die tägliche Praxis der Amnioskopie muß aber hieraus gefolgert werden, daß es auch bei den leichten EPH-Gestosen auf eine intensive Überwachung im Hinblick auf eine fetale Sauerstoffmangelsituation ankommt.

Hypertension 99% (diast.)	Ödeme 83%	Proteinurie 38%
90–100 mmHg: 77% 105–110 mmHg: 12% 115–120 mmHg: 8% ≥125 mmHg: 2%	≤ + : 63% ++ : 15% +++ : 4% ++++ : 2%	0,5‰ : 34% 0,5–0,75‰ : 3% ≥ 0,75‰ : 1%

Abb. 5. Symptome und Grad der EPH-Gestose bei FW-Verfärbung (bei 1100 Fällen, n. *Reichwein*)

In der Zeit seit Einführung der Amnioskopie, 1961 bis Ende 1969, wurden bei uns 19 713 amnioskopische Einzeluntersuchungen bei 7597 Frauen durchgeführt (Abb. 6). In 60 dieser Fälle war die Indikation zur Fruchtwasserbeurteilung der Verdacht auf ein Infans mortuus, in 281 Fällen ein fraglicher Blasensprung. Daher wurde die Amnioskopie nur bei 7256 Schwangerschaften als Methode zur Überwachung des erhöht gefährdeten Kindes eingesetzt. Bei einer Zahl von 23 130 Entbindungen im Zeitraum von 1961 bis 1969 ergibt sich daraus, daß etwa 31% der Schwangeren und z. T. auch Gebärenden amnioskopisch überwacht wurden. In dem Kontingent von 7256 amnio-

Zahl der Entbindungen	23 130
Zahl der amnioskopischen Einzeluntersuchungen	19 713
Zahl der amnioskopierten Frauen gesamt	7 597
davon	
wegen Verdacht auf Inf. mortuus	60
wegen fragl. Blasensprung	281
Zahl der amnioskopisch überwachten Fälle	7 256 (= 31,4%)

Abb. 6. Durchgeführte Amnioskopien an der Städt. Frauenklinik Berlin-Neukölln von 1961–1969

skopisch überwachten Schwangerschaften verstarben 101 Kinder (Abb. 7), dies bedeutet eine perinatale Mortalität von 1,39%; ante partum verstarben 0,15%, sub partu 0,39% und post partum 0,85%.

	Todesfälle	Mortalität
gesamt	163	
davon		
wegen Verdachts auf Inf. mortuus	60	
wegen fragl. Blasensprung	2	
Amnioskopisch überwachte, perinatal verstorbene Kinder	101	1,39%
davon		
ante partum verstorben	11	0,15%
sub partu verstorben	28	0,39%
post partum verstorben	62	0,85%

Abb. 7. Übersicht über die perinatalen Todesfälle bei 7597 amnioskopierten Fällen

Eine Übersicht (Abb. 8) über die 11 ante partum verstorbenen Feten ergibt, daß zwei ante-partum-Todesfälle durch eine vorzeitige Lösung der normal sitzenden Plazenta eintraten. Bei zwei ante-partum-Todesfällen handelte es sich jeweils um den zweiten Zwilling. Bei einem Kind wurde trotz amnioskopisch positivem Befund wegen des sehr niedrig eingeschätzten Gewichtes keine Geburtseinleitung vorgenommen, so daß das Kind verstarb. Bei den restlichen 6 Fällen lag unserer Ansicht nach ein methodisches Versagen der Amnioskopie vor. Auf die 7256 amnioskopisch überwachten Feten

2 mal	Vorzeitige Lösung der normal sitzenden Plazenta
2 mal	zweite Zwillinge
1 mal	trotz grünen FW wegen niedrig geschätzten Geb. gew. keine Geb.-Einleitung; klin. Fehlteurteilung, tatsächliches Geb. gew. 1660g
6 mal	methodische Versager

Abb. 8. Aufteilung der 11 Ante-partum-Todesfälle

beträgt die Versagerquote der Amnioskopie demnach 1:1209 (Abb. 9). Zweimal kam es im Rahmen der Überwachung einer Schwangeren mit EPH-Gestose zu methodischem Versagen, wobei einmal ein Diabetes mellitus vorlag.

1.	1963	Rh-AK-Titer 1:1024
2.	1966	Diabetes mit EPH-Gestose
3.	1965	Terminüberschreitung
4.	1967	Terminüberschreitung
5.	1969	EPH-Gestose
6.	1965	Amnioskopie wegen fraglicher KHT; normaler FW-Befund; Rö Abd. o. B.; Abd. EKG fragl. kindl. Aktionen; 5. Amnioskopie FW-Befund positiv – Geburt eines Kindes mit Maz. Zeichen 1. Grades

Abb. 9. Übersicht über die 6 methodischen Versager bei 7256 amnioskopisch überwachten Fällen (Versagerquote 1:1209)

Für die Bewertung der Amnioskopie als Überwachungsmethode bei EPH-Gestose ist der Vergleich der Ante-partum-Mortalität in den Kollektiven vor Einführung und nach Einführung der Amnioskopie in den geburtshilflichen Routinebetrieb von Bedeutung. An unserer Klinik betrug die Ante-partum-Mortalität von Kindern, deren Mütter in der Spätschwangerschaft an einer EPH-Gestose erkrankt waren, vor dem Einsatz der Amnioskopie, d. h. von 1956 bis 1960, 3,48% (Abb. 10). Errechnet man die perinatalen Todesfälle nur der amnioskopierfähigen Frauen, d. h., jener Frauen, deren Schwangerschaft älter als 34 Wochen war, so betrug die Ante-partum-Mortalität vor Einführung der Amnioskopie 2,26%. In den Jahren 1964 bis 1967, also nach Einführung der Amnioskopie, lag die Ante-partum-Mortalität der Kinder von amnioskopierfähigen Frauen bei 0,33%. Die Senkung der Ante-partum-Mortalität von 2,26% auf 0,33% ist der Amnioskopie und der sich zwangsweise ergebenden sehr viel intensiveren Überwachung der Schwangeren zuzuschreiben.

	im Gesamtgeburtengut		im Kollektiv von Müttern mit EPH-Gestose *(Reichwein)*	
	vor	nach	vor	nach
	Einführung der Amnioskopie		Einführung der Amnioskopie	
	(1958–1960)	(1961–1969)	(1956–1960)	(1964–1967)
Ante-partum-Mortalität	0,97%	0,68%	3,48%	0,33%
Sub-partu-Mortalität	0,69%	0,31%	3,31%	0,33%
Post-partum-Mortalität	3,16%	2,34%	1,39%	1,14%
Perinatale Mortalität	4,83%	3,33%	8,19%	1,80%

Abb. 10. Mortalitätsraten verschiedener Kollektive an der Städt. Frauenklinik Berlin-Neukölln

Courbe de croissance du diamètre biparietal dans la Gestose

E. De Mot, G. Müller, E. Calicis, G. Boog, R. Gandar

Hospices Civils de Strasbourg, Clinique Gynécologique et Obstétricale, Strasbourg, France

La gestose est de loin la cause la plus fréquente de retard de croissance du foetus. Le mécanisme de ce trouble de croissance est partiellement élucidé: il s'agit d'une réduction du débit sanguin sur le versant maternel du placenta. L'importance du retard de croissance dépend à la fois de l'intensité de la vasculopathie, elle-même en corrélation avec le degré de l'hypertension artérielle, et de la durée d'évolution de la maladie. Actuellement, la détermination du diamètre bipariétal foetal, par échographie ultrasonore, est la seule méthode directe d'appréciation du développement du foetus. Il convient cependant de noter que lorsque s'installe un retard de croissance in utero, c'est d'abord le poids, puis la taille qui sont atteints, et seulement en dernier le développement du périmètre crânien.

Matériel et méthode

Nous avons suivi la courbe de croissance du diamètre bipariétal foetal par échographie ultrasonore chez 27 femmes présentant une hypertension artérielle associée ou non à de l'albuminurie ou à de l'oedème.

Grâce à la tomoéchographie, les premières mesures du diamètre bipariétal peuvent être effectuées couramment dès la 20ème semaine d'aménorrhée. En raison de l'innocuité de la méthode, les mesures peuvent être répétées à volonté. Nous avons effectué, pour les 27 cas, 114 mesures, soit en moyenne 4 mesures par cas. Les premiers examens ont été pratiqués dès la 24e semaine, les plus tardifs à la 42e semaine. Chaque examen, dont la durée n'excède pas 10 minutes, doit être pratiqué dans l'ignorance des valeurs bipariétales antérieures et de préférence par 2 ou plusieurs examinateurs.

Pour évaluer nos résultats, nous avons rapporté chacune des 27 courbes sur une courbe de référence qui représente la croissance normale. Cette dernière a été établie précédemment en fonction des valeurs moyennes du diamètre bipariétal pour chaque semaine de grossesse. Elle est grossièrement linéaire; cependant elle présente 3 inflexions physiologiques: la première au début de la 29e semaine, la deuxième au début de la 37e semaine et la troisième au début de la 40 semains. Les taux de croissance que nous considérons comme normaux sont:

2,5 mm par semaine entre 24 et 28e semaines
2 mm par semaine entre 29 et 36e semaines
1,5 mm par semaine entre 37 et 39e semaines
1 mm par semaine à partir de la 40e semaine

Nous avons reporté le poids des enfants à la naissance sur le graphique de Gruenwald, indiquant le poids moyen et ses déviations standard en fonction de la durée de l'aménorrhée. Nous considérerons comme hypotrophique sévère chaque enfant dont le poids à la naissance est inférieur à la deuxième déviation standard négative, et comme hypotrophique modéré chaque enfant dont le poids est situé entre la 1ère et la 2ème déviation standard négative.

Résultats

Sur les 27 courbes, établies sur des foetus de mères hypertendues, 12 reproduisent un potentiel de croissance normal. Les poids de ces nouveau-nés sont tous normaux pour l'âge gestationnel.

En analysant nos 15 courbes pathologiques, nous avons noté 3 catégories bien distinctes:

1ère catégorie (2 cas): la courbe de croissance du diamètre bipariétal est parallèle à la courbe de référence, mais elle est située bien plus bas entre la 1ère et la 2ème déviation standard de cette courbe de référence. Tout se passe comme si le placenta, travaillant d'emblée à un niveau inférieur à la normale, fonctionnait cependant suffisamment pour assurer un taux de croissance normal. C'est pourquoi nous parlons dans ces cas „d'insuffisance placentaire compensée".

Les deux enfants de cette catégorie présentent une hypotrophie modérée.

2ème catégorie (8 cas): Ici la croissance du diamètre bipariétal a d'abord été normale, mais précocément vers la 35e–36e semaine s'installe un ralentissement, voire un arrêt

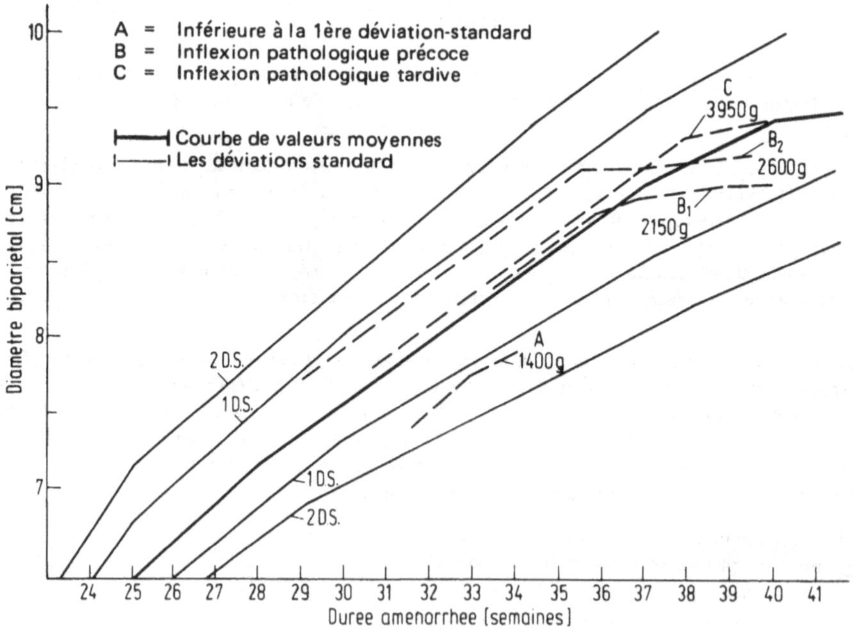

de croissance. Cinq de ces enfants sont hypotrophiques: 1 cas d'hypotrophie sévère et 4 cas d'hypotrophie modérée.

Les 3 cas restants ont un poids normal. Dans ces 3 cas on relève un cas de diabète compliqué par une prééclampsie. L'enfant, mort-né à la 38e semaine, a un poids de 3900 g.

3ème catégorie (5 cas): Dans ce groupe, l'aplatissement de la courbe de croissance est tardive, située près du terme, voire après dépassement du terme. Les 5 enfants de ce groupe ont un poids normal, ce qui n'est pas surprenant, étant donné que le trouble de la croissance ne se manifeste que près du terme. Il est néanmoins remarquable que 3 de ces enfants ont un aspect déshydraté. Enfin il est intéressant de noter que le liquide amniotique est méconial dans 4 cas, qu'il existe des anomalies de la fréquence cardiaque foetale dans 3 cas et que le score d'apgar à 1 minute est inférieur à 7 dans 3 cas.

Tous ces symptômes montrent bien que le ralentissement tardif de la croissance du diamètre bipariétal est également un indice d'insuffisance placentaire.

Commentaire

Ce travail montre bien l'intérêt de suivre la courbe de croissance du diamètre bipariétal dans les syndromes gestosiques. En effet, plus de la moitié de nos courbes se sont avérées pathologiques. Lorsque l'arrêt de la croissance se manifeste précocément, ou lorsque la courbe, tout en restant harmonieuse se situe en-dessous d'une déviation standard négative, les chances d'avoir à la naissance un enfant hypotrophique sont grandes (7/10). Lorsque l'arrêt de croissance se situe près tu terme, le retentissement pondéral semble évidemment nul, mais il existe une pathologie foetale du type de celle que *Gruenwald* décrit dans l'insuffisance placentaire subaiguë.

Résumé

Les auteurs ont étudié les courbes de croissance du diamètre bipariétal par la méthode ultrasonore dans 27 cas d'hypertension artérielle associée ou non à l'albuminurie ou de l'oedème. 15 courbes se sont avérdes pathologiques:

2 courbes ont une évolution parallèle à la courbe de référence mais sont situées en-dessous d'une déviation standard négative. Les 2 enfants sont hypotrophiques.

8 courbes présentent un ralentissement précoce de la croissance. Les 5 enfants sont hypotrophiques.

5 courbes indiquent un ralentissement tardif de la croissance. Dans 3 cas on relève des signes de déshydration foetale.

Der Step-Test, eine frühzeitige Diagnose der antenatalen Bedrohung der Frucht bei EPH-Gestose

Z. Stembera

Research Institute for the Care of Mother and Child, Prague-Podoli, CSSR

Der Step-Test gehört zur Gruppe der Untersuchungsmethoden, durch welche mit Hilfe der fetalen Toleranz die Dysfunktion der Plazenta in den letzten Schwangerschaftswochen festgestellt wird. Die Untersuchungsmethode geht von der Feststellung aus, daß ein – beispielsweise durch EPH-Gestose hervorgerufener – chronischer Distreß bei der Mutter – sofern er eine Dysfunktion der Plazenta hervorruft und so die intrauterine Entwicklung der Frucht bedroht –, der durch einen weiteren akuten, bei der Mutter experimentell hervorgerufenen Distreß ergänzt wird, vorübergehend die bereits vorhandene Dysfunktion der Plazenta potenziert. Bei der Frucht, deren Toleranz gegenüber Hypoxie durch den chronischen Distreß bei der Mutter schon herabgesetzt war, ruft dann dieser weitere akute Distreß eine typische Reaktion im Zirkulationssystem hervor, wie wir sie bei Hypoxie der Frucht antreffen. Die Methode des Step-Tests benützt als akuten Distreß die Arbeitsbelastung, die bei der Schwangeren durch ein drei Minuten dauerndes Steigen auf zwei Stufen in einem Rhythmus von 80 Schritten pro Minute (gemessen mit Hilfe des Metronoms) entsteht. Den Grad der fetalen Toleranz beurteilen wir nach der Veränderung der Herzfrequenz der Frucht unmittelbar nach dem Step-Test im Vergleich zur Frequenz vor dem Step-Test. Die Veränderungen der Frequenz werden entweder „beat to beat" oder in Intervallen von fünf Sekunden gewertet. Ihre objektive Aufzeichnung wird mit Hilfe des Phonokardiographs Hewlett-Packard durchgeführt. Für die Abteilungen, denen kein Phonokardiograph zur Verfügung steht, haben wir einen vereinfachten Step-Test ausgearbeitet, der durch bloßes Abhorchen der fetalen Herztöne ohne phonokardiographische Aufzeichnung durchgeführt werden kann und dessen Auswertung verhältnismäßig einfach ist.

Die Durchführung des vereinfachten Step-Tests

Der Arzt zählt die fetalen Herztöne in Intervallen von fünf Sekunden während zweier Minuten vor und zweier Minuten unmittelbar nach dem Step-Test. Die festgestellten Werte werden von der Hebamme aufgezeichnet. Da der Arzt nicht gleichzeitig jede fünf Sekunden die festgestellte Anzahl der Herztöne melden und dabei schon die Herztöne des folgenden fünf-Sekunden-Intervalls zählen kann, bedient er sich, um sich mit der Hebamme zu verständigen, eines vereinbarten Kodes: Erheben eines Fingers – 11 Herztöne/5 Sek., d. i. 132 Herztöne/Min.; Erheben von zwei Fingern – 12 Herztöne/5 Sek. usw.; kein erhobener Finger, also geschlossene Faust – 10 Herztöne/5 Sek. Bei Bradycardie, wo die Anzahl der fetalen Herztöne auf 9/5 Sek., d. i. 108/Min. und weniger absinkt, kann der Arzt diese Zahl schon melden und gleichzeitig die Herztöne im folgenden 5-Sekunden-Intervall zählen.

Auswertung der Veränderungen in der Frequenz der fetalen Herztöne

Die endgültige Auswertung der verschiedenen Abweichungen der Frequenz der fetalen Herztöne wurde auf Grund von 300 Step-Tests ausgearbeitet, bei denen wir die Bedeutung der einzelnen Abweichungen aus dem weiteren Verlauf der Schwangerschaft, der Geburt, aus verschiedenen, den Zustand der Frucht während der Geburt anzeigenden klinischen Symptomen, den klinischen Zustand des Neugeborenen eine, fünf und zehn Minuten nach der Geburt resp. während der ersten sieben Tage nach der Geburt beurteilten. Bei der Auswertung der ermittelten Abweichungen der Frequenz der fetalen Herztöne werden sieben verschiedene Kennziffern beurteilt.

Als günstige Toleranz der Frucht betrachten wir einen Step-Test mit 0–2 Punkten, als herabgesetzte Toleranz der Frucht betrachten wir einen Step-Test mit 3 und mehr Punkten.

Die Verläßlichkeit des Step-Tests erhöht sich, wenn er in einem Intervall von 1–3 Tagen wiederholt wird. Das Andauern des erhöhten Punktwertes oder sogar eine weitere Erhöhung steigert die Wahrscheinlichkeit der Gefährdung der Frucht. Dagegen zeugt das Andauern eines niedrigen Wertes, ev. das Absinken von einem erhöhten Punktwert auf 0–2 Punkte und das weitere Andauern dieses niedrigen Punktwertes von einer normalen Entwicklung, ev. von einem vorübergehenden Distreß, der für die Frucht keine weiteren Folgen hat.

Obschon die Verläßlichkeit des Step-Tests nach diesen unseren Erfahrungen 80% beträgt, ergänzen wir ihn zum Zweck der endgültigen Beurteilung des Zustands der Frucht und der Entscheidung über einen ev. Abschluß der Schwangerschaft – entweder durch Einleitung der Geburt oder primären Kaiserschnitt – noch durch weitere Methoden – Schwangerschaftszytologie, Östriolspiegel, Amnioskopie –, da die Kombination mit diesen wiederholt applizierten Methoden die Sicherheit der Diagnostik des fetalen Distreß in den letzten Wochen der Schwangerschaft erhöht.

Klinischer Zustand des Neugeborenen (der Frucht)	Step-Test negat. (0–2 Punkte)	Step-Test posit (≥ 3 Punkte)
1. gesund	27	9
2. gesund Bradikardie Mekonium	6	19
3. Apgar seore ≤ 8/1 Min.	0	8
4. Apgar seore ≤ 8/5 Min.	1	7
5. perinatal gestorben	0	1
	34	44

Punkt-Auswertung des Step-Tests

A. Etappe von 24 fünf-Sekunden-Intervallen vor dem Test

Absolute Frequenz:	1. Bradykardie 2 × 9 oder weniger	1
	2. Tachykardie 3 × 9 oder mehr	1

Frequenzschwankungen:	(Differenz zwischen ermittelter niedrigster und höchster Frequenz)	
	3. Differenz 2 × um 3	1
	oder	
	Differenz 2 × um 4 ev. mehr	2
	oder	
	unveränderte Frequenz (sog. „silence") d. i. mindestens 20 × gleicher Wert	2

B. Etappe von 24 fünf-Sekunden-Intervallen nach dem Test

Absolute Frequenz:	4. Bradykardie 3 × 10	1
	oder 2 × 9	2
	oder 2 × 8 oder weniger	3
	5. Tachykardie 3 × 14 oder mehr	1
Frequenzschwankungen:	6. „silence" d. i. 20 × gleiche Frequenz	2

Absinken der unteren Frequenzgrenze der fetalen Herztöne nach dem Test im Vergleich zur unteren Grenze vor dem Test (oder Erhöhung der oberen Grenze):

7. 2 × um 1	1
oder	
mehrmals um 1	2
oder	
2 × um 2	2
oder	
mehrmals um 2	3

The Placenta and its Bed in EPH-Gestosis

Mohamed B. Sammour, B.Sc. (Oxford), F.R.C.S., M.I.A.C.,
Abd-el-Kader S. Fahmy, D.G.O., *A. R. Ammar,* M.Ch.,
M. Mahran, M.R.C.O.G., F.R.C.S., Ph.D., *M.Sherif,* M.D.

Department of Obstetrics and Gynecology, Department of Pathology,
Ain Shams University, Faculty of Medicine, Cairo, UAR

Introduction

The placenta of EPH-Gestosis shows an accentuated maturation of the chorionic villi, marked syncytial degeneration and proliferated Langhans' layer, together with proliferative endarteritis of the foetal vessels. The placental bed on the other hand, shows organic changes in its vessels when the course of pregnancy is complicated by EPH-complex [1, 2, 3, 4]. The extent of these changes is directly related to the clinical severity of the disease. From this point we attempted to confirm the clinical diagnosis of EPH-Gestosis by establishing the pathological changes in the placenta and its bed after delivery. Besides supporting the already present process of toxaemia during pregnancy, this examination also helps in the future prognosis and after-care of the patient particularly in connection with the future pregnancies.

Material and methods

This study was carried on 103 cases classified as follows:

1. 26 women with normal uncomplicated pregnancy as control group.
2. 65 patients suffering from EPH-gestosis.
   This group included:
   a) Twenty four patients with mild EPH-gestosis.
   b) Thirty three patients with severe EPH-gestosis.
   c) Eight patients with severe EPH-gestosis complicated with abruptio-placentae.
3. Twelve patients suffering of chronic hypertensive vascular disease, without EPH-gestosis.

The description of these different groups is detailed in Tab. 1.

Of the 103 cases under study, 98 patients were delivered by lower segment caesarean section, while the remaining five cases were managed by caesarean hysterectomy, four because of ruptured uterus and one case because of severe concealed accidental haemorrhage. The biopsies were collected at caesarean section from the placental bed and from the placenta and they were placed at once into 10% neutral buffered formol saline solution. The blocks from the placenta and placental tissue were processed taking care to align the tissues so that both myometrium, decidua and placental tissue were included in the sections. A minimum of 8 serial sections were cut from each block. All the sections were stained by the following methods:

1. *Harris* hematoxyline and eosin as a routine stain.
2. *Heidenhain's Azen* stain for connective tissue.
3. *Van Gieson* stain for fibrous tissue.
4. *Van Gieson* Verhoeff's stain for elastic tissue.
5. Periodic acid-*schiff* stain for basement membranes.

Tab. 1. The full description of 103 cases of EPH-gestosis including 26 normally pregnant women as a control.

Group	No. of cases	Mean age in years	Primigr. %	Grand multipara %	Average parity	Mono-symptom-atic EPH-gestosis	Poly-symptom-atic EPH-gestosis	Gestosis Index
Control normal	26	27.3	26.9	23.0	2.8	–	–	–
Mild EPH-gestosis	24 (31.1%)	25.7	37.5	20.8	1.7	15.3%	84.7%	2.4
Severe EPH-gestosis	33 (42.9%)	26.8	39.4	21.4	2.1	6.5%	93.5%	7.8
EPH-gestosis with abruptioplacentae	8 (10.4%)	32.5	37.5	25.0	2.5	12.5%	87.5%	8.9
Chronic hyperten-sive vascular disease	12 (15.6%)	35.6	16.7	41.7	3.4	–	–	–

Results

Examination of all sections collected from the 103 cases under study were compared in the different groups according to the following pathological findings:

1. The villous maturity comparing the incidence of mature, premature and hyper-mature villi (Fig. 1 and 2).

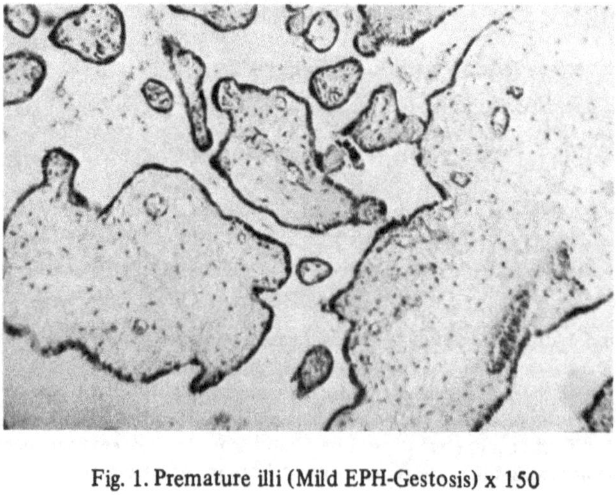

Fig. 1. Premature illi (Mild EPH-Gestosis) x 150

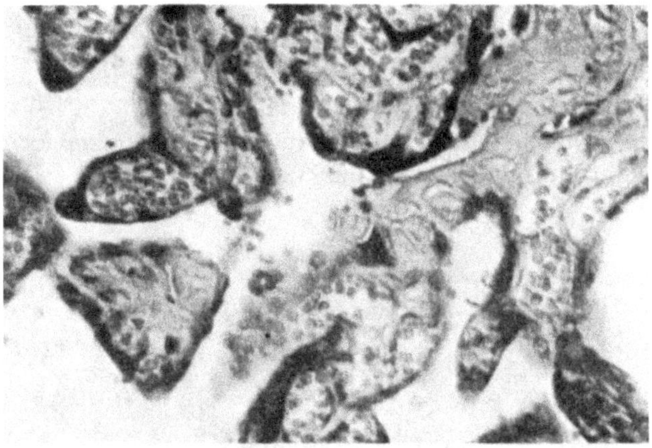

Fig. 2. Hypermature villi with syncytial degeneration (severe EPH-Gestosis)

2. The syncytial changes, considering its thinning, loss of continuity, nuclear-knots and syncytial sprouts (Fig. 3 and 4).

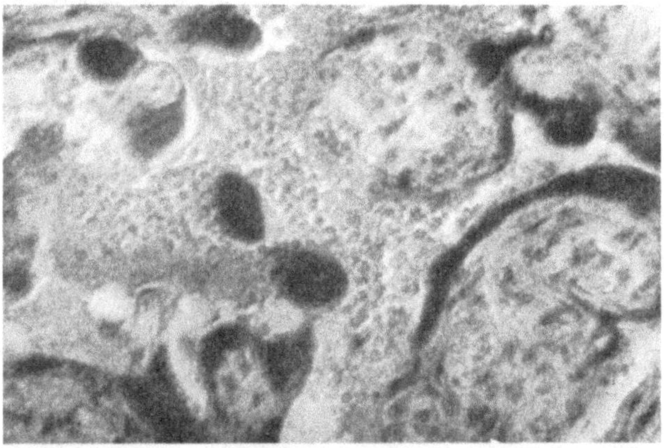

Fig. 3. Premature fibrosis in villi, multiple syncytial sporuts x 150

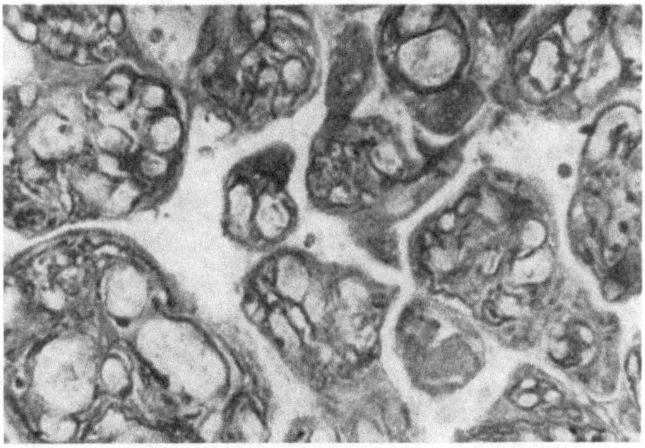

Fig. 4. Thickened basement membranes of the Cytotrophoblast and the foetal capillaries x 150

3. Changes in the Langhans' layer.
4. Basement membrane (Fig. 4).
5. Changes in the villous stroma in the form of collagenous and increased density together with fibrosis of the villi (Fig. 5).

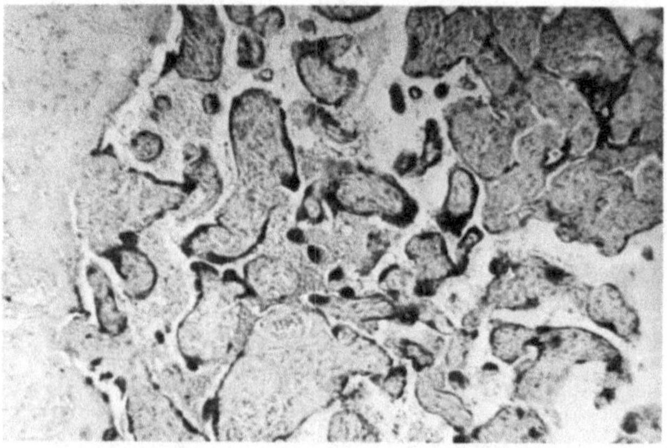

Fig. 5. Mature villi showing increased stromal density, nuclear knots and syncytial sprouts x 150

6. Villous congestion.
7. Increased fibrin deposition in the intervillous space with the formation of intervillous thrombi (Fig. 6 and 7).

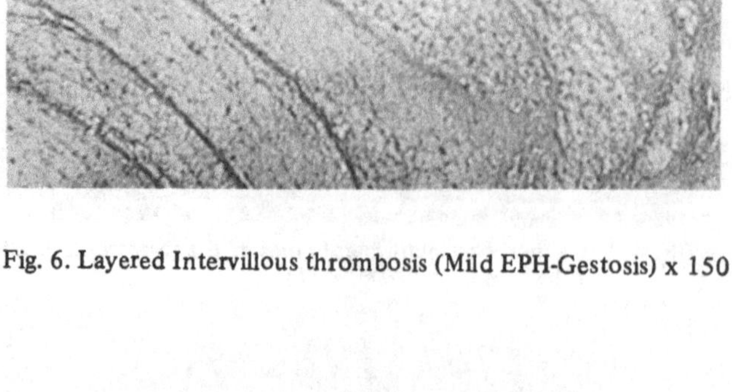

Fig. 6. Layered Intervillous thrombosis (Mild EPH-Gestosis) x 150

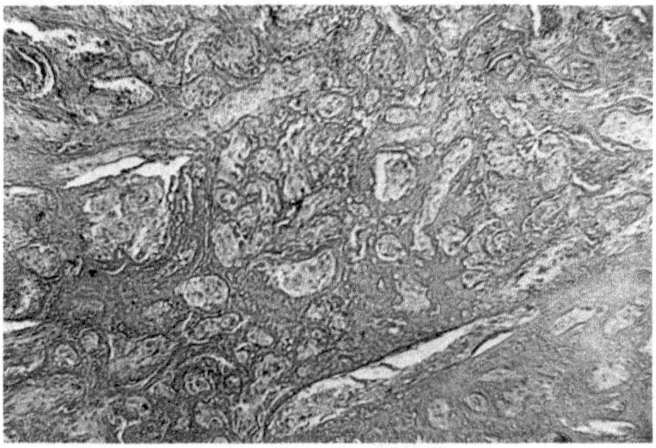

Fig. 7. Perivillous fibrin deposition (Mild EPH-Gestosis) x 150

8. Decidual hematomata (Fig. 8).

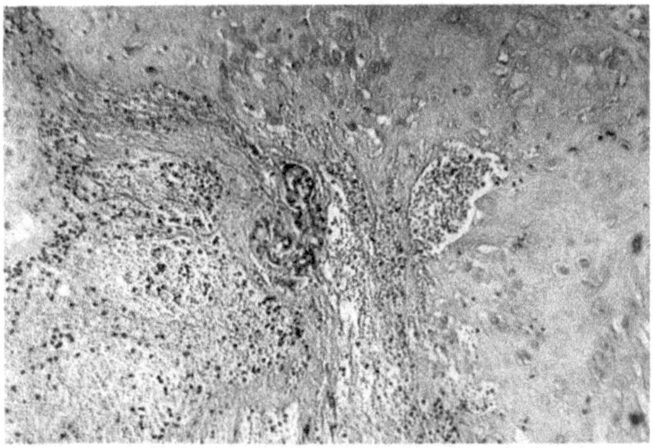

Fig. 8. Decidual hematoma (severe EPH-Gestosis) x 150

9. Endarteritis of foetal vessels in the villous stalks (Fig. 10 and 11).
10. Fibrinoid necrosis of the villi seen as a mass of structureless homogenous, acidophilic, strongly PAS positive material around the periphery of which were few degenerate syncytial nuclei (Fig. 12).
11. Changes in decidual vessels in the form of:
    a) Denudation of endothelium.
    b) Proliferation of the intimal cells.
    c) Growth of connective tissue fibres from the vessels wall straight into the lumen.
    d) Precipitation of blood components.
    e) Absorption of soft fibrinoid material into the arterial wall.
    f) Deposition of fat with foam cell infiltration in the decidual spiral arterioles.
    g) Necrosis and solid thrombosis or damage with layered thrombosis.

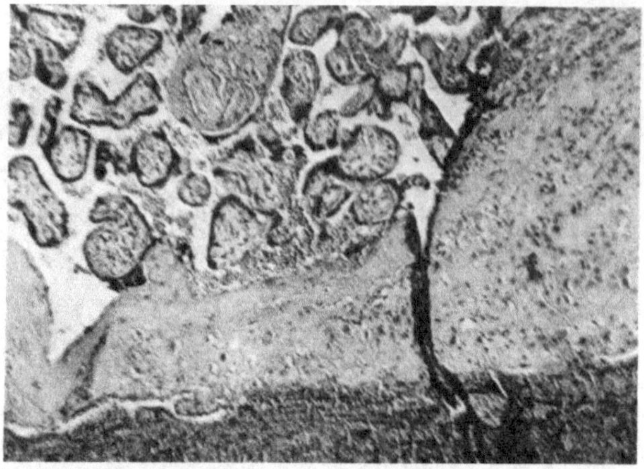

Fig. 9. Retroplacental hematoma (severe EPH-Gestosis complicate with abrutio-placentae) x 150

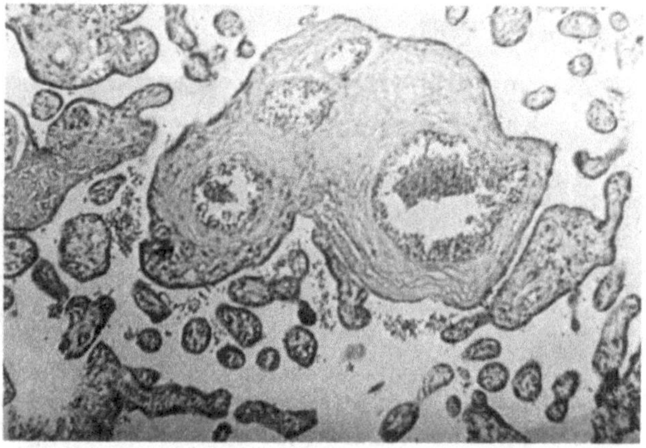

Fig. 10. Villous stalk (normal full time pregnancy) x 150

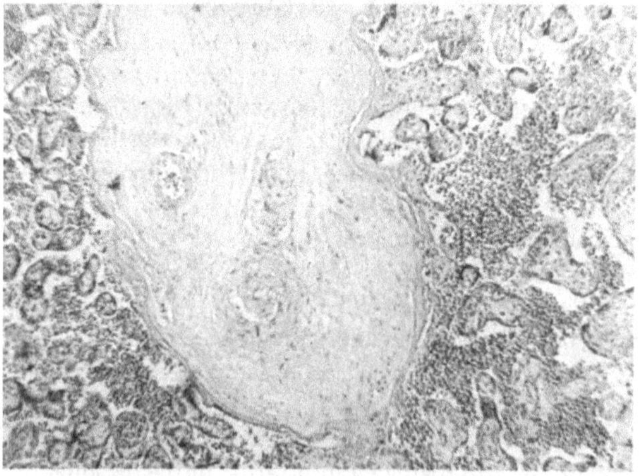

Fig. 11. Villous stalk with vascular thickening and abliterative changes with stromel fibrousis (severe EPH-Gestosis) x 150

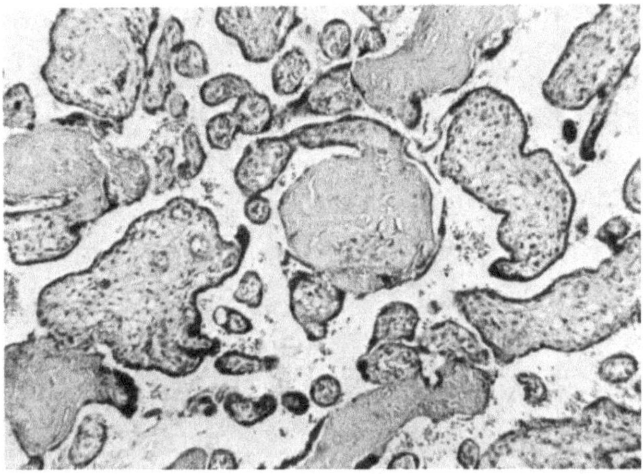

Fig. 12. Fibrinoid degeneration of villi other villi are premature (severe EPH-Gestosis) x 150

Tab. 2 summarizes the results in the different groups examined.

Conclusions

Comparison of the placentas and placental beds from normal gestations and patients with mild EPH-gestosis, severe EPH-gestosis, EPH-gestosis complicated with abruptio-placentae and chronic hypertensive vascular disease with pregnancy shows that well defined pathological alterations take place in these conditions:

1. Premature ripening of the chorionic villi.
2. Degeneration of the syncytium.
3. More prominent nuclear knots.
4. More frequent syncytial sprouts.
5. Persistence of the Langhans' cell layer.
6. Thickening of the basement membrane.
7. Fibrosis and collagenous transformation of the villous stroma.
8. Congestion of the villous capillaries and prevention of sinusoid formations.
9. Proliferative endarteritis of the foetal vessels in villous stalks.
10. Increased incidence of intervillous fibrin deposition.
11. Increased incidence of fibrinoid degeneration of villi.
12. Increased incidence of small decidual hematomata.

Tab. 2. The pathological changes in the component of the placenta and its bed in 103 cases of EPH-gestosis including 26 normally pregnant females as a control group.

Pathology	Control	Mild EPH-gestosis	Severe EPH-gestosis	Abruptio placentae	Hypertensive Vascular dis.
1. Villous Maturity	88.6% mature 7.6% premat. 3.8% hypermat.	62.5 mature 44.2% premat. 33.3% hypermat.	21.4 mature 7.1% premat. 71.5% hypermat.	50% mature 25% premat. 25% hypermat.	33.3 mature 8.3% premat. 5.8% hypermat.
2. Syncytial changes	normal degeneration	grossly thinned with nuclear knots	syncytial sprouts	syncytial sprouts	no greater degeneration
3. Langhans' layer	Flattened & Irregular cells	Cellular Proliferation with variation	Cellular Proliferation	Cellular Proliferation	Less Proliferation
4. Basement membrane	Normal	Thickened	Thickened intensely PAS + ve	Thickened	Thickened
5. Villous stromal density and fibrosis	Not increased	increased in 41.7%	increased in 67.8%	increased in 50%	increased in 41.7%
6. Congestion of villi	in 3.8%	in 8.3%	in 52.1%	in 50%	in 41.7%
7. Increased fibrin deposition in the intervillous space	in 7.6%	in 62.5%	in 60.7%	in 37.5%	in 50.0%
8. Decidual haematomata	in 3.8%	in 4.2%	in 42.5%	in 62.5%	in 25.0%
9. Endarteritis of fetal vessels	in 0.0%	in 8.3%	in 37.5%	in 25.0%	in 58.3%
10. Fibrinoid necrosis of villi	in 0.0%	in 12.5%	in 16.3%	in 12.5%	in 8.3%
11. abnormal decidual vessels	in 0.0%	in 91.7%	in 89.3%	in 100%	in 100%

13. The maternal spiral decidual vessels pass through the following different pathological processes.
    a) denudation of endothelium with formation of fibrin and red blood cell flakes (Fig. 14).
    b) Intimal proliferation (Fig. 13).
    c) Growth of connective tissue from the wall with incorporation of blood components.
    d) Precipitation of blood components in the lumen.

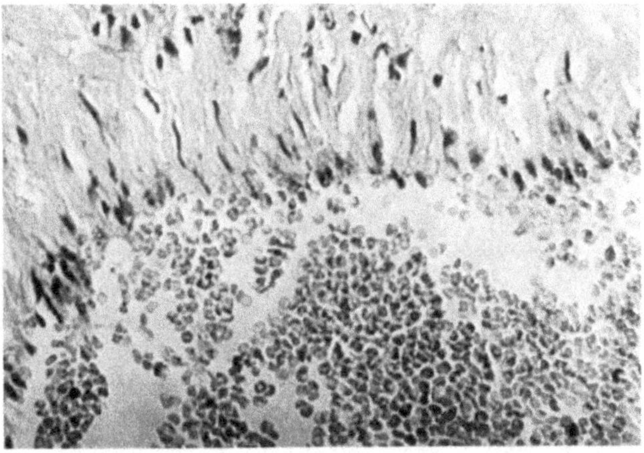

Fig. 13. Fibroblastic intimal response of spiral arterioles (Mild EPH-Gestosis) x 150

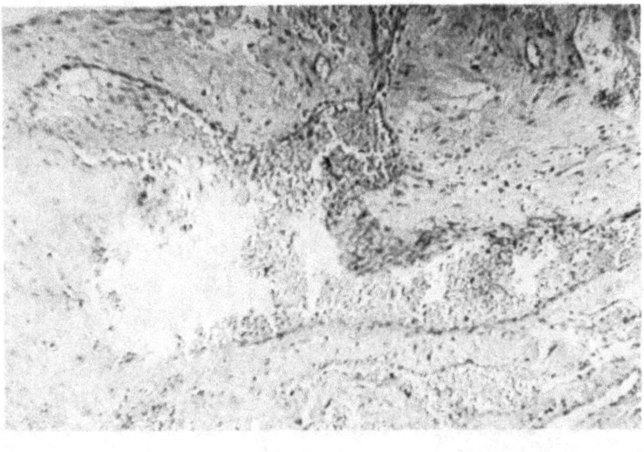

Fig. 14. Decidual vessel with partially denuded epithelium at one sit and intimial sclerosis at another site (severe EPH-Gestosis) x 150

e) Absorption of fibrinoid material in the wall (Fig. 18).
f) Deposition of fat with foam cell infiltration in the wall (Fig. 15).
g) Necrosis of the wall with thrombosis in the lumen (Fig. 16 and 17).

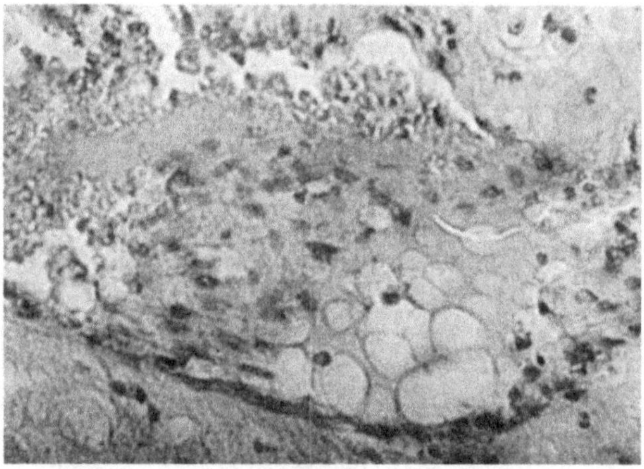

Fig. 15. Decidual vessel with foam-cell infiltration ot its wall (severe EPH-Gestosis) x 825

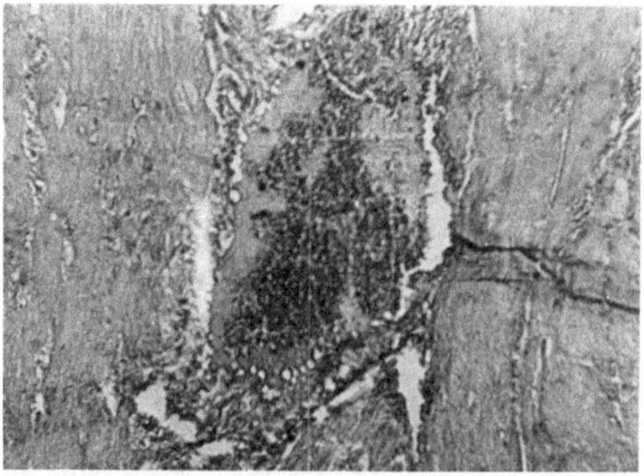

Fig. 16. Extensive thrombosis in a decidual vessel (severe EPH-Gestosis) x 150

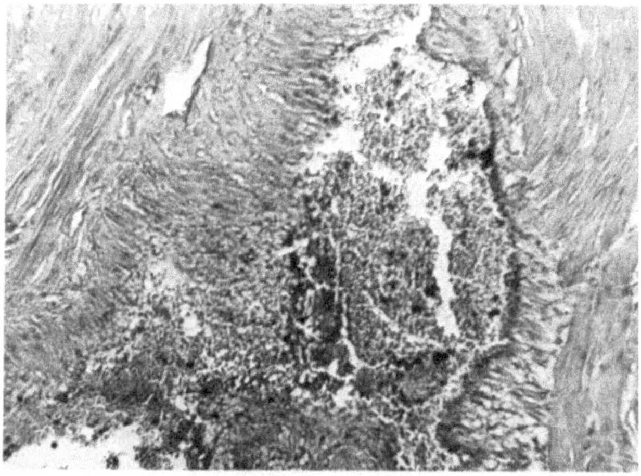

Fig. 17. Acute necrosis of decidual arterial wall, rupture of the wall with exudation of red blood cells (severe EPH-Gestosis) x 150

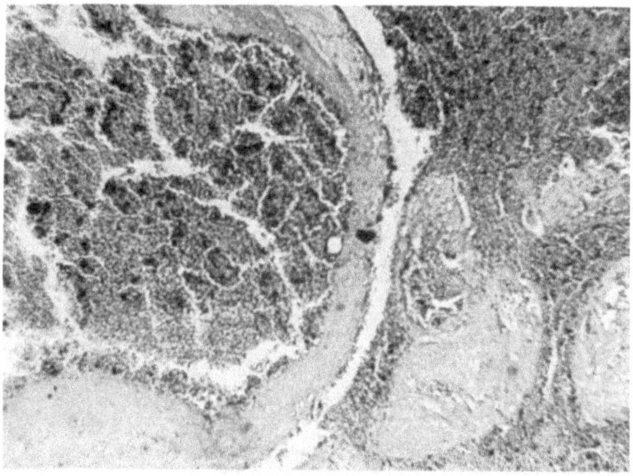

Fig. 18. Fibrinoid degenration in a decidual vessel with a decidual hematoma (severe EPH-Gestosis with abrouptio-placentae) x 150

The frequency of the above alterations depends upon the severit of the disease. We guess that we can formulate a placental score or index from the above 10 pathological findings in the placenta and its bed, thus one can correlate the clinical signs of gestosis with the pathology of the placenta.

References

[1] *Fox, H.:* Fibrinoid necrosis of placental villi. J. obstet. Gynaec. Brith. Cwlth 75 (1968) p. 448–452.

[2] *Marais, W. D.:* The clinical evaluation of normal and abnormal spiral arterioles of placental lesions. J. Obstet. Gynaec. Brit. Cwlth 70 (1963) p. 77–786.

[3] *Salvatore, C. A.:* The placenta in acute Toxaemia. Amer. J. Obstet. Gynaec. 102 (1968) p. 347–353.

[4] *Wigglesworth, J. S.:* Morphological variations in the insufficient placenta. J. Obstet. Gynaec. Brit. Cwlth 71 (1964) p. 871–884.

Diagnostic Value of Cytological Examination in EPH-Gestosis

Mohamed B. Sammour, B.Sc. (Oxford), F.R.C.S., M.I.A.C.

Department of Obstetrics and Gynecology, Ain Shams University, Cairo, UAR

Introduction

Exfoliative vaginal cytology is a good reflection of the balance of the female hormones. Its procedure is simple and could be easily performed in the antenatal clinic without any inconvenience to the patient.

Pananicolaou in 1925 [1] was the first to describe the navicular cells in the vaginal smears of pregnant women. The navicular cell is intermediate between the superficial and the basal cell, has a dense cytoplasm and an elongated nucleus with dark thickened borders. *Sammour* [3] in his study of the vaginal smear during pregnancy has described 4 stages:

1. The smear of early pregnancy up to sixteen weeks when the placenta becomes established; The cell morphology, the smear back ground and the phenomena of cytoloysis were similar to the picture of the smear during the late secretory phase of the menstrual cycle. The navicular cells were scarce and the karyopyknotic index varied from 25% to 12% (Fig. 1).
2. The placental phase which covers the duration from 16–38 weeks: all smears showed a similar picture described as "the typical pregnancy smear". The chief influence appeared to be a progesterone domination. More than 80% of the cells were of the navicular type arranged in compact grouping. The karyopycnotic index never exceeded 15%, the background of the smear is full of mucous and leucocytes and cytolysis is a feature in 70% of smears collected during the second half of the pregnancy (Fig. 2 and 3).
3. The antepartum phase covering the last two weeks of pregnancy: The sequential changes observed in smears collected during this phase showed that the navicular cell was no longer predominent and it was replaced by the intermediate cell; the cells tend to be discrete, the background showed gradual clearing with fewer bacteria and leucocytes and cytolysis has markedly disappeared from the smear (Fig. 4 and 5).
4. The "at term" smear is characteristic of pregnancy which has reached term. The changes are those of the antepartum phase, but, are greater in degree. The cells are intermediate, discrete or in small groups, clean background and absent cytolysis (Fig. 6).

The purpose of this study is to describe the vaginal smear in EPH-Gestosis and to correlate it with the expected hormonal inbalance as a result of the placental insufficiency.

Material and Methods

The vaginal smear was collected by scraping of the lateral vaginal wall using the dry wooden spatula and after applying a bivalve speculum. The patient was advised not to do any vaginal wash the morning the smear was collected. The smear was immediately spread on a dry clean glass slide and fixed in a mixture of 3% acetic acid in 95% ethyl alcohol, then stained by the Papanicolaou stain using Harris haematoxyline as counter-stain. The collection of vaginal smear was repeated every 2–3 weeks until the onset of labour. We examined 850 smears, collected from 372 patients suffering from EPH-gestosis. The duration of the pregnancy varied between 30 and 36 weeks.

The discription of these patients is detailed in Tab. 1. The smears were examined mainly for:
1. The dominant type of cells.
2. The cellular arrangement.
3. The karyopycnotic index.
4. The background of the smear.
5. Cytolysis.

Tab. 1. The description of 372 patients suffering for EPH-gestosis.

Type of EPH-gestosis	No. of cases	average Age (years)	primi-para %	grand multi-para %	average No. of deliveries	Mono-sympto-matic	Poly-sympto-matic	Mean value gestosis Index
Mild EPH-gestosis	177	23.9	41.6	11.2	1.6	14.7%	85.3%	2.4
Severe EPH-gestosis	195	25.3	32.1	16.5	3.1	0%	100%	8.1

Results

The cytological picture deviated from the typical smear of pregnancy in 85.7% of the cases of mild EPH-gestosis and in 97.5% of the cases of severe EPH-gestosis. The following are our findings:

1. *The type of cell:* the navicular cell was replaced by the superficial intermediate cell and the navicular index ranged between 35–50% in all slides examined. The appearance of some superficial squames with eosinophilic cytoplasm was frequently encountered.

2. *Cellular arrangements:* the cells were discrete or in small groups in 75% of the specimens examined, while in 25%, the cells were arranged in thick groups (Fig. 7 and 8).

3. *The karyopycnotic index:* it remained unchanged in most of the specimens examined. The smears which showed marked discrete arrangement of the cells demonstrated a mild rise in the karyopycnotic index.

4. *The background of the smear:* it was clear, showing no infiltration with non-cellular elements in 65% of the specimens examined, while in 35% of cases, the smear was full of leucocytes, histiocytes, mucus, debris and bacteria.

5. *Cytolysis:* the pheomena of cytolysis was absent in 60% of the specimens. The cells had a well defined outline and well developed cytoplasm with clear background of the smear. In the remaining 40%, cytolysis was present but not so marked as in the typical pregnancy smear (Fig. 9).
Tab. 2 summarizes the cytological results in the 850 smears collected. From the table the difference in the smear description is slightly variable between the mild and the severe EPH-gestosis. Most of the 850 smears collected conform to the picture of the "at term" smear which could be simply described as being composed of discrete intermediate and navicular cells, clear background of the smear, limited or no cytolysis and a slight rise in the karyopycnotic index.
Basal cell infiltration of the smear was encountered in eleven of the 372 cases of EPH-gestosis examined. This basal cell infiltration is considered as a serious sign in the smear as far as the foetal salvage is concerned (Fig. 10). Fig. 1–9 can be looked into at the author's.

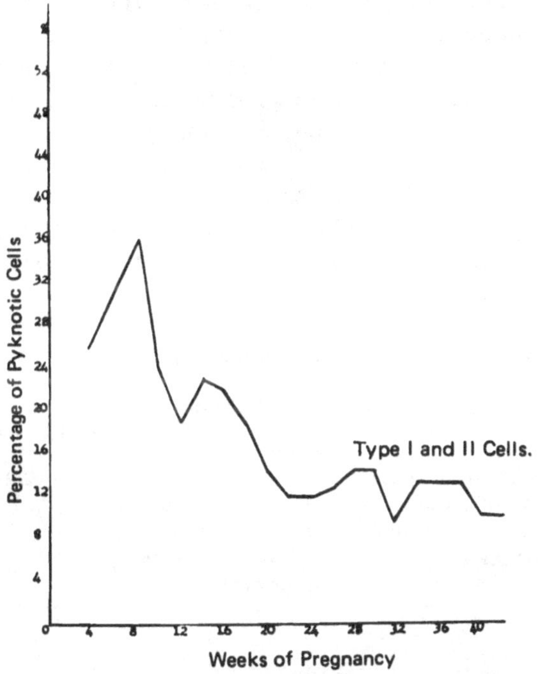

Fig. 10. A smear at 38 weeks from a pregnancy complicated with severe EPH-Gestosis, pregnancy ended in Stilbirth, note the basal cell infiltration. x 450

Tab. 2. The cytological findings in 850 smears collected from 372 pregnant women (30–36 weeks) suffering from EPH-gestosis.

Type of EPH-gestosis	Type of cell	Cellular arrangements	Karyopy-cnotic index	Background of the smear	Cytolysis
Mild EPH-gestosis (410 smears)	Navicular cell index varied from 40–50%	discrete in 60%, clumps in 40%	15–20%	mainly clean	absent in 50%
Severe EPH-gestosis (440 smears)	Navicular cell index varied from 25–40%	discrete in 80%, clumps in 20%	25–30%	always clean	absent in 85%

Discussion

There is good reason to suppose that vaginal cytology can now be added to the diagnostic procedures in EPH-gestosis and it is an established test as far as the foetal prognosis is concerned. The picture of the normal typical pregnancy smear is well defined and variation from the normal would certainly mean some defect in the hormonal production from the placenta [2, 4]. Such a simple test might well save many babies from intrauterine or perinatal death. This could be demonstrated in Tab. 3. The rise in the foetal loss is corresponding markedly to the changes in the vaginal smear. One can safely state that vaginal cytology provides a new and a comparatively simple method of selecting those for whome induction of labor is required to avoid placental insufficiency. The changes in the cells making the distinctive pattern of the insufficient placenta in EPH-gestosis are qualitative and not quantitative and in particular the pyknotic index per se is of little value in this assessment. More than one smear collected at an interval of at least one week are necessary for describing the smear pattern.

Tab. 3. The relation of the foetal mortality and the atypical picture of the vagial smear in 372 patients suffering from EPH-gestosis.

Type of smear	No. of cases	Perinatal Mortality
1. Normal typical smear	52	2.9%
2. "at term" smear	308	13.6%
3. Basal cellular infiltration in the smear	11 (six intrauterine deaths)	54.5%

Summary

The vaginal smear was examined in 372 patients of EPH-Gestosis. The cytological picture deviated from the typical smear of pregnancy in 85.7% of the cases examined.

The karyopycnotic index was of no much significance. The discrete arrangement of the cells, the disappearance of cytolysis and the abundent superficial squames were the essential characters of the smear in EPH-gestosis.

References

[1] *Papanicolaou, G. N.:* The diagnosis of early human pregnancy by the vaginal smear method. Proc. Soc. Exper. Biol. & Med. 22 (1925) p. 436.

[2] *Pundel, J. P.:* Vaginal Cytology as prognostic method in pregnancy disorders. Acta cytol. 3 (1959) p. 231.

[3] *Sammour, M. B.:* Vaginal cytology during normal pregnancy, its role in determination of the approximate date of confinement, obst. Gynec. 24 (1964) p. 682.

[4] *Von-Haam, E.* and *R. Schwallenberg:* Symposium on hormonal cytology during pregnancy and the postpartum period. Acta cytol. 3 (1959) p. 218.

Die rechtzeitige Zytodiagnostik der Gefährdung des Kindes bei EPH-Gestose

Z. Zidovsky

Research Institute for the Care of Mother and Child, Prague-Podoli, CSSR

Die vaginale Zytodynamik am Ende der normalen Schwangerschaft

Vom 3. Schwangerschaftsmonat an findet sich im Zytogram ein typisch uniformer Schwangerschaftsabstrich, der mit dem *Vaginalabstrich der „fortgeschrittenen Schwangerschaft"* identisch ist.

In der Periode unmittelbar vor der spontanen Geburt ändert sich dieses uniforme Schwangerschaftsbild deutlich:

1. Die Zahl der navicularen und austerförmigen Schwangerschaftszellen (cellules en forme d'hûitre) nimmt ab, manchmal verschwinden sie ganz.
2. Die Zahl der Oberflächen- und Intermediärzellen steigt an.
3. Vermehrt Leucocyten und Schleim. (Leucocyten haben nur bei Abwesenheit einer pathologischen Vaginalflora diagnostische Bedeutung.)
4. Manchmal schlechte Färbbarkeit des Plasma – die Zellen haben ein „verwaschenes" oder „schmutziges" Aussehen.
5. Oft findet man eine ausgesprochene „Östrogenisation", d. h. der Eosinophilieindex erreicht bis 25%, der kariopyknotische Index maximal 45%.

Diese Veränderungen erlauben festzustellen, ob sich die Schwangere dem Geburtstermin nähert, oder sich schon am Termin befindet. Den Geburtstermin bestimmen wir zytologisch mit Hilfe der 4 Vaginalzytotypen:

Zytotypus I = „fortgeschrittene Schwangerschaft"

Vorwiegend Navicularzellen, welche charakteristische Zellgruppen (Clusters) bilden. In geringer Zahl findet man die eigentlichen Intermediärzellen. Die Navicularzellen können auch eine rundliche Form annehmen (= Austerförmige Schwangerschaftszellen). Das Verhältnis von Navicularzellen zu intermediären Zellen beträgt in diesem Bild 3:1. Oberflächenzellen fehlen ganz, oder sind nur vereinzelt anzutreffen. Keine Leucocyten, kein Schleim. Das Plasma ist meist basophil, die Umrisse sind kontrastreich und gut angefärbt. Der Karyopyknose- und Eosinophilie-Index ist praktisch gleich Null.

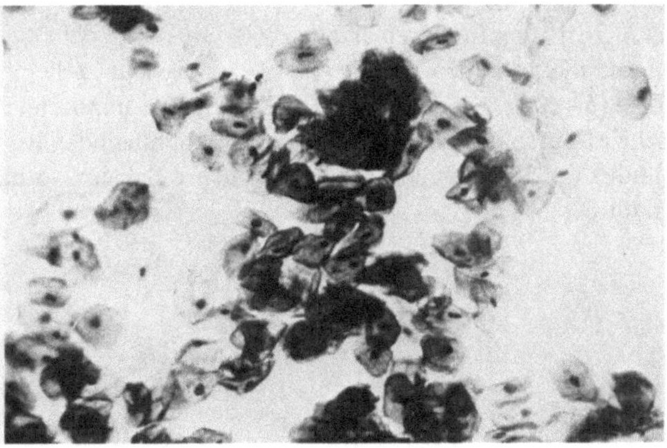

Abb. 1

Zytotypus II = „kurz vor dem Termin"

Dieser Typ unterscheidet sich vom vorhergehenden bes. durch das Verhältnis von Navicularzellen zu eigentlichen Intermediärzellen, das jetzt nicht mehr 3:1, sondern 1:1 ist. Die Basophilie bleibt bestehen – die Zahl der Oberflächenzellen nimmt zu. Leucocyten in geringer Zahl, kein Schleim. Der Eosinophilieindex liegt bei 2–3%, der Karyopyknoseindex unter 7%. Die Anfärbbarkeit des Plasmas und der Kerne ist noch immer gut, die Zellgrenzen sind kontrastreich und scharf. Die typischen Gruppen von Navikularzellen fangen an zu zerfallen.

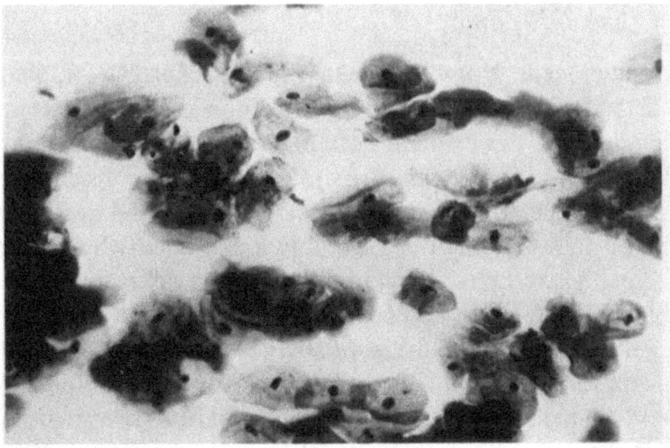

Abb. 2

Zytotypus III = „am Termin"

Überwiegen der eigentlichen Intermediärzellen (60–80%) und der Oberflächenzellen mit vesikulären und pyknotischen Kernen (20–40%). Navicularzellen in deutlich verminderter Zahl (5–10%). Die Zellen sind isoliert, liegen einzeln und bilden nicht mehr die typischen Haufen wie bei I und II. Der Eosinophilieindex liegt um 10%, der Karyopyknoseindex um 20%. Leucocytenzahl vermehrt, Schleim vorhanden, schlechtere Anfärbbarkeit der Zellen.

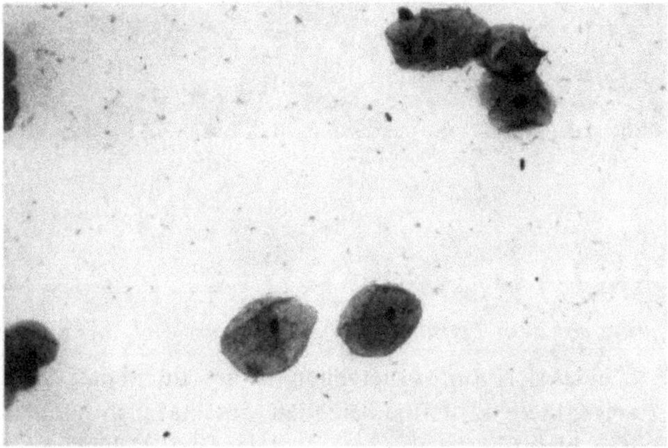

Abb. 3

Zytotypus IV = „klar am Termin"

Keine Navicularzellen mehr. Vorwiegend Oberflächenzellen (40–80%), gelegentlich eosinophile, vollständig verhornte Zellen ohne Kern, wie „rote Schatten" aussehend (Cornified Cells), der Rest des Epithels besteht aus eigentlichen Intermediärzellen. Das Plasma färbt sich oft sehr schwach an, ist sehr kontrastarm und sieht „schmutzig" und „verwaschen" aus. Deutliche Vermehrung der Leucocyten und des Schleims. Eosinphilieindex kann bis 25% erreichen, der Karyopyknoseindex schwankt zwischen 20–45%. Manchmal bilden Leucocyten und Schleim im mikroskopischen Bild charakteristische Gebilde. Manchmal finden sich auch Cervixzellen in typischen Gruppen und Erythrocyten, welche sicher aus dem Cervikalkanal stammen (Cave Artefakte, welche von unvorsichtigem Einführen der Scheidenspecula stammen können). Wenn im Scheidenbild bei Fehlen von Leucocyten und Schleim superfiziale eosinophile Zellen mit pyknotischen Kernen vorherrschen, sprechen wir von einem oestrogenen Aussehen des Scheidenbildes.

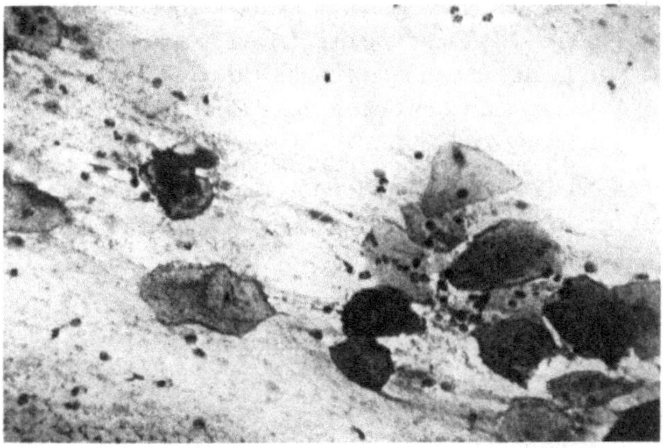

Abb. 4

Der *Zytotypus I hat eine Zeitabgrenzung von 10 und mehr Tagen, der Zytotypus II 4–9 Tage* vor der spontanen Geburt. Die Gültigkeit dieser Zeitabgrenzungen besteht nur bei dynamischer Verfolgung der Veränderungen im Zytotypus, d. h. daß bei einem wiederholten Befund dieser Zytotypen die Zeitabgrenzung dauernd perseveriert. *Bei Vorliegen eines Zytotypus I und II können wir sagen, daß die Schwangere noch nicht für die Geburt bereit ist* – die Schwangerschaft geht weiter.

Beim Zytotypus III und IV ist die Zeitabgrenzung nicht mehr fakultativ, wie bei den vorhergehenden Zytotypen I und II. Eine zeitliche Überschreitung bei dynamischer Verfolgung weist auf eine Bedrohung der Frucht hin.

Der *Zytotypus III hat eine Zeitabgrenzung von 1–6 Tagen,* der Zytotypus IV ist mit 0–3 Tagen begrenzt. Diese „Terminzytotypen" besagen, daß die Schwangere biologisch zur Geburt „reif ist", die Schwangerschaft geht zu Ende.

Die rechtzeitige Diagnostik der EPH-Gestose

Bei Spätgestose sind die Früchte potentiell bedroht. Es kommt zu pathologischen Veränderungen in der Placenta, Stoffwechselstörungen etc. Metabolische Veränderungen in der Placenta, die während der Schwangerschaft als Haupthormonproduzent angesehen werden muß, haben einen Einfluß auf den Hormonspiegel und das Schwangerschaftsgleichgewicht. Diese hormonalen Veränderungen finden ihren Ausdruck im Vaginalabstrich. Sie sind den Veränderungen ähnlich, die wir gegen den Geburtstermin hin antreffen. Sie äußern sich in den bekannten Veränderungen der „Östrogenisation" des Vaginalabstriches.

Aus unseren Ergebnissen geht hervor, daß in Fällen von pathologischer Schwangerschaft in denen es *zu einer Veränderung* des Vaginalabstriches vom Zytotypus I resp. II (Schwangerschaft im Laufe) in den Zytotypus III resp. IV (Schwangerschaft am Ende) *noch vor der 38. Schwangerschaftswoche kommt,* die Früchte in den meisten Fällen bedroht oder gar geschädigt sind.

Deshalb kann man bei *dynamischer* Verfolgung der Vaginalabstriche den Zustand der Schwangerschaft bei den potentiell bedrohten Graviditäten wie bei EPH-Gestose erkennen.

The Cardinal Signs of EPH-Gestosis: Determination, Pathophysiology, Implications

Weight Gain in Pregnancy

N. A. M. Bergstein

Dept. Obstetrics and Gynaecology, Ziekenhuis, Zevenaar, Holland

This reports deals with a series of continuing investigation about weight gain during pregnancy.

The material is constituted by 97 women having a normal pregnancy. They were selected according to the following criteria:

1. Their history gave no reason to believe that they had any disease before pregnancy.
2. During this pregnancy there was no reason to prescribe a diet or any medication.
3. Normal values for hemoglobine, creatinine, uric acid and liver-function were obtained.

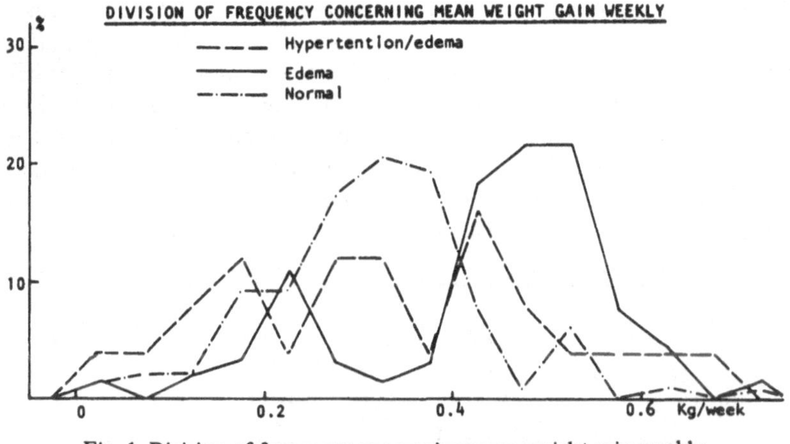

Fig. 1. Division of frequency concerning mean weight gain weekly

The group "edema" in pregnancy comprised 65 women.
They had a weight gain exceeding one, three or more times 500 g in two weeks. At the end of pregnancy blood pressure was 130/90. During pregnancy they had no therapy; all of them delivered in time.

In group "hypertension-edema" there were only 25 women.
This group is so small because it is very difficult to find women who did not have any therapy if in pregnancy hypertension and edema is noted.

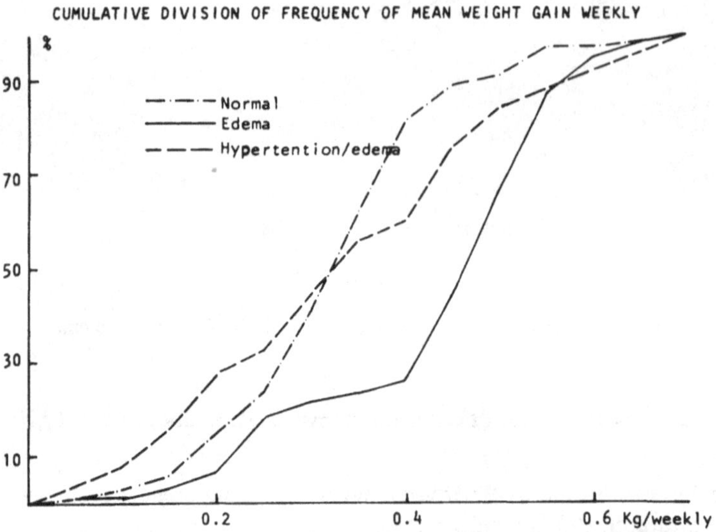

Fig. 2. Cumulative division of frequency of mean weight gain weekly

In these women blood pressure from the start of pregnancy on was 140/100 or 130/90. Considering weight gain, one can distinguish three groups. A niveau-difference in weekly weight-gain is apparent comparing the three groups. In group 2 (edema) it seems that one has to do with two categories of women:

One with a weight gain of 0,5 kg weekly and one with 0,25 kg of weight gain weekly. Because many women came to our policlinic being pregnant, their pre-pregnancy weight remained unknown. Therefore we asked the computer, what the probable weight in the 20th week of pregnancy could possibly have been. The computerized weight-gain curve of these women gave a curve of "best-points". It tells what the probable weight might have been at 20 weeks of pregnancy. In this consideration this time is very critical, because then the uterus muscle is at its maximum; from then on it gets thinner, and as the uterus grows, becomes distended (Fig. 3 and 4).

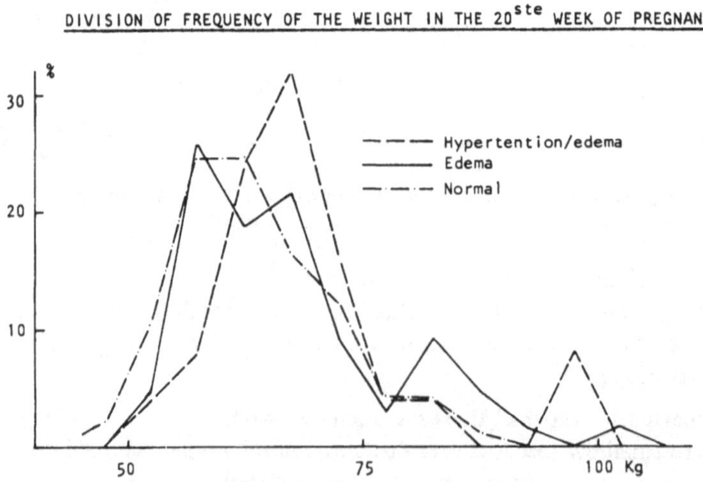

Fig. 3. Division of frequency of the weight in the 20ste week of pregnancy

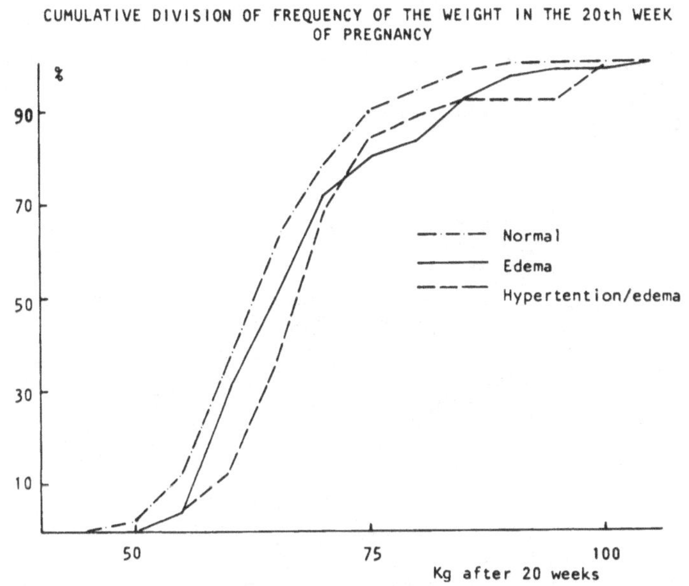

Fig. 4. Cumulative division of frequency of the weight in the 20th week of pregnancy

One can see that the "edema"-group has a higher weight at 20 weeks of pregnancy.

It appears that the "hypertension-edema"-group is made up of two sub-groups: One showing a weight of 75 kg, and another showing 95 kg.

In the "edema"-group one can distinguish those women with 62 and those with about 80 kg.

In the group of normal pregnancies one finds a weight of 60 kg at 20 weeks. The difference between the weight of normal pregnancies and the other two groups is about 4 kg.

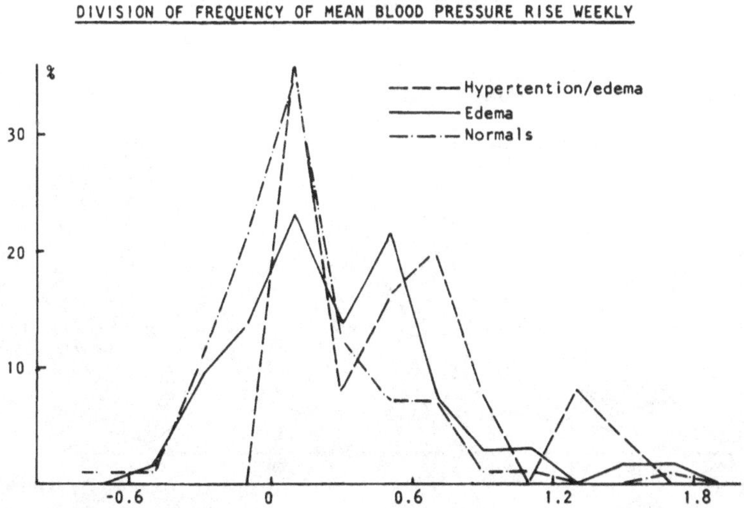

Fig. 5. Division of frequency of mean blood pressure rise weekly

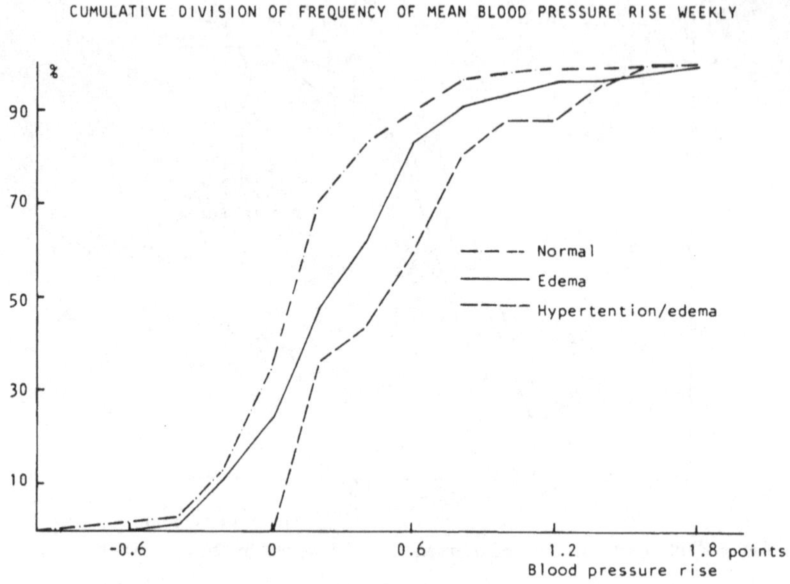

Fig. 6. Cumulative division of frequency of mean blood pressure rise weekly

Blood pressure

In normal pregnancy the mean diastolic value was 75 mm/Hg. The "edema"-group seems to have two peaks, and the "hypertension-edema"-group three peaks.

Fig. 7 and Fig. 8 show the differences between the three groups at 20 weeks pregnancy.

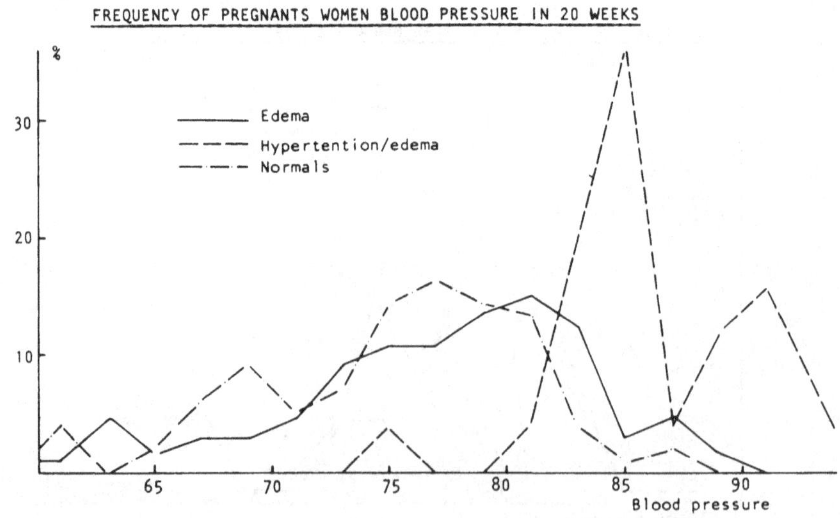

Fig. 7. Frequency of pregnants women blood pressure in 20 weeks

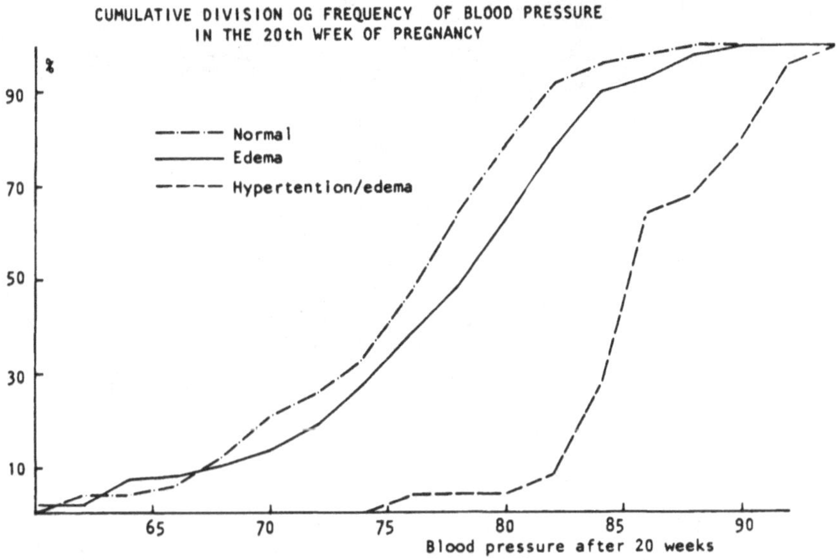

Fig. 8. Cumulative division og frequency of blood pressure in the 20th week of pregnancy

Considering the birth-weights of the children from these women, one finds (Fig. 9 and Fig. 10) that patients with edema have heavier children than the other two groups.

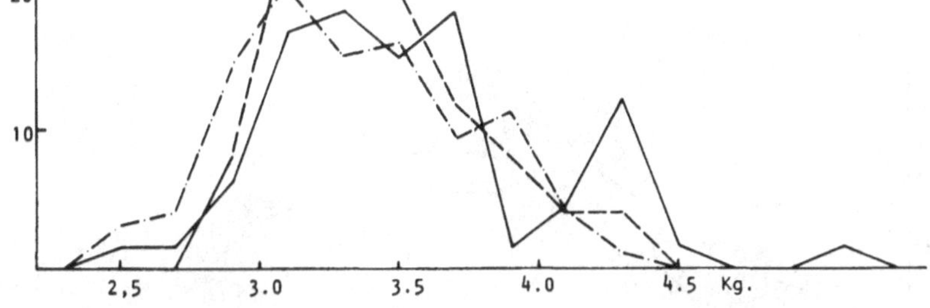

Fig. 9. Division of frequency of birth weight

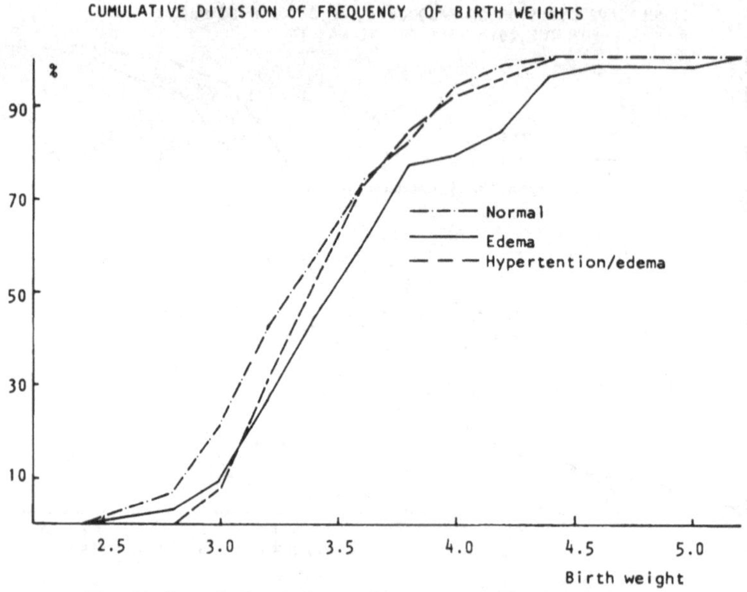

Fig. 10. Cumulative division of frequency of birth weights

The greatest weight of the placenta was found in the "hypertension-edema"-group. The ratio child-weight/placenta-weight (index) has also been investigated. A higher index was seen in the "hypertension-edema"-group. But even in this group one can notice wide variations (Fig. 11 and 12).

Furthermore the weight-gain-curve from normal pregnancies was analysed: It shows an S-shape. Up to the 10th week of pregnancy weight-gain is not important (Fig. 13). From the 10th till the 15th week the curve becomes steeper, and after week 15 till week 30 there is an almost constant weight-gain of 370 g/week. After the 30th week the weight gain decreases and at the 40th week it is only 100 g/week.

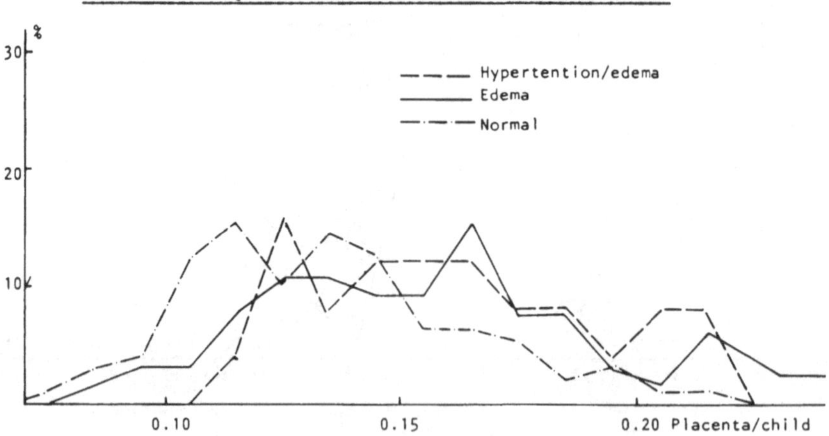

Fig. 11. Division of frequency of hie ratio of placenta/child weight

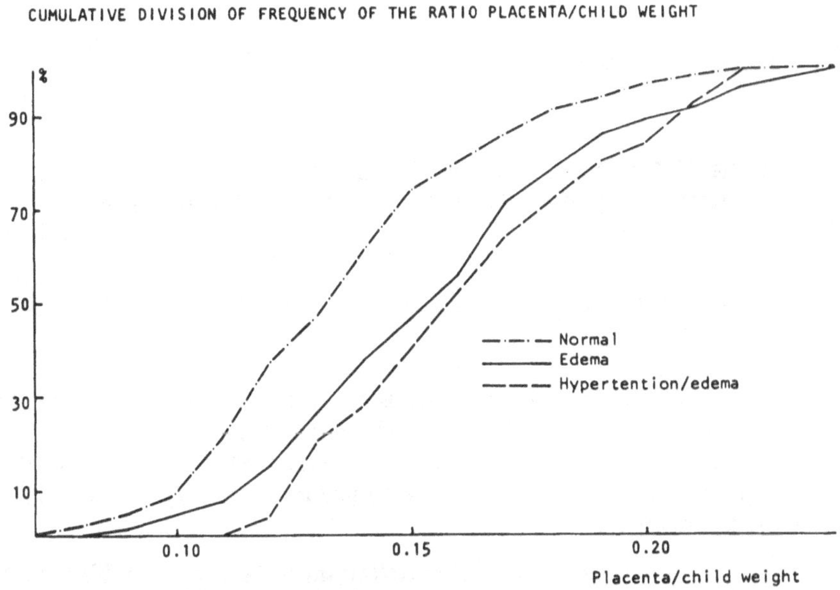

Fig. 12. Cumulative division of frequency of the ratio placenta/child weight

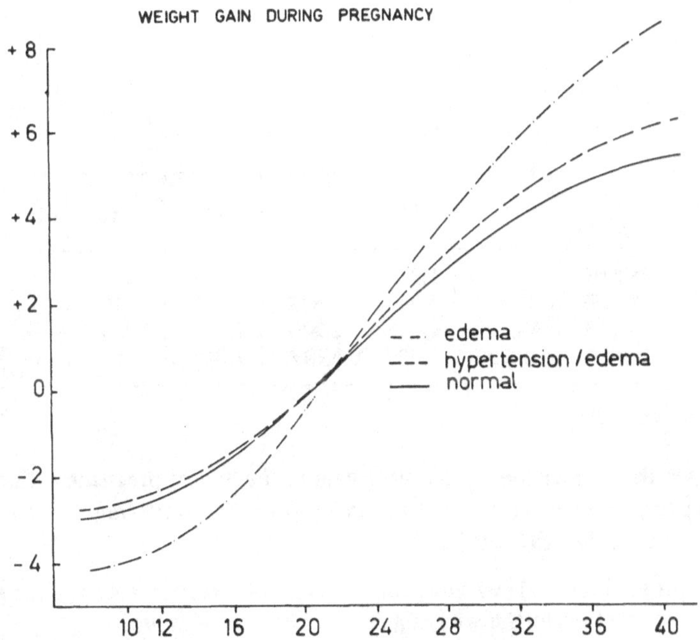

Fig. 13. Weight gain during pregnancy

The increase of diastolic blood pressure values also showed a S-shaped curve. There is a rise till the 25th week of 1 to 2 mm/Hg. Thereafter it seems to remain constant. There is a second rise after the 35th week of 2 mm.

The Interrelationship between Weight Gain, Weight of Placenta, Birth Weight of the Fetus and EPH Symptoms

B. Vedra

Institute for the Care of Mother and Child, Prague 4, Podoli, CSSR

It is well known that women with EPH-gestosis have a greater total weight gain at the end of pregnancy. This fact is usually explained by an abnormal salt and water retention. The increased salt and water retention is explained as a consequence of the disease. Silently it has been accepted that the disease is the primary, the salt and water retention the secondary phenomenon.

Let us try to observe the interrelationship between the weight gain and EPH-gestosis from an opposite point of view: EPH-gestosis as a consequence of "abnormal" weight gain.

Tab. 1. $X^2 = 125{,}42$.

weight gain in kg	no EPH-symptoms	E	EP	EH	EPH	total	P	H	PH
0–10	78,51%	18,75%	1,95%	0,78%	0,00%	256	2	–	1
11–15	64,25%	27,34%	3,97%	2,80%	1,64%	428	3	–	–
16–20	40,68%	48,73%	4,66%	2,97%	2,97%	236	–	2	1
20–	17,65%	62,75%	5,82%	7,84%	7,84%	51	1	–	–

Tab. 1 shows: the greater the total weight gain at the end of pregnancy, the less frequent are the pregnancies without any symptoms, the more frequent are the pregnancies with E, EP, EH, EPH symptoms.

The symptoms P, H and PH (without edema) were observed in a very small number of patients. No correlation to the weight gain can be demonstrated.

The conclusion of Tab. 1:
The greater is the weight gain, the more frequent are the symptoms of EPH-gestosis and vice verse. The correlation is highly significant, but it does not tell anything of what is a primary phenomenon and what a secondary one.

Tab. 2. A healthy controls
B EPH symptoms present in the last weeks of pregnancy
C EPH symptoms in twin-pregnancies in the last weeks of pregnancy
n number of measurements
Kg relative weight gain

week		15.	20.	25.	30.	35.
A	n	105	132	151	162	220
	Kg	2,07	3,87	6,26	7,94	10,62
B	n	23	26	34	37	50
	Kg	3,30	5,86	8,90	12,65	15,41
C	n	16	23	22	31	55
	Kg	7,78	5,34	9,10	12,58	15,17

The data of the Tab. 2 were used for linear regression analysis. The equations for the regression lines of the regression lines of the average weight gains and the regression lines are shown in Fig. 1.

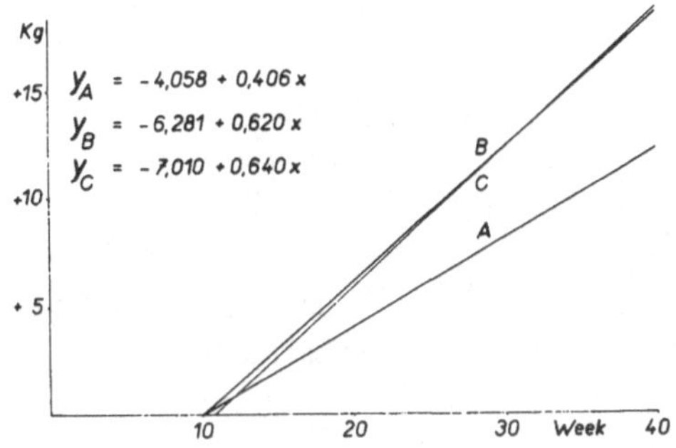

The conclusion of the regression analysis of the weight gains: the difference of the weight gains at the end of pregnancy between the healthy controls and patients with EPH symptoms is developing linearily from the end of the I. trimester.

The conclusion of Tab. 1 and Fig. 1:
The greater weight gain preceeds the development of the EPH symptoms. The above-average weight gain predisposes for EPH-gestosis. It is not the consequence but the condition.

Tab. 3 shows that there is a correlation between the total weight gain at the end of pregnancy and the weight of placenta. The greater the weight of placenta, the greater the total weight gain in the group of edema and in the group of EP, EH, EPH-gestosis. In controls the weight of placenta is also increasing with the exception of the weight gain over 20 kg.

Tab. 3.

Weight gain in kg	Controls	Edema	EP–EH–EPH
	weights in placenta in g		
0–10	484 n = 194	486 n = 47	473 n = 6
11–15	487 n = 272	490 n = 116	486 n = 35
16–20	505 n = 91	513 n = 112	504 n = 24
> 20	476 n = 9	520 n = 32	533 n = 10

In another group of 203 pregnant individuals the objectively measured weight gain/ 24 hours was correlated to the weight of placenta: the equation for the correlation between the weight gain/day and weight of placenta is given in the Tab. 4.

Tab. 4.

$y = 476 + 0{,}6\,x$
y weight of placenta
x weight gain g/day

The data of Tab. 4 when used for the calculation of the weight gain for a concrete weight of placenta show the following interrelationship:

weight gain in g/day	weight of placenta in g
24 g	490 g
67 g	517 g
111 g	543 g

The conclusion of the Tab. 3 and 4:
The greater the weight of placenta, the greater the weight gain. It is difficult to accept the opposite interpretation that the weight gain itself would influence the weight of placenta.

The conclusion of the Tab. 3, 4 and 1:
The greater is the weight of placenta, the greater is the weight gain in pregnancy and the greater is the frequency of E and/or EP, EH, EPH symptoms.

Tab. 5.

weight gain in kg	controls	E	EP–EH–EPH
	birth weight in g		
0–10	3307 n – 201	3351 n – 48	3112 n – 6
11–15	3365 n – 274	3363 n – 117	3417 n – 36
16–20	3549 n – 96	3523 n – 115	3575 n – 25
20	3322 n – 9	3563 n – 32	3571 n – 10

The conclusion of Tab. 5:
The greater the total weight gain, the greater the birth weight of the newborn.

Summary

Between the weight gain in pregnancy (both the total weight gain at the end of pregnancy and weight gain/day), the weight of placenta, the birth weight of the newborn and the frequency of EPH symptoms a linear correlation exists.

The following interpretation could be offered: the greater the placenta, the greater the production of some placental hormones which influence both the growth of the mother and the fetus. At the same time the physiological retention of fluid in the tissues is influenced. The greater is the weight gain (and the physiological hydration), the greater is the probability of EPH symptoms.

Proteinuria in Pregnancy

H. P. McEwan

University Department of Obstetrics and Gynaecology, Royal Maternity Hospital, Glasgow, UK

Proteinuria in pre-eclampsia has always been regarded as a serious prognostic sign representing deterioration of the condition and an indication by many obstetricians for premature induction. Thus it is important to determine the accuracy of protein concentration in the urine.

Considerable variation in protein concentration of the non pregnant urine in the same patient has been found to occur (*Altmann* and *Stellate,* 1963). The purpose of this paper is to establish the extent of variation in protein excretion in pregnancy, to determine whether there is a period of maximal protein excretion, and its relation to blood pressure.

Materials and methods

A group of normal patients awaiting operative delivery for mechanical obstetric reasons, such as a variable lie and previous caesarean section, collected their urine for a period of 5 days. Each 24 hours was divided into four six hourly periods and urine excreted during these times was collected in separate containers. The total amount of protein in the 24 hours and in each of the six hourly periods was determined and related to the urinary output. Protein estimations were performed by the Biuret Method.

Two further groups of patients were similarly studied. These were patients with moderate pre-eclampsia defined as a blood pressure over 130/90 mm/Hg plus proteinurea developing after the 28th week of pregnancy, and cases of essential hypertension, patients known to be hypertensive without pregnancy. Twenty one normal patients were studied, 23 with hypertension and 25 with pre-eclampsia.

Results

The mean amount of protein in 24 hours during the five day periods in the normotensive, hypertensive and pre-eclamptic groups was as follows. The mean normal level was

0.36 g with a slightly lower level in the hypertensive group of 0.33 g. The mean range of protein in the pre-eclampsia patients was between 1.6 g and 2.0 g (Tab. 1).

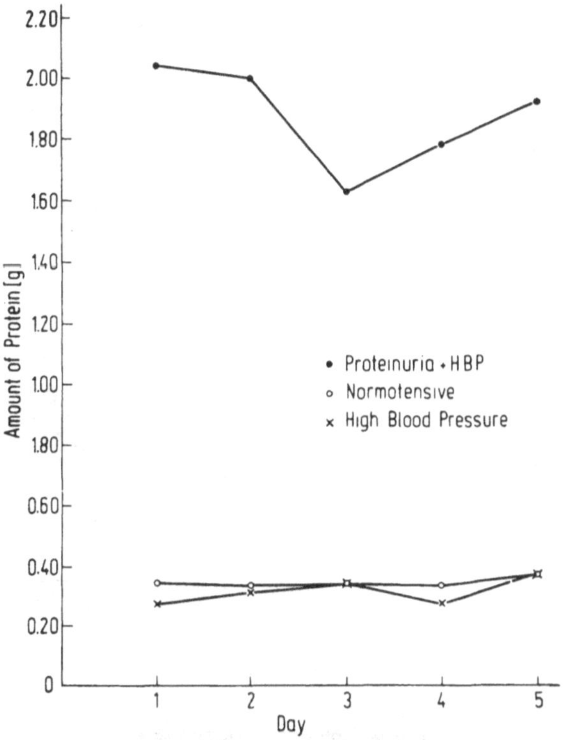

Tab. 1. Amount of protein (g)

When urinary volume was considered, the mean normal protein concentration range was between 0.04 g % and 0.07 g %, the hypertensive group again being lower between 0.02 g % and 0.04 g %. The lower protein concentration in the hypertensive group is due to the increased urinary output in these patients. The mean concentration of protein excreted in the pre-eclamptic patients again was higher than that of the normal and hypertensive patients, the range being 0.15 and 0.24 g % (Tab. 2). When the total amount of protein in each of the four six hourly periods was examined, some variation was found to occur especially in the second period of the day between 14 and 20 hours (Tab. 3). Even when this figure was adjusted for urinary volume and the result expressed as a percentage, this peak was still present (Tab. 4). Although in the normal cases this is not statistically significant further studies in pre-eclamptic patients are at present being undertaken to determine whether this trend persists.

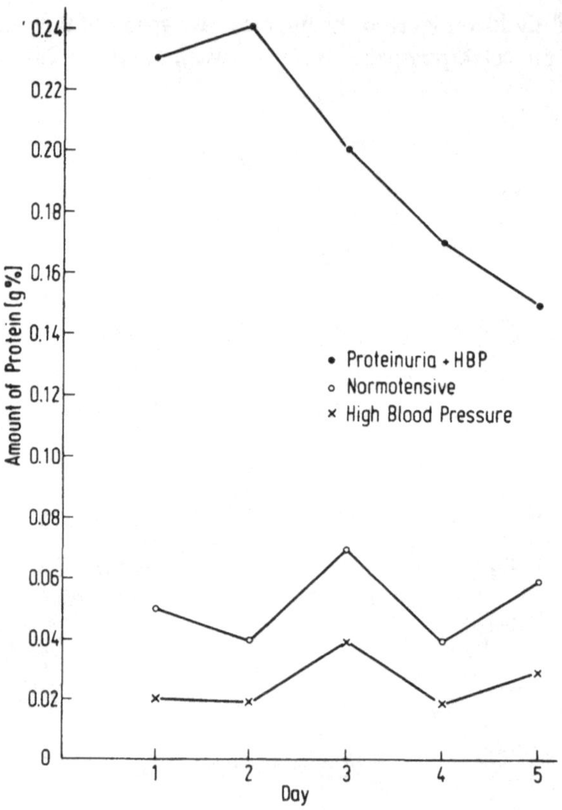

Tab. 2. Amount of protein (g%)

Blood pressure was charted in relation to the daily amount of protein excretion in the three groups. There was no relation between blood pressure readings in the normotensive or hypertensive patients in relation either to total output or concentration of protein (Tab. 5–8).

In the pre-eclamptic group there was a fall in total protein output on the second day which was followed by a progressive rise in protein output accompanying a rise in blood pressure on days 4 and 5 (Tab. 9). Curiously although total output of protein increased the concentration per 100 ml continued to fall (Tab. 10).

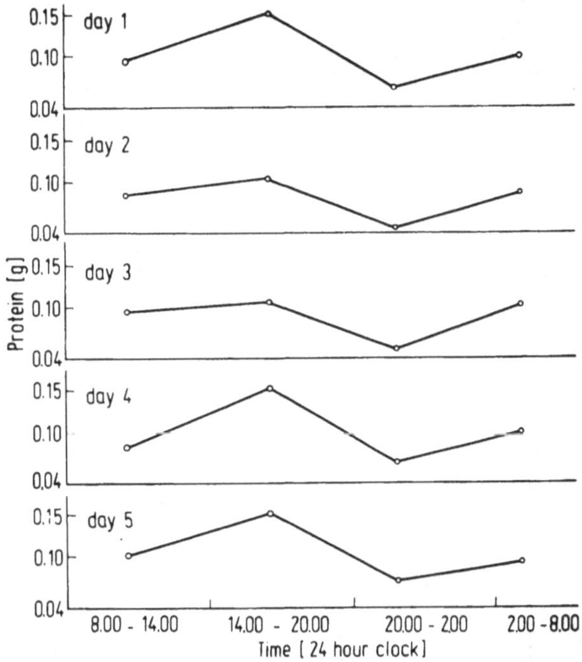

Tab. 3. Variation in protein excretion with time

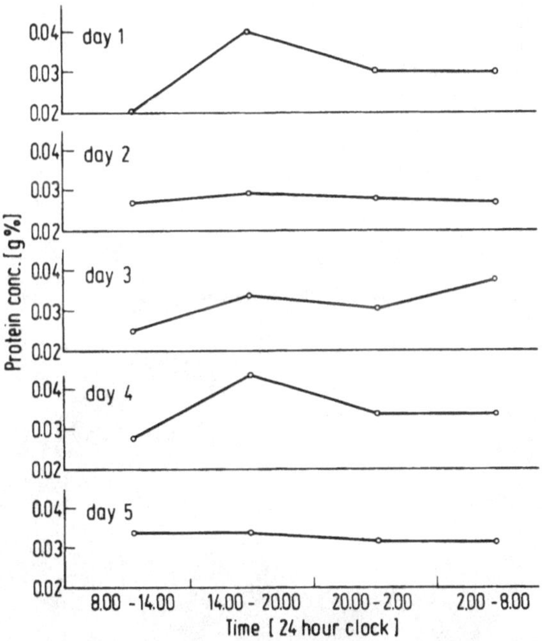

Tab. 4. Variation in protein concentration with time

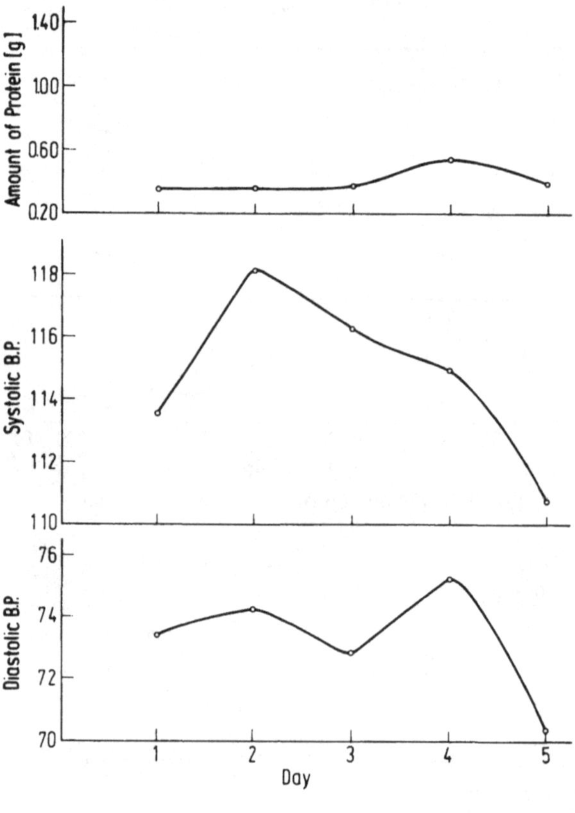

Tab. 5. Normotensive

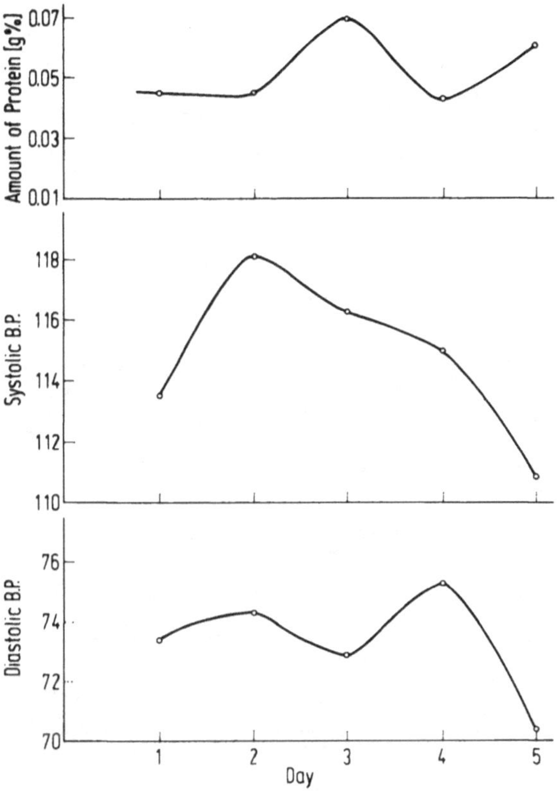

Tab. 6. Normotensive

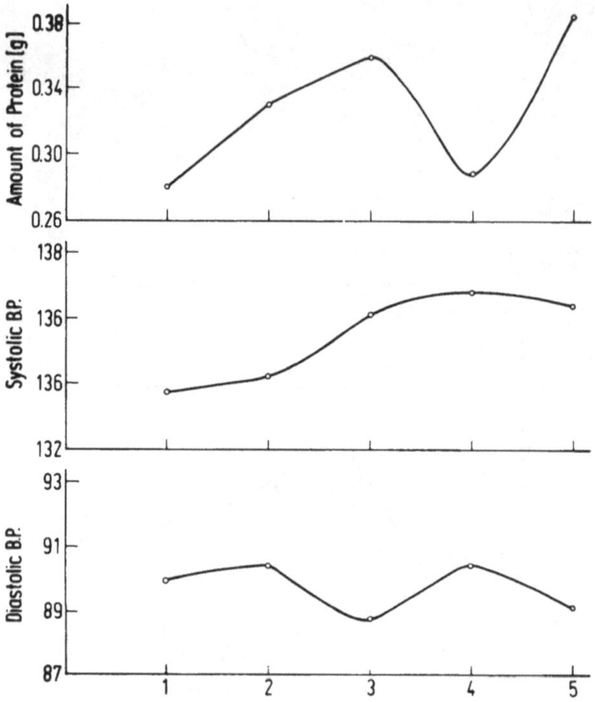

Tab. 7. High blood pressure

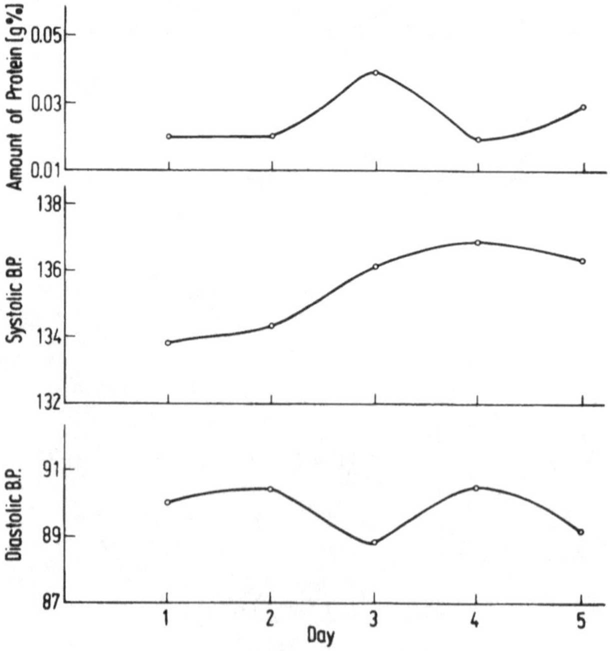

Tab. 8. High blood pressure

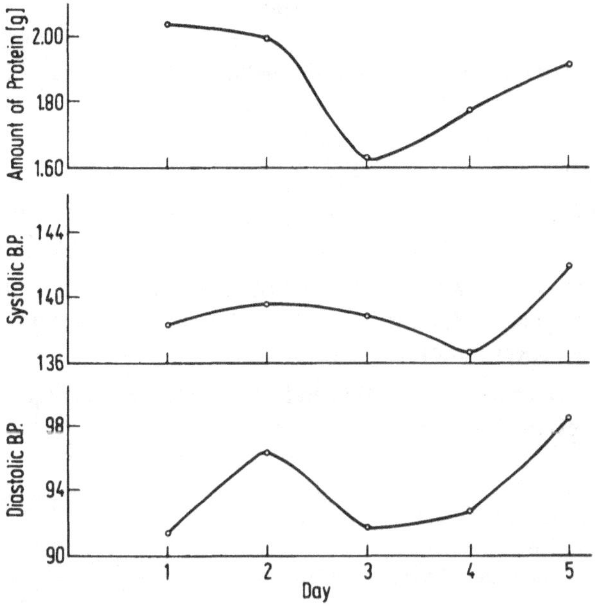

Tab. 9. Proteinuria + H. B. P.

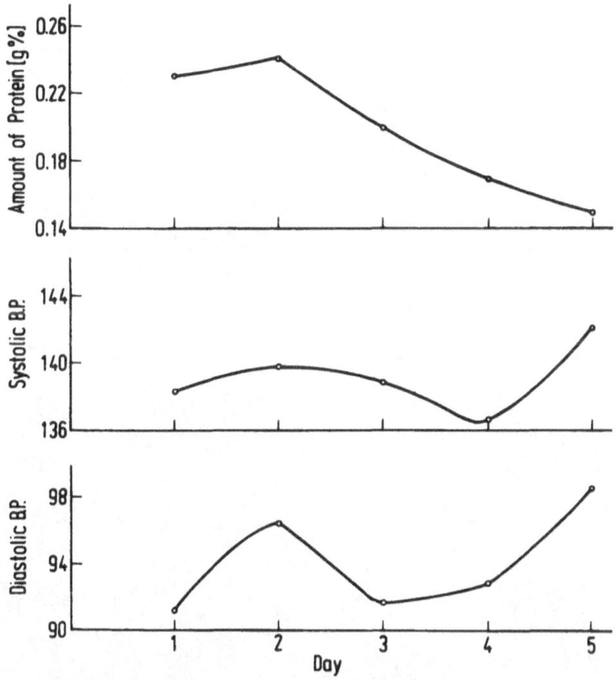

Tab. 10. Proteinuria + H. B. P.

Summary

1. Random specimens are only of qualitative value and give no indication of the amount of protein excreted, and it is doubtful whether examination of the early morning specimen is clinically useful. Only by estimating the total daily output can one hope to gain insight into the renal function in pregnancy.
2. In essential hypertension associated with pregnancy total protein excretion and concentration is within normal limits and is not affected by the blood pressure level.
3. In moderate pre-eclampsia the main effect of an increase in blood pressure is to raise the urinary volume thus increasing the total protein excretion although diminishing the concentration.

This has been a preliminary investigation and further studies will require to be carried out especially in severe pre-eclampsia.

Reference

Altmann, K. A., R. Stellate: Clin. Chem. 9 (1963) p. 63.

Differential Protein Clearance and Selectivity in the Proteinurias of Pregnancy

M. Simanowitz

Institute of Obstetrics and Gynaecology, Hammersmith Hospital, London W. 12, Great Britain

This paper is concerned mainly with some pathophysiological concepts associated with pregnancy proteinuria.

An investigation was set up to study protein clearance patterns in pregnancy and to try and relate differential clearances in pregnancy proteinuria to the selectivity index previously described by other investigators. Renal protein selectivity as a measure of glomerular membrane permeability has been found to be a useful guide to the nature of the glomerular lesion in the nephrotic syndrome. Selectivity in this context refers to the clearance of large molecular weight plasma proteins expressed as a percentage of the clearance of low molecular weight proteins, the ratio increasing as the membrane becomes more permeable to larger molecules. Thus a high selectivity ratio is found in more advanced forms of renal disease, whereas patients with "minimal change" renal lesions tend to exhibit a very low ratio.

In this investigation a total of 44 patients with noninfective proteinuria in pregnancy were studied. Forty-one were associated with hypertension.

Serum/urine protein ratios of 7 proteins were estimated for each patient, with a range of molecular weights from 69 000 (albumin) to 960 000 (Ig M gamma globulin). Each clearance ratio was expressed as a percentage of the albumin and transferrin (MW 88 000) clearance. In this way, urine volume becomes unimportant and untimed serum and urine could be collected, avoiding the more cumbersome 24-hour urine collection ($^{uv}/_{p} \div {}^{uv}/_{p}$ so that v cancels out).

Individual proteins in serum and urine were measured by radial immuno-diffusion as described by *Mancini*.

Selectivity in each case was expressed, both as the slope of the regression line of protein clearance on molecular weight and as the Ig G/transferrin clearance ratio of *Cameron* and *Blandford*. The latter ratio provides a simpler working index and, since a reasonably good correlation was found between the two indices, Ig G/transferrin was used as the main selectivity index in this study.

Results

Selectivity in pregnancy is compared to a similar investigation of nephrotics from a variety of aetiologies. It will be seen that the highly selective pattern of protein excretion (less than 0.1) characteristic of patients with "minimal change" glomerulonephritis is virtually never found in pregnancy. Pregnancy proteinurias appear to be poorly selective whatever the aetiology, many of the selectivities approaching those found in patients with advanced renal disease. Of interest in this regard were three patients with chronic renal disease in pregnancy found to have a poorly selective proteinuria. Six weeks after delivery, protein excretion had become highly selective and renal biopsy in one of these cases showed a "minimal change" renal lesion. The contention of some investigators that the selectivity ratio is a constant feature of a patient's particular disease clearly does not apply to pregnancy proteinuria.

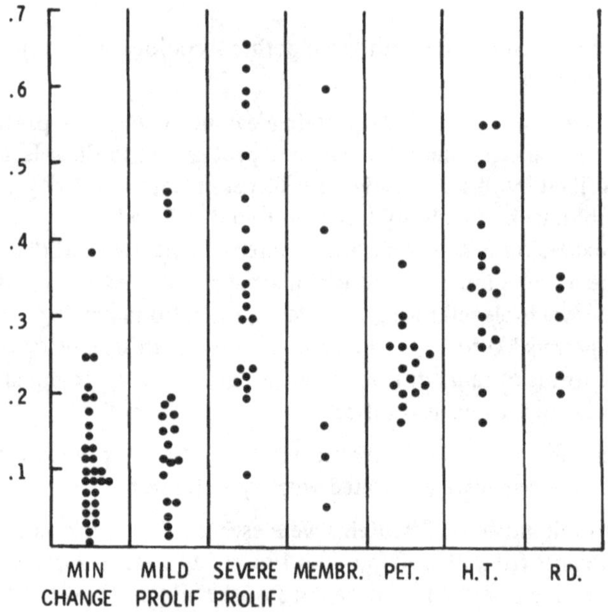

Simanowitz, M.
Differential Protein clearance etc . . .

Slide I = Fig I

Abreviations:

Min. change = minimal change glomerulonephritis.
mild prolif. = mild proliferative glomerulonephritis.
severe prolif. = severe proliferative glomerulonephritis.
membr. = membranous glomerulonephritis.
PET = preeclampsic toxemia
HT = hypertension
RD = renal disease in pregnancy.

Fig. 1. Selectivity patterns in proteinuria in pregnancy compared with non pregnant nephrotics: of Cameron & Blandford (1966)

A histogram of the range of selectivities found in the patients studied is shown (Fig. 2). It would seem that whatever the mechanism of protein filtration in pregnancy proteinuria may be, it can not be on the basis of glomerular basement membrane damage as found in patients with renal disease. This, of course, is supported by renal biopsies done in patients with EPH-gestosis where the basement membrane has been found to be characteristically intact. Some form of ischaemic mechanism would seem to be a more likely explanation where temporary ischaemic damage to the glomerular basement membrane permits a free leakage of protein without any permanent damage being caused. This ischaemic process is relieved by the conclusion of the pregnancy, with immediate disappearance of protein from the urine.

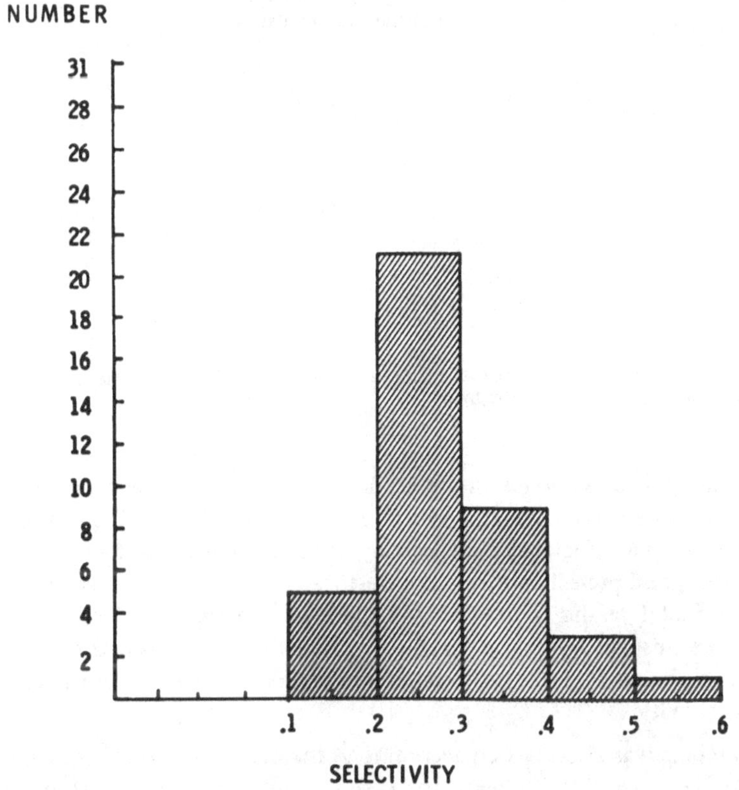

Fig. 2

An attempt to apply the Gestosis Index to protein selectivity was non-contributory. There was no correlation between Gestosis Index and selectivity. This was to be expected since we are dealing with a group of patients where a high Gestosis Index is almost implicit in the criteria for inclusion in the study. Thus, of the 44 patients studied, only 4 had a Gestosis Index of less than 5 and 26 had a Gestosis Index of 9 and above.

If we look at EPH-gestosis from an aetiological standpoint we find certain trends emerging with regard to protein selectivity. Thus patients whose blood pressures were raised (140/90 and above) in the first trimester (essential hypertensives) were compared as a group with patients who developed EPH-gestosis for the first time in the second and third trimesters (pre-eclampsia). Poorer selectivity patterns were a feature of the "essential hypertension" group. Although there was a considerable overlap, the difference between the mean selectivity for each group was significant at the 1% level. There were no differences in any other parameters of renal function between the two groups (Fig. 3).

Renal function. A comparison of mean values found in PRE-Eclampsia with those found in essential hypertension (in Pregnancy)

Renal function. A comparison of mean values found in PRE-Eclampsia with those found in essential hypertension (in Pregnancy)

	PRE-Eclampsia	Hypertension	Student ‚t‘
Blood urea	28.3 mgs. per 100ml. (± 12.0)	27.2 mgs. per 100ml. (± 5.4)	not significant
Blood uric acid	6.8 mgs. per 100ml. (± 1.7)	6.5 mgs. per 100ml. (± 1.3)	not significant
Creatinine clearance	86.2 ml. per min. (± 37.1)	75.7 ml. per min. (± 21.9)	not significant
Selectivity	0.25 (± .05)	0.35 (± .11)	P < .01

Fig. 3. Renal function. A comparison of mean values found in PRE-Eclampsia with those found in essential hypertension (in Pregnancy)

With regard to foetal outcome, interpretation must necessarily be guarded in such a small series. There was an overall perinatal foetal loss of 23.3% (10 out of 43, with one hydatidiform mole). Foetal loss was equally divided between the two above groups (hypertensives and pre-eclamptics). The Gestosis Index, however, was 9 and above in 8 of the 10 foetal deaths. In other words, there was a perinatal loss of 8 out of 25 where the Gestosis Index was 9 and above (32.0%) and a loss of 2 out of 18 where the index was below 9 (11.1%). There was no correlation between perinatal loss and protein selectivity.

Foetal outcome was also assessed according to the degree of intra-uterine growth retardation. Birthweights fell below the 10th percentile in 11 out of 16 patients in the „hypertensive" group. This "small for dates" syndrome appeared to be unrelated to the duration of proteinuria. In the pre-eclamptic group 6 out of the 17 infants had birthweights below the 10th percentile. However, in 10 of these patients where proteinuria had been present for less than 2 weeks, only one infant was small for dates. Five out of the seven infants were dysmature where proteinuria had been present for more than 2 weeks.

Applying the Gestosis Index, the incidence of dysmature infants was exactly the same whether the index was above or below 9 (55.5%).

Immunologische Untersuchungen der Serum- und Urineiweißkörper in EPH-Gestose und bei Nierenerkrankungen

B. Zsolnai, M. Toth

II. Frauenklinik der Medizinischen Universität, Budapest, Ungarn

Bei Schwangerschaft ist die Differenzierung der reinen EPH-Gestose und der Pfropfgestose keine einfache Aufgabe. Außer den bereits bekannten Verfahren (Nierenfunktionsproben, Isotopennephrographie, Nierenbiopsie), kann aufgrund theoretischer Erwägungen auch die mit immunologischen Methoden erfolgende Untersuchung gewisser Proteine des Serums und des Urins zur Differenzierung der zwei Formen der EPH-Gestose verhelfen.

In Fällen von EPH-Gestose und verschiedenen Nierenkrankheiten untersuchten wir im Serum und im Urin die Konzentration des Transferrins, des Immun-γ-G-Globulins (IgG) und des Immun-γ-M-Globulins (IgM). Diese Globuline verschiedenen Molekulargewichtes wurden teils mit semiquantitativer Immunelektrophorese nachgewiesen, teils bestimmten wir der Methode von *Mancini* gemäß, deren Konzentration im Serum und im Urin. Den Grad der durch die Nieren erfolgenden Ausscheidung des IgM und IgG wurde auf das Transferrin bezogen, d. h. die Untersuchungen wurden dem *Mancini'*scher. Verfahren gemäß aufgrund des IgG/Transferrin- bzw. IgM/Transferrin-Quotienten vorgenommen. Unsere Untersuchungen nahmen wir an 34 gesunden Gravidae in der 39.–40. Woche der Schwangerschaft vor, ferner bei 16 schweren EPH-Gestosen, sowie in 6 Fällen von Pyelonephritis und in 7 Fällen von Nephrose. Die Nierenkranken gehörten zur Abteilung für künstliche Nieren der Urologischen Klinik und zur Nephrologischen Abteilung der Kinderklinik.

Abb. 1 veranschaulicht das Bild, das mittels Immunelektrophorese von den Sera einer gesunden Gravida in der 39. Schwangerschaftswoche, ferner einer an EPH-Gestose und einer an Nephrose leidenden Kranken erzielt wurde. Im immunoelektrophoretischen Bild besteht zwischen den verschiedenen Sera kein Unterschied, obgleich sich das Serum-Protein-Bild bei EPH-Gestose und bei Nierenkrankheit verändert.

Wenn man jedoch z. B. bei an Nephrose leidenden und gesunden Gravidae die Transferrin-IgG- und IgM-Konzentration im Serum mit Hilfe der *Mancini*'schen halbierenden Verdünnungsreihe vergleicht, so sind die quantitativen Veränderungen augenfällig (Abb. 2). Die Abbildung zeigt, daß im Serum im Verhältnis zur Kontrolle der Spiegel des IgM mit großen Molekülen ansteigt und der des IgG und Transferrins abnimmt. Die Erhöhung des IgM-Spiegels ist – der verstärkten Ausscheidung von Proteinen geringen Molekulargewichtes zufolge – gewiß das Resultat eines Kompensationsmechanismus.

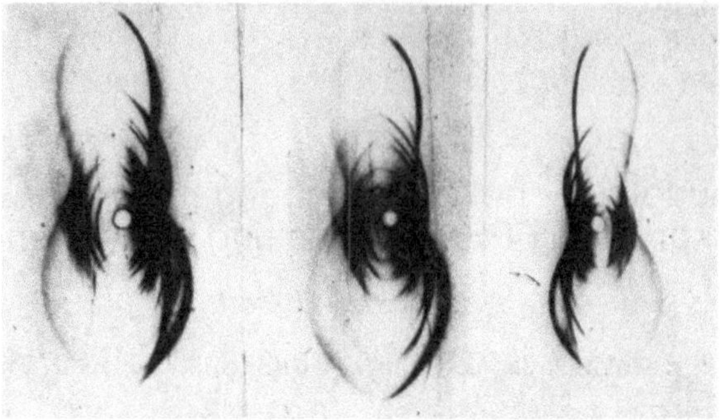

Abb. 1

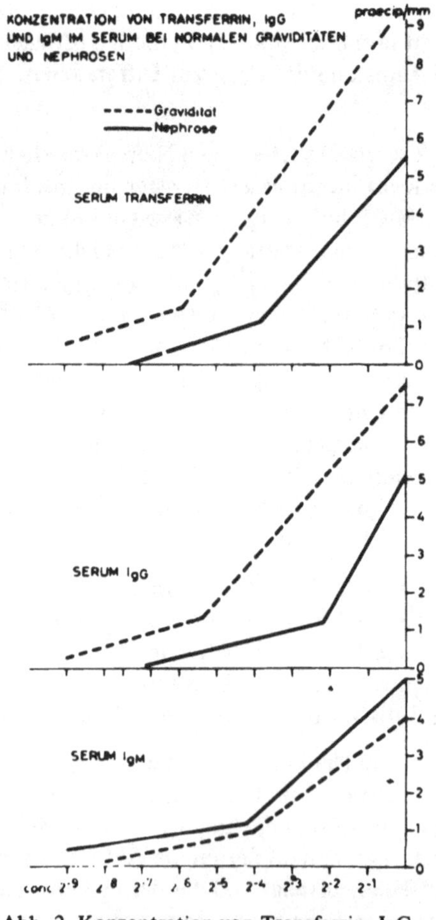

Abb. 2. Konzentration von Transferrin, IgG und IgM im Serum bei normalen Graviditäten und Nephrosen

Auch bei der mittels semiquantitativer Immunelektrophorese vorgenommenen Untersuchung der Urinproteine ist der Unterschied zwischen den Gesunden und den an Gestose und Nephrose leidenden Gravidae in Bezug auf das Urinproteinbild gut wahrnehmbar. Bei EPH-Gestose und Nierenkrankheiten ist nämlich – wie die Abb. 3 veranschaulicht – nicht nur die Zahl der Fraktionen im Urin erhöht und hat sich nicht nur die Intensität der Konturbogen verstärkt, sondern ist auch deren von der Mittellinie gemessene Entfernung größer geworden.

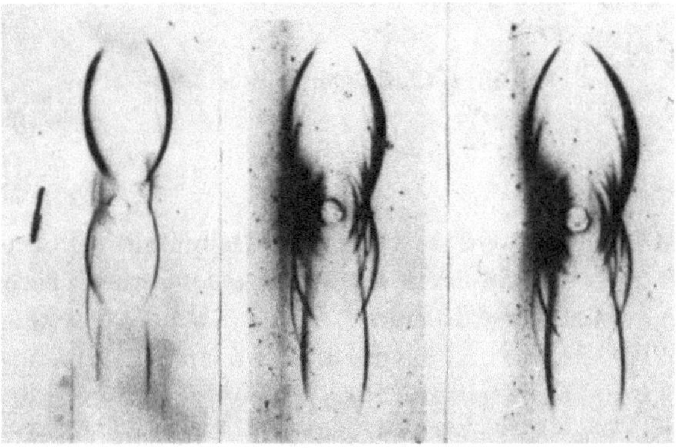

Abb. 3

Bekanntlich läßt sich mit der *Mancini'*-schen Methode mit der radialen, direkten Immundiffusion die Clearance jedweden durch die Niere ausgeschiedenen Proteins bestimmen. Dies scheint bei EPH-Gestose hinsichtlich der Beurteilung der Nierenfunktion von besonderer Bedeutung zu sein. Im Verlauf unserer Untersuchungen wurden bei 2 Immunoglobulinen, dem IgG und IgM das Ausmaß der durch die Nieren erfolgenden Ausscheidung aufgrund des Quotienten der Transferrin-Clearance festgestellt. Hierdurch läßt sich nämlich die mit der künstlichen Einkonzentrierung des Urins einhergehende große Fehlermöglichkeit vermeiden. Dies ist besonders dann ein wesentlicher Gesichtspunkt, wenn – wie auch im Falle der quantitativen Bestimmung der untersuchten Proteine – der Urin auf das 500–600-fach vaporisiert werden muß.

Wie Abb. 4 veranschaulicht, beträgt bei reiner EPH-Gestose und im Nephrose-syndrom die IgG-Ausscheidung etwa den 0,3 bis 0,5-ten Teil der Transferrinausscheidung und die IgM-Ausscheidung nur deren 0,01–0,05-ten Teil. Dem gegenüber ist bei EPH-Gestose, welche mit Pyelonephritis einhergeht, nur die IgG-Ausscheidung mit der Vorigen identisch, während die IgM-Ausscheidung stark erhöht ist.

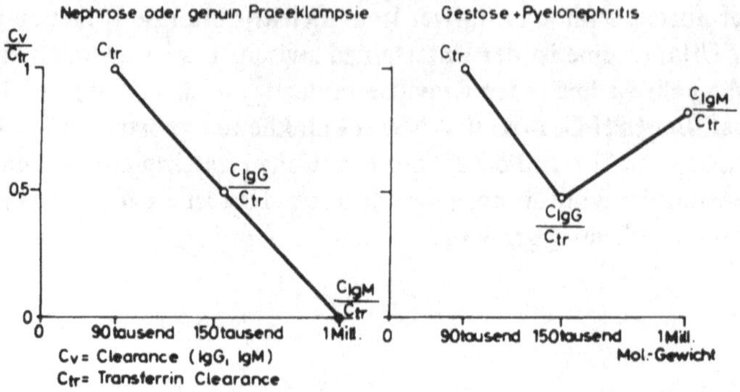

Abb. 4. C_v/C_{tr} Quotient bei EPH-Gestose

Der erhöhte IgM-Gehalt des Urins ist auch mit der Immunreaktion gut nachweisbar. Auf Abb. 5 sind oben die IgM-Präzipitationsringe des Serums, darunter von rechts nach links die Präzipitationsringe wahrnehmbar, welche bei der gesunden Gravida, bei der klinisch reinen EPH-Gestose und bei der an Pyelonephritis leidenden Kranken den IgM-Gehalt darstellen. Die Dicke der Ringe ist zur IgM-Konzentration proportional. Während man bei reiner EPH-Gestose das IgM im Urin nur in Spuren wahrnehmen kann, ist bei Pyelonephritis und bei Schwangerschaftskomplikationen der IgM-Spiegel signifikant erhöht. In solchen Fällen läßt sich die Erhöhung des IgM-Spiegels um so eher erwarten, als dieses Protein bei bakteriellen Infektionen bekanntlich der empfindlichste Antikörper ist.

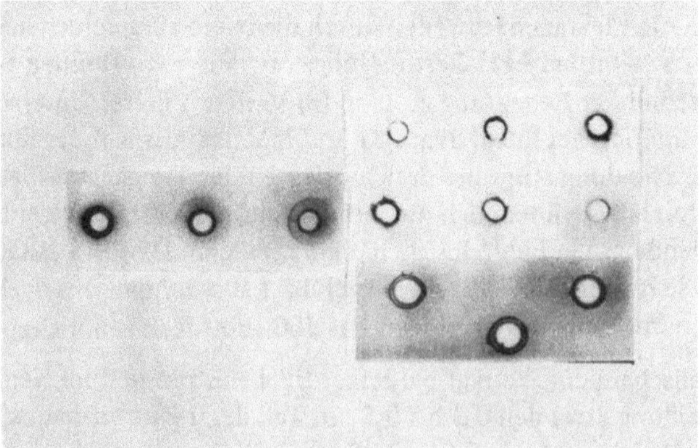

Abb. 5

Zusammenfassung

Auch unsere immunologischen Untersuchungen bestärken die aufgrund von Nierenbiopsien und elektronenmikroskopischen Untersuchungen gemachten Beobachtungen, laut welchen bei reiner EPH-Gestose fast ausschließlich die Veränderung des glomerulären Systems im Vordergrund steht. So ist die Proteinausscheidung, wie auch unsere Untersuchungen erwiesen, vom Grad der glomerulären Membranveränderungen und der Molekulargröße des Proteins abhängig.

Bei Pfropfgestosen, bzw. im Falle von Pyelonephritis und Schwangerschaftskomplikation erhöht sich die IgM-Ausscheidung und ist der IgM-Gehalt des Urins hoch.

Der Nachweis der signifikanten Bakteriurie und die Bestimmung des IgM-Gehaltes des Urins scheinen innerhalb der Pfropfgestose zum Erkennen der Pyelonephritis verhelfen zu können.

A Hypothesis of the Etiology of Hypertension in Pregnancy

C. Goecke

Universitäts-Frauenklinik, Würzburg, BRD

Hypertension is present in 10% of all pregnant women and in about 90% of EPH-gestosis. In 20–25% the hypertension is pre-existing, sometimes in form of a latent essential hypertension. I want to limit the etiologic considerations on hypertension to those forms which cannot be traced back to a renal or vascular basic disorder.

Two causal factors of the essential hypertension should be mentioned:

1. Changes of the electrolyt content of the vessel wall.
2. Insufficient uterine blood supply probably leading to an increased production of a vascoconstrictory substance, and a decrease of placental hormones, especially progesterone.

In hypertension of non-pregnant patients it is suggested that a rise of sodium within the smooth muscle cells of the vessels leads to a decrease of the gradient between the intra- and extracellular sodium concentration and to a rise of the vessel tone.

Experiments performed to reduce the blood supply of the uterus by pinching off the vessels caused a reversible hypertension in pregnant animals. In parabiosis experiments with pregnant rats it was possible to rise the blood pressure in the parabiotised animal, indicating that a vasoconstricory substance was produced. Hitherto, the identification of this substance has not been possible. The effectiveness depends upon pregnancy with an altered sensibility of the vessels. In gestosis there seems to be an increased response of the vessels especially to angiotensin.

We were interested to learn, whether there could be an altered sensibility of the arterioles, resp. of smooth muscle cells during pregnancy, to get an explication for the etiology of hypertension in pregnancy. Studies on the muscles of the human vessels are until now technically impossible. Thus, the changes of the arterioles can only be explained analogously by smooth muscle cells of other organs.

We therefore performed investigations on the human uterine muscle. Some figures will give an idea that there seems to be an analogue of the uterine muscle and the vessel-muscle reaction to physiologic and pharmacologic stimuli. Dr. *Babenerd,* Würzburg, was so kind to place a few slides to our disposal.

Isolated human uteri of pregnant and non-pregnant women were perfused by a method, inaugurated by *Mosler* and the intravascular perfusion pressure were recorded simultaneously (Fig. 1). Equal changes were found under physiologic conditions (Fig. 2) and certain drugs (Fig. 3). It could be seen that the intravascular pressure precedes the intrauterine pressure. So we may assume that the increase of the perfusion pressure is not due to uterine contraction. After a period of time it was shown (Fig. 4) that the response of the uterine muscle decreases, while the response of the vessels is preserved for a longer period of time. These investigations are going on. They show that the results, attained with the uterine muscle probably can be transfered to the smooth muscles of the vessels.

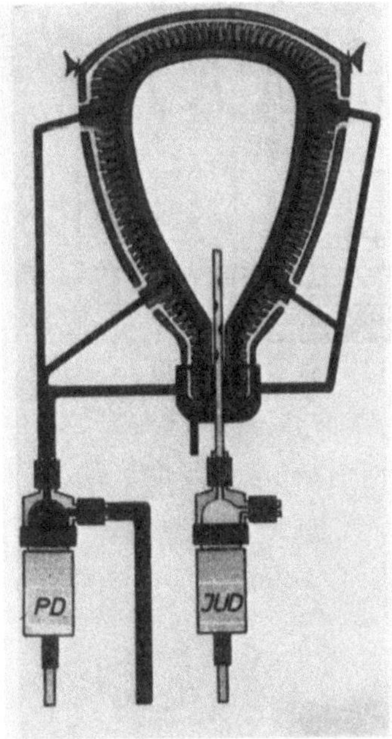

Fig. 1

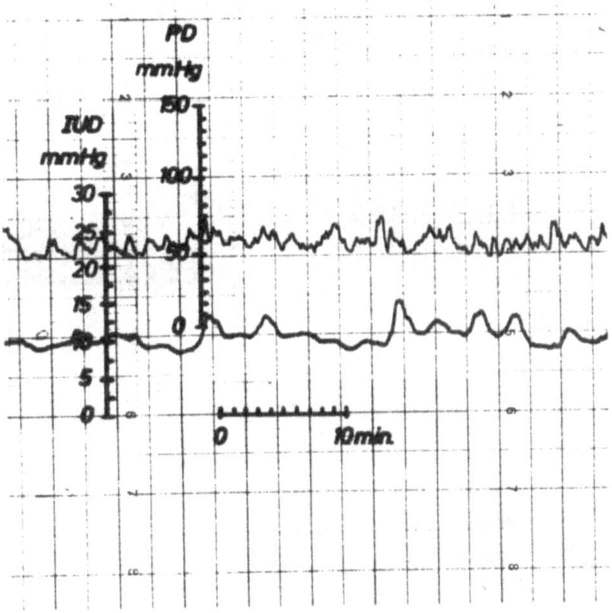

Fig. 2

To find out, whether there is a change in muscular cation content, we determined the intra- and extracellular sodium and potassium concentration in the uterus of non-pregnant women and pregnant women during several stages of gestation. The extracellular cation concentration did not change significantly. On the other hand, the intracellular cation concentration – taking into account the extracellular inulin-space – presents marked changes. We have to stress, however, that there were no changes in the concentration of intracellular potassium related to 1 l cell water (Fig. 5). The figure presents the results we got from the uteri of non-pregnant women (N), pregnant women in the 3–4th month of gestation (I), and of women shortly before the onset of labor (II), and during labor (III). Significant changes were found only in the intracellular sodium concentration (Fig. 6). During pregnancy – conpared with non-

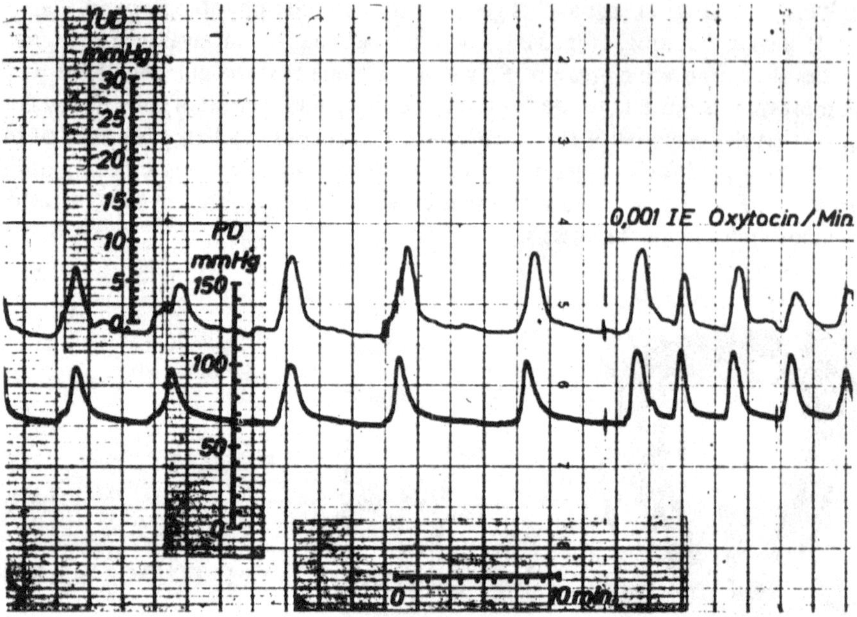
IUD
mmHg
30
25
20
15
10
5
0
PD
mmHg
150
100
50
0
0,001 IE Oxytocin/Min
0
10 min

Fig. 3

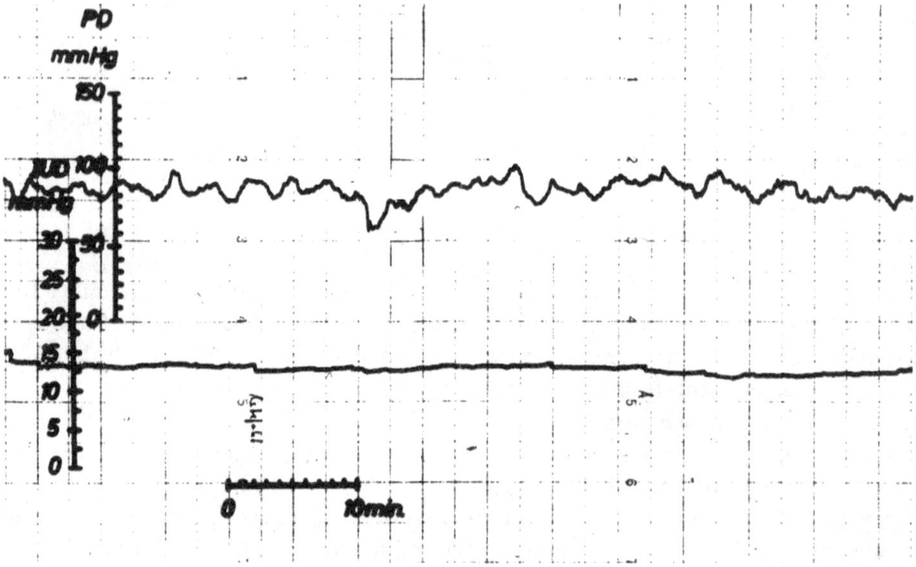
PD
mmHg
150
100
50
0
IUD
mmHg
30
25
20
15
10
5
0
0
10min

Fig. 4

pregnant women – the intracellular sodium concentration rises markedly; during delivery there is a significant fall of the intracellular sodium concentration. It should be mentioned, that on the placental side there is no increase of intracellular sodium during pregnancy.

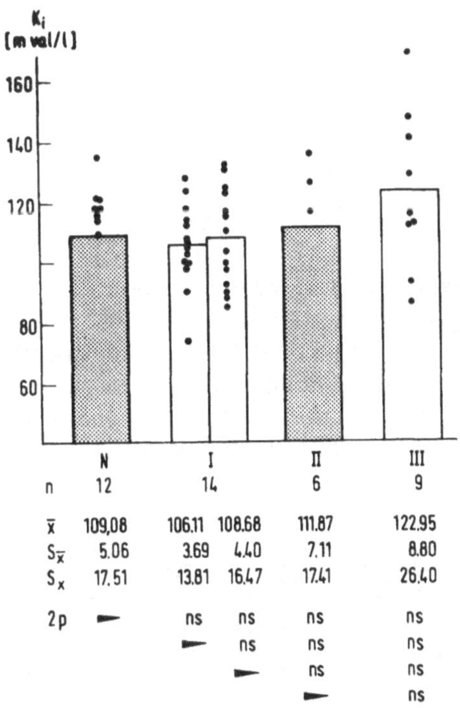

Abb. 5. Corpus

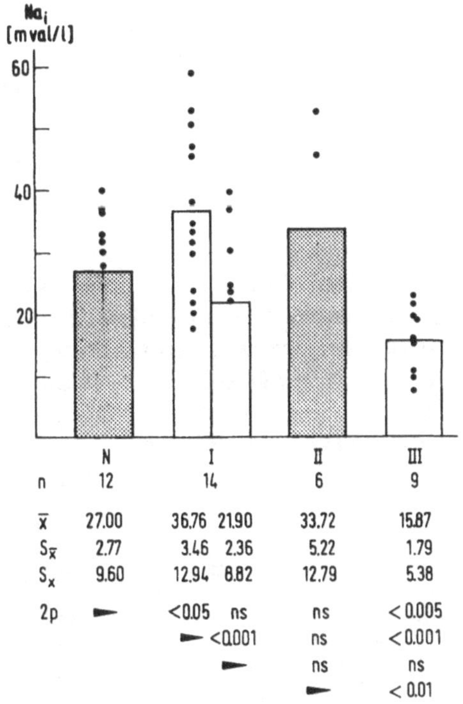

Abb. 6. Corpus

For the better understanding of these results I should like to give a schematical presentation of a muscle cell with its intracellular and extracellular distribution of electrolytes (Fig. 7). Normally we find a low sodium concentration and a high potassium concentration within the muscle cell, while ouside the cell the sodium concentration is higher. Due to these differences in cation distribution there is a membrane potential of about-80 mV which can be calculated too by the potassium concentration. To maintain these differences in concentration between the interior and the exterior compartments, an active cation transport is necessary. Sodium is shifted against the concentration gradient out of the cell, and potassium into the cell.

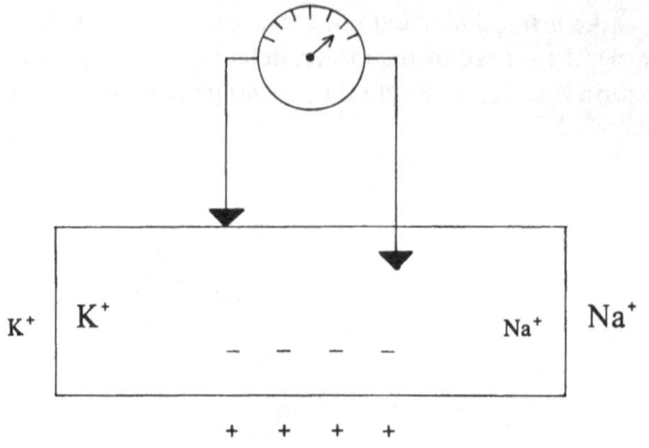

Abb. 7

The feature of these active cation transports which is independant of the osmotic water flow, is the intracellular sodium/potassium quotient. The decrease of this quotient represents an activation and the increase an inhibition of the cation transport (Fig. 8). You will see, that the corpus uteri as well as the isthmus uteri presents a higher quotient during pregnancy, i. e. an inhibition of the cation transport, and during delivery we see an increase of the transport process. Simultaneous investigations on the rectus muscle did not show these changes.

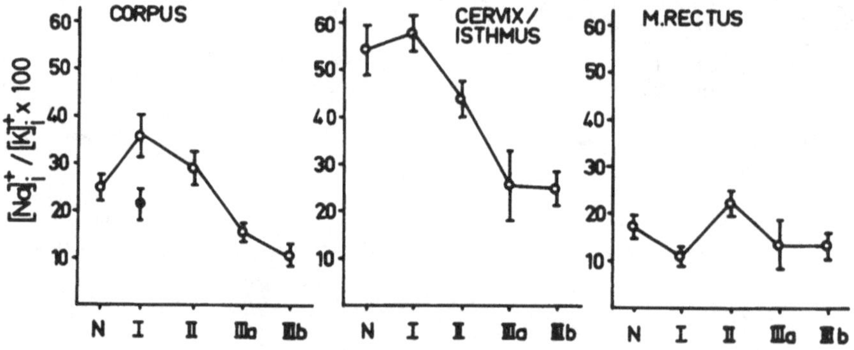

Abb. 8

The following figure may hypothetically explain these effects on the cation transport mechanism (Fig. 9). The intracellular space, the cell membrane and the extracellular space of the muscle cell are shown. Independent of the water shifts, the smooth muscle presents an increase of the intracellular sodium concentration during pregnancy which is on one hand due to an increased diffusion of sodium into the intracellular space, probably caused by changes in permeability, and on the other hand due to a reduced sodium transport against the concentration gradient out of the cells. The main reason for this intracellular sodium increase is an inhibition of the active transport mechanism through the cell membrane which is influenced by a calcium activated

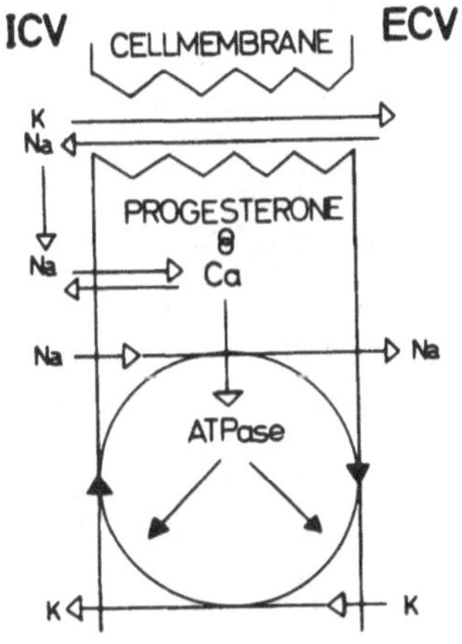

Abb. 9

membrane-ATPase. We know that a higher calcium concentration (0,5–1 mMol/1) inhibits the membrane-ATPase, and thus the active cation transport. Furthermore, it was proved, that progesterone is able to fix calcium into the cell membrane. Thus, we can see, that during pregnancy due to the increasing amount of progesterone, there is a higher fixation rate of calcium causing an inhibition of the active cation transport which leads to the rise of intracellular sodium.

On the other hand it could be proved that a sufficient rise in intracellular sodium concentration is able to mobilize calcium out of the cell membrane. This seems to be the fact at the end of pregnancy. The increasing intracellular sodium concentration mobilizes calcium and leads to an activation of the ATP-ase and to an activation of the cation transport. Sodium leaves the cell and potassium is shifted into the cell.

Aldosterone has an influence on the cation transport too by stimulating the transport mechanism. In placental insufficiency there is a decrease of progesterone as well as a relative preponderonce of its antagonist aldosterone, both effecting the transport mechanism by activation.

For a number of substances, for example oxytocin, vasopressin and probably angiotensin, such an activated cation transport seems to be necessary to inhibit again this transport mechanism. This acute inhibition of the cation transport is followed by a rapid escape of potassium out of the cell leading to a contraction of the smooth muscle cell. Simultaneously, the intracellular sodium concentration rises again, resulting in a circulus vitiosus.

Thus, in essential hypertension of pregnancy, resp. arteriolar spasm, the following features could be involved:

1. An increase of the intracellular sodium concentration in the muscle cells.
2. A decrease of the progesterone level due to placental insufficiency altering the fixation rate of membrane-bound calcium.
3. Mobilization of membrane calcium.
4. A relative hyperaldosteronism (refered to progesterone).
5. Activation of the cation transport as a pre-supposition for substances which inhibit the transport mechanism.
6. Acute inhibition of the cation transport by vasoconstrictory substances leading to a decrease of the membrane potential of the muscle cells.

The following figure (Fig. 10) illustrates hypothetically the consequences of a reduced placental blood supply and placental insufficiency. Relative hypoplasia of the uterine

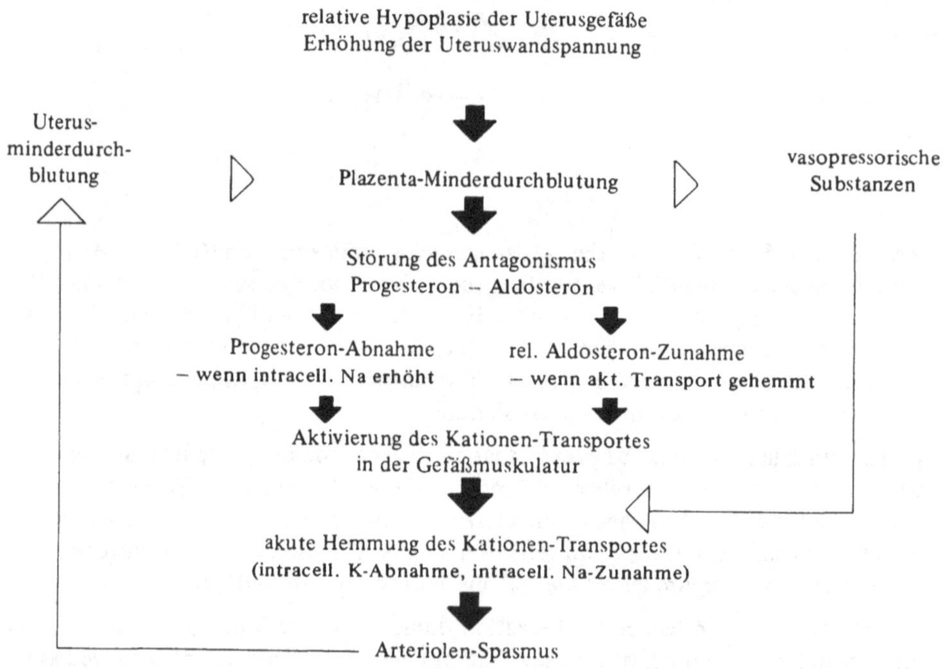

Abb. 10

vessels or increased tension of the uterine wall for example may cause a reduction of the placental blood supply; what happens is:

1. a release of a vasopressoric substance,
2. a disturbance of the progesterone-aldosterone-antagonism.

If during pregnancy, the intracellular sodium concentration of the muscle cells is elevated, the cation transport of the vessel muscle is more easily activated by a decrease of progesterone and a reduction of Ca-fixation to the cell membranes as well as by a relative surplus of aldosterone. The acute inhibition of this activated cation transport mechanism by vasopressor agents results in an intracellular decrease of potassium leading to a reduction of membrane potential which will cause an arteriolar spasm.

This hypothesis on the etiology of essential hypertension in pregnancy leaves many questions open. To prove this hypothesis, experiments in patients with hypertension in pregnancy and EPH-gestosis are in progress.

Arterial Blood Pressure after Late Toxemia of Pregnancy

B. D. Bozhkov

Wissenschaftl. Institut für Geburtshilfe und Gynäkologie, „Christo Smirnenski", Sofia, Bulgarien

Many authors think that a connection exists between late toxemia of pregnancy and the hypertension, renal and vascular diseases in later age, although this interrelationship is still discussed [2, 4, 6, 7, 10, 11, 12, 13].

We examined arterial blood pressure in women, who had suffered from late toxemia of pregnancy, and compared this pressure with the arterial pressure of women, who had normal pregnancies.

Material and Method

121 Bulgarian women from the town of Sofia were examined, who were delivered of a baby at our clinic 13 years ago. 60 of them – 25 primigravidas and 35 multigravidas, suffered from late toxemia which was described in the case-histories by at least two of the three cardinal symptoms: elevated arterial blood pressure over 140/90 mm/Hg and proteinuria and/or edema, occurring during the second half of pregnancy. In this study women who had suffered from eclampsia were not included. In the toxemia-group the the mean age at the time of delivery was: for primigravidas 23.9 years with standard deviation σ 4.1 and final deviations from 19 to 30 years, but for multigravidas 28.8 years with σ 6.1 and final deviations from 20 to 43 years. The remaining 61 women – 24 primigravidas and 37 multigravidas, were our control-group which differed from women with toxemia only in that respect, that at delivery they had a normal arterial blood pressure, no proteinuria and no edema, and that in later pregnancies there were no symptoms of late toxemia. The time-interval between pregnancy and the control-examination was on the average 13 years as the mean age of the primigravidas with toxemia was 36.9, but for multiparas with toxemia 41.8 years. Standard deviation in all groups was unchanged. In this way each woman, who had suffered toxemia, had her counterpart as a control.

The control measurement of arterial blood pressure under standard conditions was carried out according to the method recommended by the WHO. The results obtained were compared and estimated for statistical significance with the t-test.

Results and discussion

The results of our study are given in Tab. 1 and Fig. 1.

Tab. 1. Indices of the control examination.

Group	Numbers	Arterial pressure $\bar{x} \pm \sigma$	> 140/90 mm/Hg %	Age $\bar{x} \pm \sigma$
Toxemia				
Primigravidas	25	136.4 ± 19.5 / 88.8 ± 12.45	40	36.9 ± 4.1
Multigravidas	35	137.4 ± 22.89 / 89.2 ± 16.90	34.28	41.8 ± 6.1
Controls				
Primigravidas	24	117.2 ± 9.41 / 79.9 ± 7.51	4.16	36.6 ± 5.7
Multigravidas	37	120.5 ± 15.24 / 79.8 ± 7.87	5.45	40.6 ± 4.9

The arterial blood pressure of women who had suffered from toxemia during pregnancy on the average 13 years before the control study, was higher than that of the control-group and the difference was highly significant (p/t: 99.99). In 40% of the primigravidas and in 34% of the multigravidas, who had had toxemia, the arterial pressure was higher than 140/90 mm/Hg; while in the control-group the percentage was 4.16 and 5.45 respectively. In 32% of the primigravidas and 31.42% of the multigravidas who had been affected by toxemia, there was a family history of hypertension, but in none of the patients from control-group.

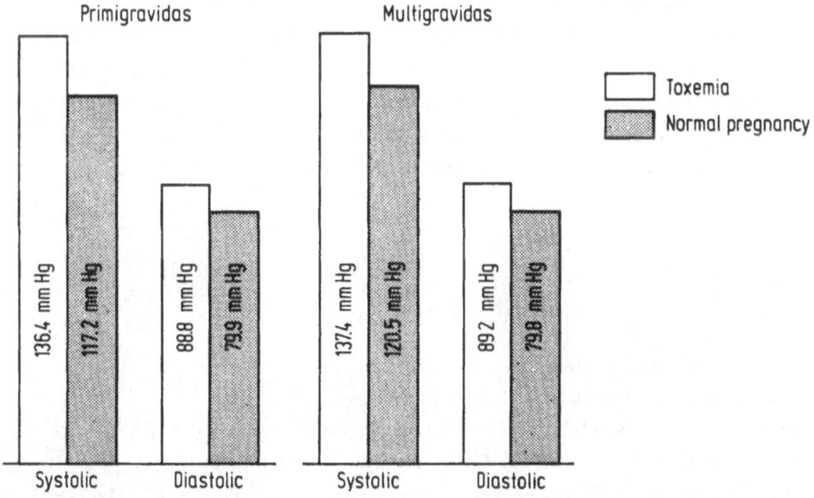

Fig. 1. Arterial blood pressure in women with toxemia and with normal pregnancy

The data proved a definite tendency toward developping hypertension in women who had had toxemia. These findings corroborate the results of other authors as well [2, 4, 6, 10, 13, 14, 16]. In our catamnestic study we found a family history of hypertension in 32% of the formerly toxemic patients, while in the control-group there were no such data. This supports the concept that women with a congenital disposition to hypertensive disease, who could develop hypertension als well, manifest their tendency to elevation of arterial blood pressure during pregnancy [1, 2, 3, 5, 8, 9, 15]. Not only anamnestically could our patients with toxemia preceeding essential hypertension be clearly distinguished with a higher probability from those with toxemia, but also because of their young age during pregnancy. To exclude a preexisting pyelonephritis was more difficult, because it could have had an asymptomatic or oligosymptomatic course.

Although clear cut interrelationship between toxemia and hypertension is difficult, it is clear from our study that women who had endured toxemia are at higher risk to develop hypertension, than women who had a normal pregnancy. This makes it imperative that those women who had suffered from toxemia be under observation by the internist many years after delivery.

Summary

Arterial pressure was measured in 121 women: 60 with late toxemia (pre-eclampsia) and 61 with normal pregnancy 13 years after delivery. In the toxemia group 25 women were primipara and 35 multipara, in the control group – 24 primipara and 37 multipara (every woman with toxemia had a counterpart in the control group). It was established that the arterial pressure in women who have had toxemia was higher than the arterial pressure in women having had normal pregnancy; the difference is statistically significant. In women who have had toxemia, hypertension (arterial pressure higher than 140/90 mm/Hg) was about eight times as common as in women having normal pregnancy. Familial history of hypertension was present in 32 per cent of the women who have had toxemia and in none of the control group.

References

[1] *Adams, E. M., A. Finlayson:* Lancet 2 (1961) p. 1375.
[2] *Adams, E. M., J. MacGillivray:* Lancet 2 (1961) p. 1373.
[3] *Barnes, C. G.:* Medical Disorders in Obstetric Practice, Oxford (1962).
[4] *Bechgaard, P., C. Andreassen, E. Hertel:* Med. Welt (1960) p. 2538.
[5] *Chesley, L. C., R. A. Cosgrove, J. E. Anitto:* Amer. J. Obst. Gynec. 83 (1962) p. 1360.
[6] *Epstein, F. H.:* New England, J. Med. 271 (1964) p. 391.

[7] *Fisgberg, A. M.:* Hypertention and Nephritis, Fifth edition, Philadelphia, Lea (1954).
[8] *Friedberg, V., J. Margale:* Med. Klinik 31 (1958) p. 1333.
[9] *Friedberg, V.:* Geburtsh. Frauenheilk. 24 (1964) p. 93.
[10] *Gibson, G. B., R. Platt:* Brit. med. J. II (1959) p. 159.
[11] *Hochuli, E.:* Zbl. Gynäk. 84 (1962) p. 885.
[12] *Hochuli, E., A. Stoeckli:* Schweiz. med. Wschr. 89 (1959) p. 901, 934.
[13] *Hosemann, H., H. Helmich, J. Heller:* Path. Microbiol. 24 (1961) p. 667.
[14] *Schreier, P. C.* and al.: JAMA 159 (1955) p. 105.
[15] *Schwarz, R. Z.:* Geburtsh. Gynäk. 160 (1963) p. 110.
[16] *Tillman, A. J. B.:* Circulation, 30, Suppl. 2 (1964) p. 76.

Epidemiological Factors in EPH-Gestosis/ Gestosis-Index

Ernährung in der Schwangerschaft und bei toxikosegefährdeten Frauen

K. Bregulla

Universitäts-Frauenklinik, Erlangen, BRD

Als optimale Ernährung für eine Schwangere wird eine ausreichende und abwechslungsreiche Kost empfohlen. Sie soll die benötigten Kalorien, Nähr- und Ergänzungsstoffe in einem ausgewogenen Verhältnis enthalten. Diese allgemeine Empfehlung läßt sich differenzieren, sie klingt aber so einfach, daß viele, die heute Schwangere untersuchen und beraten, das Problem einer richtigen Ernährung während der Schwangerschaft falsch einschätzen.

Das Übergewicht ist am häufigsten Folge einer falschen Ernährung. In der Inneren Medizin gilt der Zusammenhang zwischen dem Übergewicht und der Arteriosklerose mit ihren oft letalen Komplikationen als gesichert. Inwieweit das Übergewicht in der Geburtshilfe eine Rolle spielt, ist noch nicht ganz klar. Versucht man die Ergebnisse der bis heute publizierten Arbeiten zusammenzufassen, so scheint der Verlauf der Schwangerschaft, der Geburt und des Wochenbettes bei übergewichtigen Frauen komplizierter als bei normalgewichtigen zu sein.

Wir haben versucht, das an unserem Krankengut der letzten 4 Jahre zu überprüfen. 7180 Frauen wurden entbunden. Ihre anamnestischen Angaben und Befunde kamen in ein dokumentationsgerechtes Journal. Dadurch war eine weitere Datenverarbeitung möglich. Für die Untersuchungen haben wir aus statistischen Überlegungen Größen-, Gewicht- und Altersklassen in Anlehnung an das Durchschnitts- und Idealgewicht erwachsener Frauen formuliert. Der Paritätsstatus wurde berücksichtigt. Für die Signifikanzberechnung haben wir das Chi-Quadrat-Verfahren nach *Pearson* mit einer Irrtumswahrscheinlichkeit von $p = 0{,}05$ angewandt.

Schwangere, die ein normales Ausgangsgewicht hatten und bei denen die Schwangerschaft, die Geburt und das Wochenbett komplikationslos verlief und deren Kinder vom Pädiater als gesund beurteilt wurden, nahmen abhängig von ihrem Ausgangsgewicht, der Körpergröße und dem Alter, 8 bis 10 kg während der Schwangerschaft zu. Von den 7180 Schwangeren hatten aber nur 45% ein normales Körpergewicht, d. h. die Hälfte aller Schwangeren war übergewichtig.

Übergewicht und Sozialstatus sind korrelierbar. Frauen aus der unteren Sozialschicht waren häufiger übergewichtig als solche aus der oberen Sozialschicht. Das prozentuale Verhältnis betrug etwa 65% zu 35%.

Der Verlauf der Schwangerschaft und der Geburt war bei norm- und übergewichtigen Patientinnen unterschiedlich. Übergewichtige Frauen haben häufiger größere und schwerere Kinder geboren, wenn man für die Kinder ein Gewicht bis zu 3500 g und eine Länge bis zu 50 cm als normal annahm. Der Geburtstermin wich bei den übergewichtigen Frauen häufiger im Sinne einer Übertragung von dem errechneten Geburtstermin ab. Weitere Unterschiede waren nicht erkennbar.

Das Ergebnis entspricht nicht in allen Einzelheiten den Erfahrungen anderer Untersucher. Es zeigt aber, daß unser Hauptproblem auch während der Schwangerschaft die Überernährung, die adipösen Schwangeren sind.

Der Kalorienbedarf in der Schwangerschaft wird von den Frauen fast immer überschätzt. Er beträgt nur 10 bis 20% mehr als außerhalb der Schwangerschaft. Die meisten Frauen dürften mit 2300 bis 2700 Kalorien bei der zur Zeit herrschenden Berufssituation, die durch eine vorwiegend sitzende oder leichte körperliche Arbeit charakterisiert ist, ausreichend bilanziert sein. Das Maximum des Mehrbedarfs liegt im letzten Trimenon.

Der Kalorienbedarf der Graviden ist also definierbar. Komplizierter ist es, die Nährstoffe: Eiweiß, Fett und Kohlehydrate, die Ergänzungsstoffe: Vitamine, Mineralstoffe und die Spurenelemente qualitativ und quantitativ exakt anzugeben. Umfangreiche Bilanzuntersuchungen sind dafür noch notwendig. Es können deshalb nur Ratschläge für eine Schwangerenernährung gegeben werden, die im Moment optimal zu sein scheinen und den Empfehlungen der Deutschen Gesellschaft für Ernährung weitgehend entsprechen.

Die Ernährung in der Schwangerschaft ist in den hochindustrialisierten Ländern kalorisch fast immer ausreichend. Die Verteilung zwischen den Kohlehydraten, Fetten und dem Eiweiß ist aber selten gut. Die Zusammensetzung der Nahrung in ihrer gesamten Kalorienzahl sollte prozentual aus 17 Kalorien % Protein, aus 25 Kal. % Fett und aus 58 Kal. % Kohlehydraten bestehen. Der Proteinbedarf von 80 bis 100 g täglich ist nicht immer gedeckt. Die Nahrung ist entweder kalorisch falsch zusammengesetzt oder es wird von den Frauen, die einem falschen modischen Ideal, dem Mannequintyp, anhängen, unbewußt mit der allgemeinen Reduzierung der Nahrung zu wenig Eiweiß aufgenommen.

Die Bedeutung einer ausreichenden Eiweißzufuhr läßt sich im Tierversuch demonstrieren. Abhängig von dem Beginn, dem Umfang und der Dauer der proteinarmen Ernährung waren Ratten und Hunde infertil oder abortierten sehr früh. Bei einer nicht so drastischen Eiweißreduzierung über einen längeren Zeitraum wurden Junge mit einer makroskopisch und mikroskopisch nachweisbaren Retardierung aller Organe ausgetragen. Diese Differenz war gegenüber einem gesunden Kollektiv postnatal durch eine weitere Proteinunterbilanzierung noch zu vergrößern. Eine Verminderung der Hirnzellen um 50% war auf diese Art provozierbar.

Ergebnisse von Tierversuchen auf den Menschen zu übertragen, ist immer problematisch. Das trifft hier aber nicht zu. Beobachtungen in Südamerika, Südostasien und Afrika, in Gegenden, in denen der Proteinmangel heute für den Menschen eine bedeutende Rolle spielt, haben das bestätigt. Der Intelligenzquotient eines Kindes ist also bereits vor der Geburt beeinflußbar.

Eine Steigerung der täglichen Proteinzufuhr während der Gravidität auf das doppelte der angegebenen Werte, etwa 150 bis 200 g, ist in verschiedenen Situationen, etwa bei der Gestose mit einer hohen Albuminurie, möglich.

Mit 300 bis 400 g Kohlehydraten pro Tag ist die Schwangere meist ausreichend versorgt. Von den Kohlehydraten werden heute fast ausschließlich aufgeschlossene Produkte bevorzugt, d. h. während der Schwangerschaft ist die Kohlehydratzufuhr wohl immer ausreichend, es werden aber zu wenig Ballaststoffe mitgegessen. Das begünstigt die Obstipation. Aufgeschlossene Kohlehydraterzeugnisse erleiden, durch die Art der Aufbereitung bedingt, einen Vitaminverlust.

Der Fettbedarf einer schwangeren Frau beträgt pro Tag etwa 60 bis 80 g. Diese Menge wird bei unseren Ernährungsgewohnheiten weit überschritten, 100 bis 150 g täglich werden oft zugeführt. Wenn nicht eine Reduktion der Gesamtkalorien notwendig ist, sollte die Fettzufuhr zugunsten der größeren Kohlehydrataufnahme eingeschränkt werden.

Der Vitaminbedarf in der Schwangerschaft ist erhöht. Gesteigerte Stoffwechselprozesse sind die Ursache. Das gilt für alle Vitamine. Der größere Bedarf ist nur durch eine umfangreichere Zufuhr zu decken. Das gelingt bei der heute üblichen Zubereitung der Nahrung im Haushalt und in den Großküchen außerordentlich selten. Zusätzliche Vitamingaben sind notwendig.

In der Schwangerschaft nimmt die extrazelluläre Flüssigkeit um 4 bis 5 Liter zu. Das ist physiologisch. Dieser Bedarf an Wasser, Natrium und Chlor ist in sehr kurzer Zeit zu decken. Wir nehmen täglich etwa 10 bis 15 g Kochsalz bei einem Bedarf von nur max. 10 g auf. Der Überschuß wird bei einer entsprechenden Wasserzufuhr ausgeschieden. Eine Steigerung der Flüssigkeitszufuhr in der Gravidität ist nicht notwendig.

Die Mineralstoffe und Spurenelemente, Kalium, Magnesium, Kupfer, Mangan und Zink werden bei einer gemischten Kost in einer ausreichenden Menge aufgenommen. Das trifft für Kalzium, Eisen und Jod nur selten zu. Phosphor und Kalzium werden gemeinsam resorbiert. 1,5 g Kalzium und Phosphor werden täglich, zumindest vom 6. Schwangerschaftsmonat an benötigt. Da Phosphor in fast allen Gemüse- und Obstsorten reichlicher enthalten ist als Kalzium, ist die Phosphorbilanzierung gesichert. Der Kalziumbedarf kann nur dann befriedigt werden, wenn reichlich zusätzlich Milchprodukte gegessen werden. Latente Tetanien bei den Schwangeren lassen vermuten, daß das Kalzium sehr oft in nicht ausreichender Menge aufgenommen wird. Die Verordnung des Kalziums in Tablettenform in der zweiten Schwangerschaftshälfte ist empfehlenswert.

Der Eisenbedarf während einer Schwangerschaft wird auf 300 bis 400 mg geschätzt. Das ist etwa 1/10 des gesamten Körpereisens. Die Eisendepots können diesen Bedarf nicht decken. 15 bis 20 mg Eisen täglich per os zugeführt, sind als Angebot notwendig. Etwa 1/3 aller Graviden leidet vorwiegend im letzten Trimenon an einer Eisenmangelanämie. Der Eisenmangel der Mutter hat immer auch einen Eisenmangel des Feten zur

Folge. Dieser leidet darunter nicht nur intrauterin, der Verlust wird oft erst nach der Geburt innerhalb der ersten und zweiten Lebenswoche imponieren.

Bei einer bestehenden Anämie kann das Eisendefizit nicht durch eine entsprechende Ernährung gedeckt werden. Es muß ein Eisenpräparat eingenommen werden. Vitamin C-Gaben zusätzlich garantieren eine bessere Eisenresorption.

Das Jod ist in verschiedenen Gegenden in Deutschland in den Nahrungsmitteln immer unzureichend enthalten. Der erhöhte Bedarf in der Schwangerschaft wird durch künstliches Tafelsalz gedeckt.

Welche Konsequenzen lassen sich nun aus den vorgetragenen Fakten ziehen. Kalzium, Eisen und die Vitamine werden von vielen Schwangeren in einem zu geringen Umfang aufgenommen. Das Defizit dieser Stoffe läßt sich manchmal erst dann nachweisen, wenn bereits Schäden aufgetreten sind. Eine großzügige Verschreibung sogenannter Kombinationspräparate wäre deshalb wünschenswert.

Ich hatte Ihnen gesagt, daß jede zweite Schwangere übergewichtig ist. Wir haben versucht, Frauen die gravide waren, über ihre Eßgewohnheiten zu befragen. Es besteht kein Zusammenhang zwischen der Auffassung der Schwangeren über eine optimale Ernährung und ihrem Gewicht. Das ist interessant. Es konnte nämlich von unseren Patientinnen fast die Hälfte angeben, was wir als richtige Ernährung definieren würden. Man muß daraus folgern, daß diese Frauen ihr vorhandenes Wissen wegen ihrer Eßgewohnheiten nicht in die Praxis umsetzen können. Wir haben den Eindruck, daß es nicht reicht, wenn der Arzt bei der Schwangerenberatung den Wert der Ernährung für den gewünschten komplikationslosen Schwangerschaftsverlauf nur betont. Ob einfach gehaltene Aufklärungsschriften, an denen sich die Schwangere auch außerhalb der Praxis orientieren kann, hier wertvollere Hilfe leisten, bleibt offen. Wir gehen diesen Weg.

Viele der berufstätigen Frauen ist heute im gebärfähigen Alter. Die meisten von ihnen sind halbtags oder ganztags auf eine Massenverpflegung angewiesen. Es ist deshalb sinnlos, wenn sich der Arzt bemüht, einer Patientin zu erklären, warum möglichst kurze Kochzeiten eingehalten werden sollen und welche Vorteile die Tiefkühlkost gegenüber der Gefrierkost bietet. Wir können zwar dadurch den Schwangeren die Nachteile der in Großküchen hergestellten Mahlzeiten, die Vitamin- und Proteinarmut, erklären. Ändern ließe sich diese Tatsache aber erst, wenn die Verantwortlichen solcher Abteilungen schwangeren Frauen eine vitamin- und proteinreiche Kost anbieten würden. Es wäre ferner wünschenswert, kleinere und dafür aber häufigere Mahlzeiten zu Hause und im Betrieb einzunehmen.

Der Zusammenhang zwischen dem Übergewicht und der EPH-Gestose ist sicher, obwohl ihre Ursache letztlich unklar ist. Jede vierte unserer übergewichtigen Schwangeren litt an einer Gestose. Hier kann der Arzt präventiv wirken und behandeln. Übergewichtigen Frauen ist bereits vor Beginn der Schwangerschaft eine entsprechende Gewichtsreduzierung zu empfehlen. Kommen übergewichtige Frauen mit einer Frühgravidität zur Kontrolle, so sollten sie so beraten werden, daß sie in den ersten vier bis fünf Schwangerschaftsmonaten kaum an Gewicht zunehmen. Eine weitere Reduzierung unter das Ausgangsgewicht ist in manchen Fällen wünschenswert. Das ist mit einer täglichen Kalorienzufuhr von 1500 bis 2000 Kalorien möglich. Die Verminderung der Kalorienzahl sollte durch eine Reduktion der Fett- und Kohlehydratzufuhr erreicht werden. Die Proteinaufnahme muß immer zwischen 80 bis 120 g tätlich betragen.

Es läßt sich bei der Gestosefrequenz nicht nur eine Abhängigkeit von der Adipositas feststellen. Sie steigt auch bei einer zunehmenden Proteinverminderung steil an. Dafür hat die Geschichte der letzten sechs Jahrzehnte Beweise geliefert.

Normgewichtige Frauen, die an einer EPH-Gestose leiden, ernähren sich oft eiweißarm. Modetrends, die ich vorhin erwähnte, erklären das.

Die Behandlung der EPH-Gestose wird, abhängig von dem Schweregrad der Erkrankung, entweder abulant oder stationär erfolgen. Hungern und dursten als Behandlung sind sicher falsch. Als erste Maßnahme sollte eine salzarme Diät mit 1500 bis 2000 Kalorien gegeben werden. Über die sonst geforderte tägliche Proteinaufnahme von 80 bis 120 g muß hinausgegangen werden. 100 bis 150 g täglich sind notwendig um das bereits vorhandene Defizit und den evtl. anhaltenden Verlust etwa durch die Albuminurie auszugleichen. Vitamine und Spurenelemente sind bei gestosegefährdeten oder erkrankten Frauen fast immer unterbilanziert. Sie sollten deshalb routinemäßig gegeben werden. Erst wenn diese Voraussetzungen erfüllt sind, kann eine zusätzliche medikamentöse Behandlung wertvolle Hilfe leisten.

Vollbilanzierte Diäten zur Ernährung schwangerer Frauen sind heute herstellbar. Nahrungsmittel sind bereits teilweise synthetisch zu produzieren. Beides wird bei den noch notwendigen Stoffwechseluntersuchungen in der Schwangerschaft eine große Rolle spielen. Es scheint aber illusorisch, die Mehrheit der Schwangeren mit einem solchen Standardessen zu ernähren. Nur in bestimmten Situationen, etwa bei einer Erkrankung, wird diese Nahrungsart von Bedeutung sein. Es ist deshalb vielmehr unsere Aufgabe, auf die Bedeutung einer richtigen Ernährung während der Schwangerschaft hinzuweisen und Fehler, die heute noch gemacht werden, zu korrigieren.

Zusammenfassung

In der Universitäts-Frauenklinik Erlangen-Nürnberg wird seit dem 1. 1. 1966 mit dokumentationsgerechten Geburtsjournalen gearbeitet. Dadurch war es möglich, die Gewichtszunahme während einer normalen Schwangerschaft für diese Frauen zu ermitteln. Sie beträgt 8 bis 10 kg und ist abhängig von dem Alter und der Größe der Graviden.

Vom 1. 1. 1966 bis zum 31. 12. 1969 wurden 7180 Schwangere entbunden. Von ihnen waren 55% übergewichtig, nur 45% hatten ein Normgewicht. Übergewichtige Frauen gehören häufiger zur sozialen Unterschicht. Schwangerschaft, Geburt und Wochenbett verliefen bei über- und normgewichtigen Frauen verschieden. Schwangere (24%), bei denen Symptome einer EPH-Gestose diagnostiziert wurden, waren etwa 4,5 bis 5 kg schwerer als gesunde Schwangere. Kinder übergewichtiger Frauen wurden schwerer und größer geboren als die Kinder normgewichtiger Frauen. Weitere Unterschiede waren bei einem Vergleich der Gruppen nicht erkennbar.

Das Ergebnis dürfte, obwohl es nicht repräsentativ ist, übertragbar sein. Unser Hauptproblem, auch während der Schwangerschaft, ist die Überernährung. Unter diesem Gesichtspunkt werden die schwangerschaftsbedingten Veränderungen des Fett-, Eiweiß- und Kohlehydratstoffwechsels, des Vitamin-, Mineral- und Wasserhaushaltes beschrieben. Da der optimale Bedarf an Nährstoffen, Ergänzungsstoffen und Flüssigkeit während der Gravidität bis heute nicht ausreichend bekannt ist, sind keine quantitativen und qualitativen Angaben über eine ganz genaue Zufuhr möglich. Es wird vielmehr die heute als günstig empfohlende Aufnahme der einzelnen Substanzen, die eine komplikationslose Schwangerschaft garantieren, beschrieben.

Eine Unterernährung kommt bei uns außerordentlich selten vor. Die Überernährung ist sehr häufig. Die Konsequenzen, die sich daraus für die Schwangerenberatung ergeben, werden dargestellt.

An einer Beziehung zwischen der Adipositas und der EPH-Gestose besteht kein Zweifel, obwohl ihre Ätiologie noch unbekannt ist. Der Arzt kann durch eine gezielte Ernährungsberatung präventiv wirken. Ist eine Schwangere an einer EPH-Gestose erkrankt, so ist die diätetische Behandlung mit einer Einschränkung der Kalorien- und Kochsalzzufuhr kombiniert mit einer medikamentösen Therapie sinnvoll. Dem erhöhten Bedarf an Proteinen, Vitaminen und Spurenelementen muß in dieser Situation Rechnung getragen werden.

Bilan de 500 cas de dysgravidiés, observées en 2 ans à la Maternité du C. H. U. de Strasbourg

F. Wolff, H. Frenkel, P. Leissner, R. A. Schick

Maternité du C.H.U. de Strasbourg, Strasbourg, France

A la Clinique Obstétricale et Gynécologique II, Maternité et Ecole de Sages-Femmes du C.H.U. de Strasbourg (Direct.: Prof. *P. Muller*), 500 cas de dysgravidies ont été observés entre le 1er janvier 1968 et le 31 octobre 1969.

Dans le présent travail, les auteurs ont cherché à évaluer l'importance de différents facteurs biométriques, sociaux, éthniques et médicaux dans la genèse de cette pathologie gravidique. Ils en ont également apprécié le retentissement sur l'évolution de la gestation et l'état de l'enfant à la naissance.

Cette étude purement rétrospective a permis d'améliorer les conditions de surveillance prénatale et de diminuer la fréquence de la dysgravidie.

I. Méthode et Material d'Etude

A. *Méthode*

1. *Classification.* Nous nous sommes reportés à une classification simple qui a été élaborée avant la publication de l'indice gestosique de *Goecke* et *Rippmann.* Elle est toutefois très voisine de celles proposées par *Kyank, Friedberg, Muller*. . . (Tab. 1).

I. *Dysgravidie toxemies*

A. Formes légères

1. H.T.A. — Systolique $> 140 < 160$
   Diastolique $\geqslant 95 \leqslant 100$
2. Associée ou non à albuminurie
   à oedèmes
3. Albuminurie > 1 g
   associée à oedèmes importants sans H.T.A.

B. Formes moyennes

1. H.T.A. — Systolique $\geqslant 160 < 180$
   Diastolique $\geqslant 100 \leqslant 110$
   associée ou non à albuminurie
   à oedèmes
2. Albuminurie massive $\geqslant$ 2,5 g associée à des oedèmes

C. Formes graves
H.T.A. Systolique $\geqslant 180$
Diastolique > 110
ayant tendance à se maintenir ou même à augmenter malgré l'institution d'une thérapeutique hypotensive.
Associée ou non à
Albuminurie importante > 5 g ‰
Oligurie ou anurie
Oedèmes plus ou moins généralisés
Signes d'éclamptisme (céphalées, barre épigastrique. . .)

II. *Eclampsies et commas éclamptiques*

III. *Hypertensions chroniques*

A. Avec toxémie ou éclampsie surajoutées

B. Sans pré-éclampsie ou éclampsie surajoutées

IV. *Hypertension gravidique récidivante*

Apparues au cours d'une grossesse
1. Avec T.A. normale en dehors d'un processus gravidique
2. Avec T. A. élevée ou en dehors d'un processus gravidique

Fig. 1. Classification

C'est ainsi que nous étudierons successivement les toxémies légères, moyennes et graves en incorporant dans ces dernières les éclampsies et les comas éclamptiques. Les hypertensions gravidiques récidivantes ont été réparties dans ces 3 groupes selon l'importance de leur symptomatologie. Les hypertensions chronique ont été écartées de ce présent travail.

2. *Facteurs étudiés.* Pour chaque forme de dysgravidie, les facteurs suivants ont été étudiés:

1. Parité,
2. Age,
3. Origine éthnique,
4. Etat-Civil de la gestante,
5. Morphotype,
6. Prise pondérale,
7. Nombre de consultations prénatales,
8. Médecin consulté durant la grossesse,
9. Moment de l'accouchement,
10. Mode de l'accouchement,
11. Poids de l'enfant à la naissance,
12. Score d'Apgar à la naissance,
13. Mortalité néonatale,
14. H.T.A. résiduelle au 6e jour du post-partum.

B. *Matériel*

Ces 500 cas de dysgravidies ont été observés au cours d'une période s'étendant du ler janvier 1968 au 31 octobre 1969, au cours de laquelle sont survenus 5317 accouchements. La toxémie est une entité pathologique très fréquemment observée puisqu'elle survient chez près de 10% des gestantes venant accoucher dans notre service (durant la période étudiée).

Les 500 observations se répartissent en:

300 cas de toxémies légères
140 cas de toxémies moyennes
60 cas de toxémies graves et éclampsies.

II. Dysgravidies légères

Le problème qui se pose dans ces formes, c'est devant le peu d'importance de la symptomatologie de les considérer comme des grossesses à risques élevés.

A. *Parité*

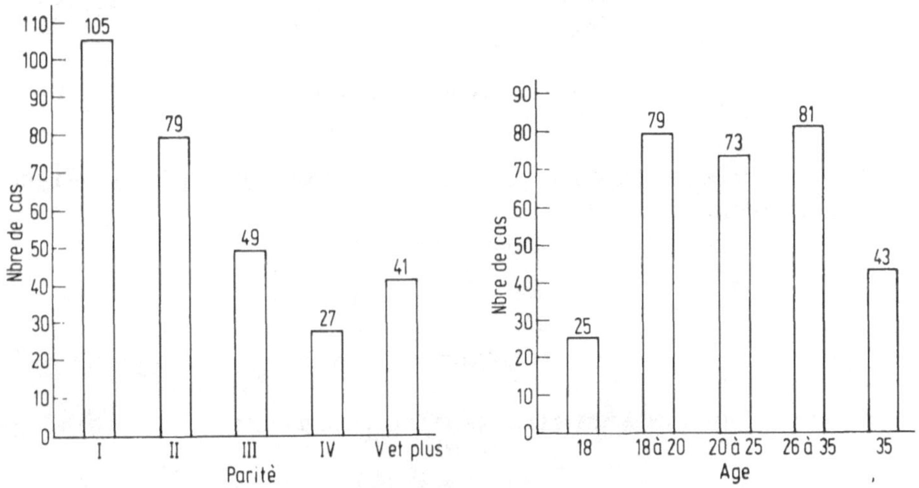

Fig. 2. Dysgravidies legeres (300)

On observe la grande fréquence des primipares (34%) et la relative fréquence des grandes multipares (13,6%) alors que pour la totalité de 5317 accouchements les primipares ne constitutent que 27% et les grandes multipares 8,7%.

B. *Age*

Si le nombre des jeunes gestantes et de celles qui ont plus de 35 ans est relativement important, la différence avec les chiffres observés sur l'ensemble des accouchées n'est pas très significative.

C. *Etat-civil*

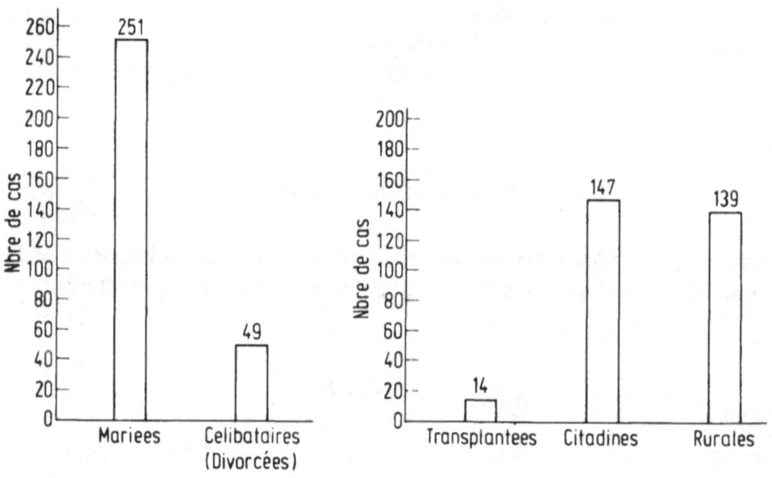

Fig. 3. Dysgravidies legeres (300)

16% des femmes de ce groupe sont célibataires ou divorcées, alors qu'il n'y en a que 7,9% dans la statistique globale.

D. *Origine ethnique*

Il n'y a pas de différence avec les chiffres de la population totale.

E. *Morphotype*

Le nombre important de femmes obèses n'est pas particulier à ce groupe de gestantes. L'alsacienne, en effet, a tendance à être plutôt de constitution généreuse.

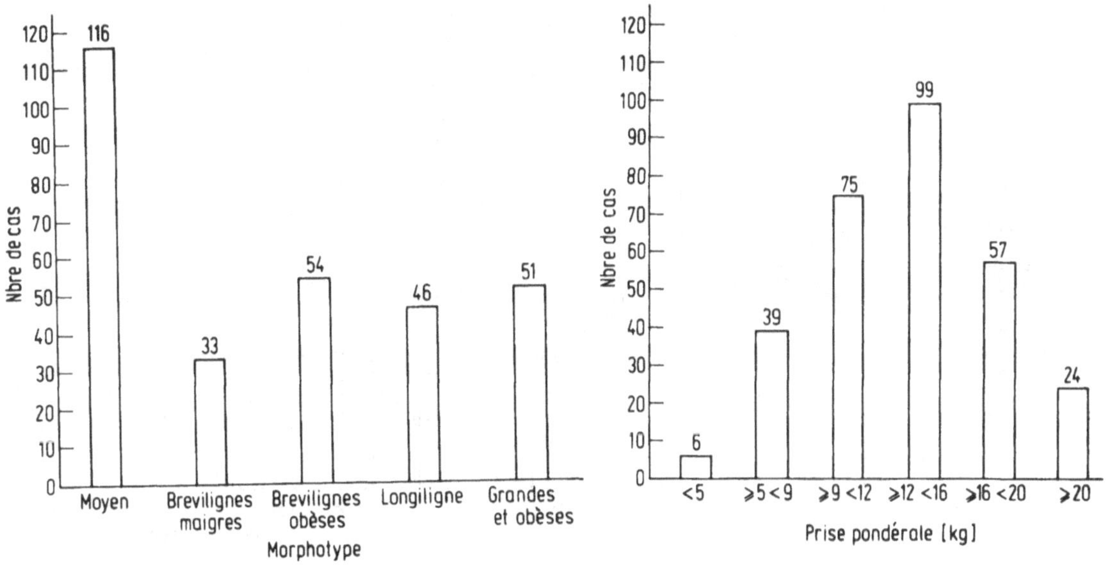

Fig. 4. Dysgravidies legeres (300)

F. *Prise pondérale*

Les prises excessives de poids constituent un facteur étio-pathogénique essentiel puisque 180 parturientes ont augmenté de plus de 12 kg durant la grossesse.

G. *Nombre de consultations*

Un facteur également important dans la genèse de la dysgravidie est l'insuffisance de surveillance prénatale puisque 25% des gestantes n'ont même pas subi les 3 consultations absolument obligatoires et que 128 d'entre elles n'ont pas eu un examen au 9e mois (42,6%) alors que celui-ci est conseillé par la loi.

H. *Médecin traitant*

Le nombre de gestantes suivies par un médecin extérieur au service est important, mais cette étude nous a également révélé les insuffisances de nos propres consultations prénatales.

I. *Moment de l'accouchement*

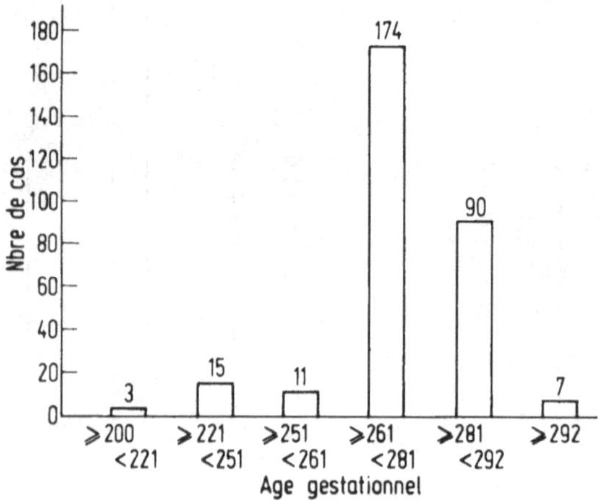

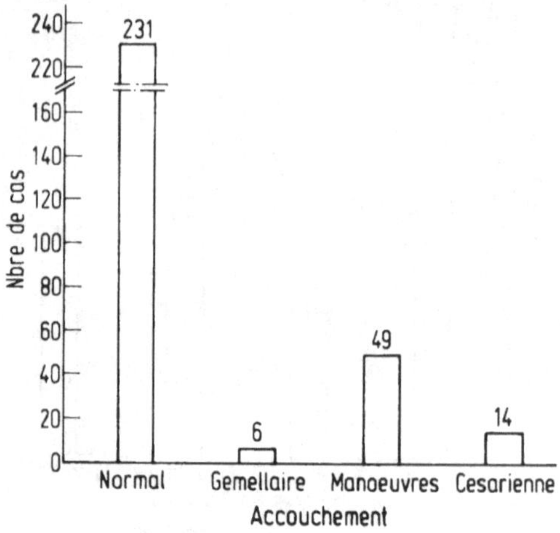

Fig. 5. Dysgravidies legeres (300)

Près de 10% de ces gestantes font un accouchement prématuré alors que ceux-ci représentent 6,8% de la totalité des accouchements durant la période considérée.

J. *Mode de l'accouchement*

14 césariennes ont été effectuées chez ces parturientes, soit près de 5%, mais la différence n'est pas très significative avec les pourcentages normaux des sections observées au service (4%).

K. *Poids de l'enfant à la naissance*

La répartition des classes de poids se fait sensiblement normalement.

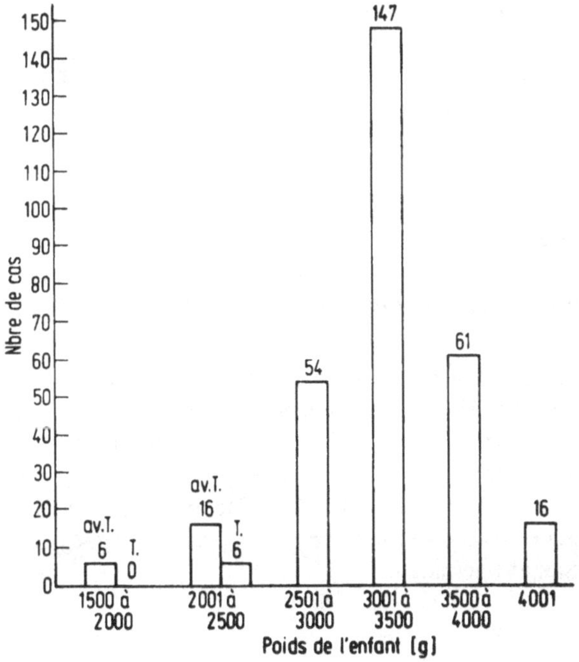

av. T. = avant terme calculé
T à terme

Fig. 6. Dysgravidies legeres (300)

L. *Score d'Apgar à la naissance*

La grande majorité des enfants est en parfait état à la naissance. Le nombre des souffrances graves et moyennes est toutefois plus élevé que dans la statistique globale (8,3%).

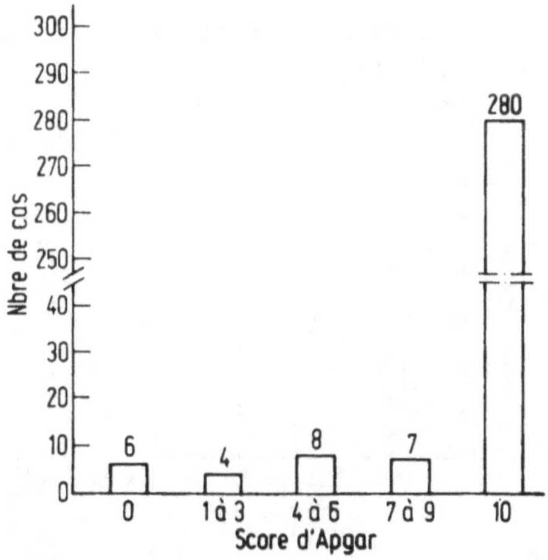

Données ultérieures

Mortalité Néonatale

Immédiate	:	6
Dans les 3 jours	:	3
Total	:	9 soit 3%

H. T. A. résiduelle chez la mère au 6e jour du post-partum: 43

Fig. 7. Dysgravidies legeres (300)

M. *Mortalité néo-natale*

Elle est plus importante que la mortalité néo-natale générale durant cette période, 3% contre 1,98%. Ce dernier taux élevé s'explique par le recrutement de notre Maternité où le nombre des grossesses pathologiques est particulièrement important.

N. *H.T.A. résiduelle au 6e jour du post-partum*

Elle est loin d'être négligeable puisque 24,3% des femmes ont encore une tension élevée au 6e jour du post-partum.

En conclusion, la toxémie dans sa forme légère constitue le type de la grossesse à risque élevé qu'il s'agit de surveiller de près. En effet, si dans la grande majorité des cas, son évolution est favorable, son retentissement sur le foetus est loin d'être négligeable (3% de mortalité). Il s'agitde surveiller tout particulièrement les jeunes primipares, les gestantes de plus de 35 ans, les grandes multipares, surtout si elles présentent une prise de poids excessive durant la grossesse. La meilleure prophylaxie sera constituée par l'augmentation du nombre des examens prénataux.

III. Toxémies moyennes

Il s'agit d'un groupe très défini et le retentissement sur le foetus est plus important.

A. *Parité-Age*

Les constatations que nous avions faites dans les formes légères de la malade se retrouvent ici avec plus de netteté: prépondérance des primipares et des grandes multipares, des très jeunes gestantes et de celles de plus de 35 ans.

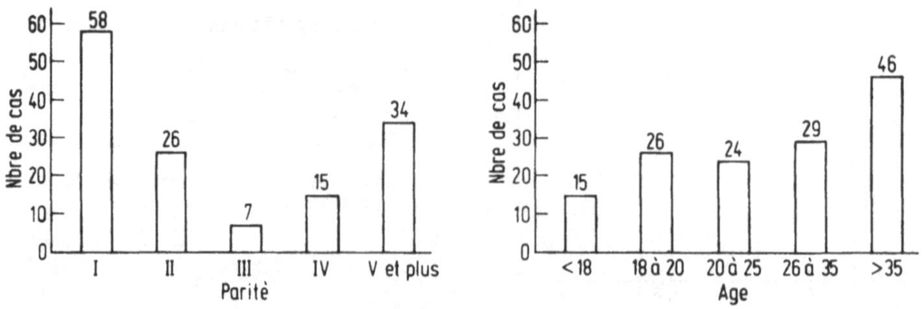

Fig. 8. Toxemies moyennes (140)

B. *Etat-Civil*

Habitat
Morphotype
Nombre de consultations
Médecin traitant

Etude de certains facteurs

Etat Civil
1. Nombre de gestantes mariées: 121
2. Nombre de gestantes célibataires ou divorcées: 19

Habitat
1. Rural: 52
2. Citadin: 77
3. Transplantées: 11

Morphotype
1. Moyen: 50
2. Bréviligne maigre: 17
3. Bréviligne obèse: 39
4. Longiligne maigre: 12
5. Grandes et obèses: 32

Nombre de consultation
1. : 15
2. : 29
3. : 101
$>$ à 3. : 5

Médecin traitant:
Extérieur à la Maternité: 96
Consultations publiques de la Maternité: 34
Consultations privées de la Maternité: 10

Fig. 9. Toxémies moyennes (140)

Les proportions sont sensiblement identiques à celles observées dans le groupe précédent. Il est toutefois à signaler l'influence du nombre des consultations.

C. *Prise pondérale*

88 gestantes, soit 62,8% ont pris plus de 12 kg durant leur grossesse.

D. *Moment de l'accouchement*

L'incidence sur la prématurité est ici plus marquée (30,7%), si l'on se réfère à l'âge gestationnel calculé selon la date des dernières règles.

E. *Mode de l'accouchement*

Le nombre de césariennes est ici nettement plus important (7,1%).

Etude de certains facteurs

C. *Prise pondérale*

< 5 kg	6
⩾ 5 < 8	18
⩾ 8 < 12	28
⩾ 12 < 16	31
⩾ 16 < 20	31
⩾ 20	26

D. *Age gestationnel*

Prématurés:	43
A terme:	92
Après terme calculé:	5

E. *Accouchement*

Normal:	81
Manoeuvre:	49
Césarienne:	10

Données ultérieures

Mortalité Néonatale

Immédiate	: 6
Dans les 3 jours	: 3
Total	: 9 soit 3 %

Hypertension artérielle résiduelle au 6e jour du post-partum: 23

Fig. 10. Toxémies moyennes (140)

F. *Poids de l'enfant à la naissance*

L'incidence de la dysgravidie sur la prématuration (14,2%) et sur l'hypotrophie foetale (4,29%) est ici manifeste. La différence entre le nombre de prématurés varit selon des critères de poids et d'âge gestationnel (20) et le nombre d'accouchements se déroulant avant le 260e jour de gestation (43) se comprend par la difficulté de recueillir des renseignements anamnestiques précis quant à la date des dernières menstruations.

G. *Score d'Apgar à la naissance*

La toxémie retentit davantage sur le devenir du foetus. On note une proportionalité nette entre le degré de la maladie et l'importance du nombre de souffrances foetales (27,1%).

Poids de l'enfant à la naissance

T à terme
A. T avant terme

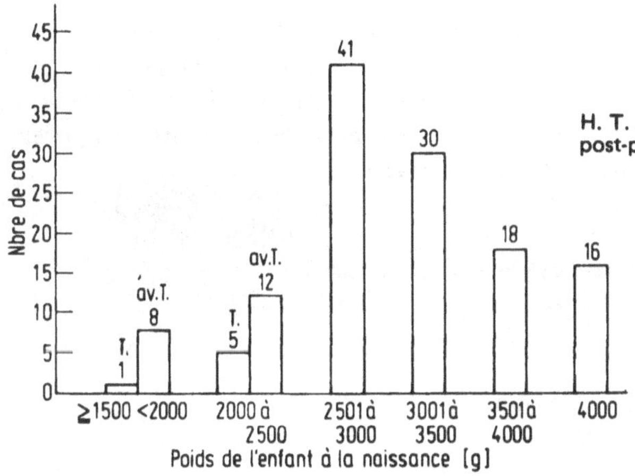

H. T. A. résiduelle chez la mère au 6e jour du post-partum:

43

Fig. 11. Toxémies moyennes (140)

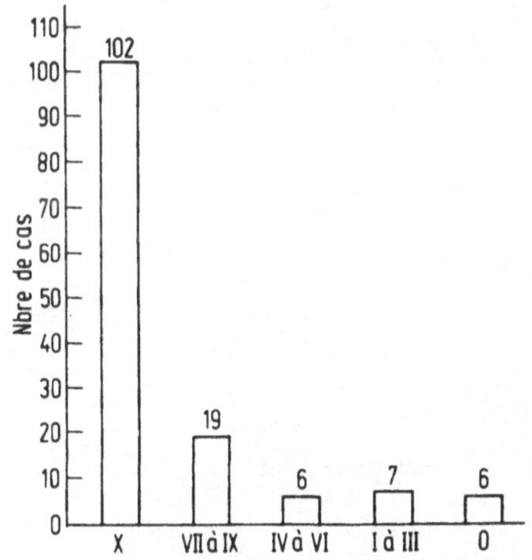

Mortalite néo-natale

6 morts in utéro ou à la naissance
2 morts dans les 3 jours après la naissance
—
8 soit 5,7%

Fig. 12. Toxémies moyennes (140)

H. *Mortalité néo-natale*

Celle-ci est nettement plus importante (5,7%) que dans le groupe précédent (3%).

En conclusion, il s'agit là, dans sa forme moyenne, d'une pathologie gravidique authentique. Elle mérite plus qu'une surveillance prénatale accrue et l'on se doit d'hospitaliser ces femmes au cours de la grossesse pour éviter une évolution fâcheuse. En effet, le nombre de prématurés, d'hypotrophies majeures, de souffrances néo-natale et le taux élevé de la mortalité sont là pour en témoigner.

III. Toxémies graves et éclampsies

Celles-ci se différencient en:

55 cas de toxémies graves,

5 cas d'éclampsie ou de coma éclamptique.

Ils ont fait l'objet d'un travail précédent.

A. *Parité-Age*

Les constatations sont ici également superposables à celles que nous avons observées dans les 2 autres groupes.

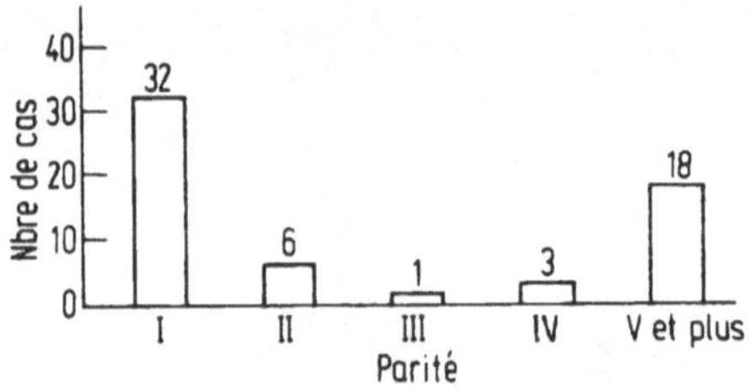

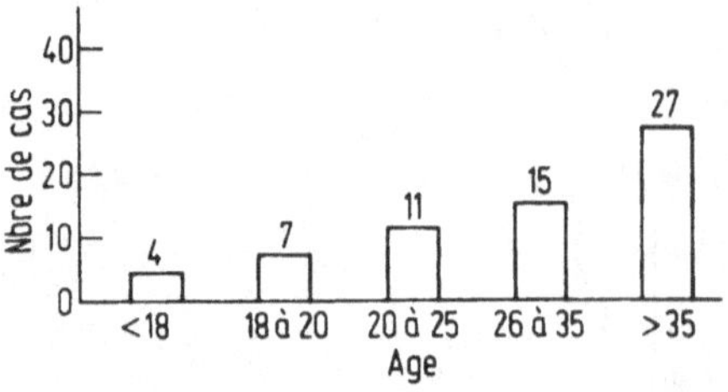

Fig. 13. Toxemies graves et eclampsie (60)

B. *Etat-civil*

Origine éthnique

Nombre de consultations

Médecin traitant

Il n'y a pas ici de particularismes par rapport aux groupes précédents.

C. *Poids de la mère à l'admission*

Les gestantes de poids faible, ainsi que les obèses constituent les groupes les plus menacés.

Etude de certains facteurs

Etat Civil
Nombre de gestantes mariées: 55
célibataires ou divorcées: 5

Habitat
1. Rural: 21
2. Citadin: 38
3. Transplantées: 1

Nombre de consultations
1. : 1
2. : 9
3. : 48
$>$ 3. : 2

Médecin traitant
Extérieur au Service: 52
Consultation publiques de la Maternité: 6
Consultation privées de la Maternité: 2

Fig. 14. Toxémies graves ou éclampsies (60)

E. *Prise pondérale*

L'incidence des prises de poids excessives est manifeste, mais il faut souligner la gravité des formes „sèche" d'éclampsie et de toxémies graves.

F. *Moment de l'accouchement*

Le nombre de prématurés vrais est très important 16 (soit 25,56%).

G. *Poids de l'enfant à la naissance*

Le nombre d'enfants de poids de moins de 2500 g est élevé. Il groupe les prématurés vrais (16), les hypotrophes à terme (6) soit 22 enfants (36,6%).

I. *Score d'Apgar à la naissance*

17 enfants soit, 28,5% ont présenté une souffrance grave ou moyenne à la naissance.

Etat foetal	6	33	21
Apgar VII–X	2 (33,3%)	19 (57,5%)	16 (76,1%)
IV–VI	1 (16,6%)	9 (27,2%)	9 (0 %)
+ né	2 (33,3%)	2 (6,0%)	3 (14,2%)
macéré	1 (16,6%)	3 (9,0%)	2 (9,5%)
	> 43–57,9	58–82,9	83–127,9

Poids en kg à l'admission de la mère comparé à l'état foetal à la naissance.

Etat foetal	20	28	12
Apgar VII–X	12 (60%)	21 (75 %)	5 (41,6%)
IV–VI	6 (30%)	2 (7,1%)	1 (8,3%)
+ né	1 (5%)	2 (7,1%)	4 (33,3%)
macéré	1 (5%)	2 (10,7%)	2 (16,6%)
	9–12	13–24	1,5–8

Prise de poids pendant la grossesse de la mère comparé à l'état foetal à la naissance.

Fig. 15

Fig. 16. voire page 201

Traitement		Apgar 0	I	II	III	IV	V	VI	VII	VIII	IX	X	Total	Décès après une semaine	Enfants vivants après une semaine
	Expectatif médicamenteux + surveillance foetale	2 4	 (14,28%)	1	1	2 5	1 (17,85%)	1	1 19	2 (67,85%)	1	15	28	8 (28,56%)	20 (71,44%)
Traitement actif	Déclenchement (perfusion ocytocique) + rupture de poche		 1	1		2 5	1	2	1 14	1	2	10	20	1 (3,84%)	25 (96,5 %)
Traitement actif	Césarienne			2 2							1 4	3	6		
Total		3	(11,53%)			5	(14,23%)		18	(69,23%)			26		

Fig. 17. Comparaison entre traitement médicamenteux avec expectative et traitement actif (déclenchement ou césarienne) et score d'Apgar à la naissance et évolution une semaine après l'accouchement

Apgar	P	P/D	D	T	G	Total			
X	2	2	1	20	4	29			
IX			1	2		3		37	
VIII	1			2		3		(68,5%)	54
VII				2		2			(100%)
VI	2	1	1			4			
V		1		1		2		10	
IV	1		1	2		4		(18,5%)	
III				1		1			
II	1		2	1		4		7	
I								(12,0%)	
0				1	1	2			
Total	7	4	6	32	5	54	90%		
Macérés	5			1		6	10%		
Total	12	4	6	33	5	60	100%		

* P prématurés vrais
* P/D prématurés et dystrophiques
* D Dysmatures
* T Foetus à terme
* G Gros enfant (4000 G.)

Fig. 16. Score d'Apgar et aspect foetal à la naissance

J. *Mortalité néo-natale*

Elle est de 13,33% si l'on se réfère au moment de l'accouchement et de 25% si l'on considère le nombre d'enfants vivants une semaine après l'accouchement.

La gravité de cette forme est suffisamment connue pour ne pas y revenir davantage. Elle justifie la réunion de ce symposium et fait comprendre la nécessité d'une prophylaxie active.

Conclusion

L'étude de 500 cas de dysgravidie nous a amenés à considérer certains facteurs étio-pathogéniques dont la surveillance permettra une diminution du nombre de toxémies observées.

Il s'agit essentiellement de facteurs péjoratifs:
- la primiparité,
- la grande multiparité,

l'âge jeune et encore l'existence d'une grossesse chez une femme de plus de 35 ans,
les prises de poids excessives,
le nombre de consultations prénatales insuffisant.

Summary

500 cases of EPH-gestosis are reported here. Different epidemiologic factors seems to have a real importance:

Primiparity,
Grand multiparity,
Teen age pregnancy,
More specially over 35 years old pregnant women,
Excessive weight gain.

The best way to prevent gestosis seems to be an increased number of prenatal exams.

Zusammenfassung

500 Fälle von Gestose sind hier zusammengefaßt. Verschiedene epidemiologische Faktoren scheinen ein Einfluß zu haben.

Primiparität,
Multiparität,
unter 18 Jahre alte Schwangere,
über 35 Jahre alte Schwangere,
die zu große Gewichtszunahme

Das beste Mittel, diese Pathologie zu vermindern, würde darin liegen, die Untersuchungen während der Schwangerschaft zu vermehren.

Environmental Temperature and the Occurence of EPH-Gestosis in a Subarctic Area

P. Ylöstalo, A. Kauppila, E. Sotaniemi

Department of Obstetrics and Gynaecology, University of Oulu, Oulu, Finnland

Environmental temperature has been found to affect the occurrence of e.g. myocardial infarctions and apoplexias in a subarctic area. It has been observed, too, that perinatal mortality, the frequency of preterm infants and low birth weight infants

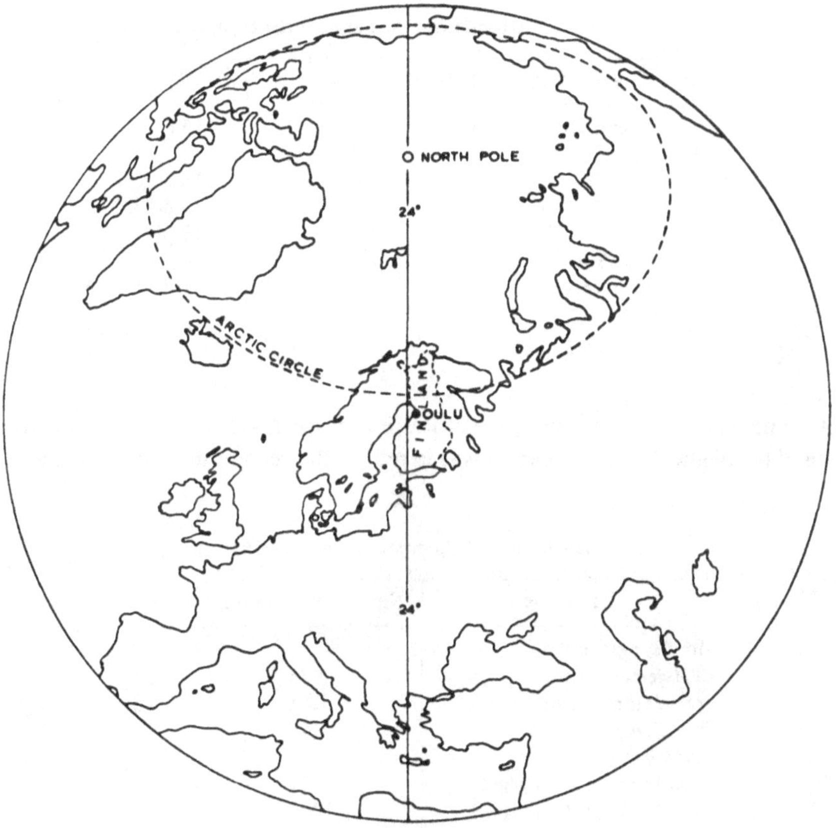

Fig. 1. The geographical situation of Oulu

are higher in the cold winter season than in the warm summer season. Environmental weather conditions, strong radiation and cold weather have been observed to influence the occurrence of eclampsia, the most serious form of toxemia.

A study has been conducted at the Department of Obstetrics and Gynaecology, University Hospital, Oulu, on the effect of environmental temperature and its variations on the admission of patients with EPH-gestosis. Oulu is (Fig. 1) on the Gulf of Bothnia in Northern Finland, almost exactly on latitude 65°N.

Material and methods

EPH-gestosis was the reason for the admission of a patient 1152 times at the Department of Obstetrics and Gynaecology, University Hospital, Oulu, in 1965–1968, and essential hypertension was the reason 209 times. The age distribution of the patients is presented in Tab. 1. Patients aged 21–25 years were in the majority, accounting for

Tab. 1. Distribution of the material by age.

Age (years)	Number of patients	%
= and under 20	185	13.6
21–25	276	20.3
26–30	248	18.2
31–35	249	18.3
36–40	248	18.2
41–45	137	10.1
over 45	18	1.3

some 20 per cent. Tab. 2 shows the distribution of the material according to diagnostic groups. The diagnostic classification was based on the recommendation of the

Tab. 2. Distribution of the material by diagnostic groups.

Diagnosis	Number of patients	%
Monosymptomatic EPH-gestosis	323	24
Pre-eclampsia levis	241	18
Pre-eclampsia gravis	342	25
Eclampsia	15	1
Superimposed EPH-gestosis	231	17
Essential hypertension	209	15
Total	1361	100

American Committee of Maternal Welfare. Pre-eclampsia gravis was the commoenest diagnostic group (342/1,361 or 25 per cent), followed by monosymptomatic EPH-gestosis in which hypertension of pregnancy accounted for 80 per cent. There were only 15 cases (1 per cent) of eclampsia. Essential hypertension was present in 209 cases. 231 patients had so-called superimposed EPH-gestosis. Fig. 2 shows the mean monthly temperature, the monthly total of admissions and the number of patients with EPH-gestosis. The figures are stated in per cent of the corresponding

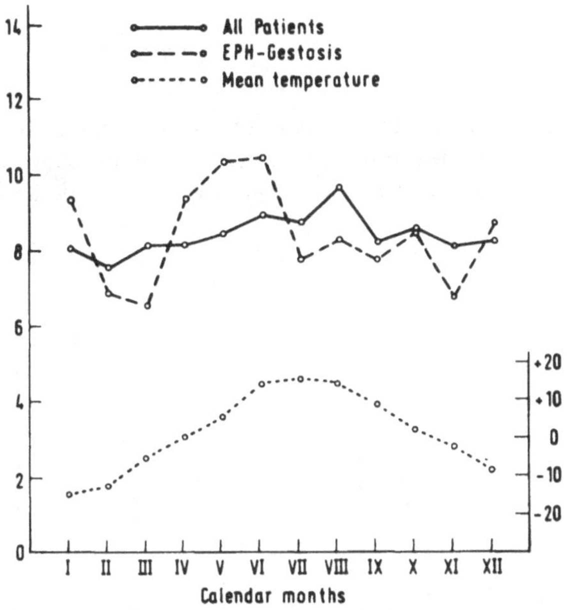

Fig. 2. Mean monthly temperature, total admissions monthly and the number of patients with EPH-Gestosis. The figures for the years 1965–1968 were combined and the monthly number of patients in per cent was calculated from the total

totals. EPH-gestosis accounted for a higher proportion of the admissions in April–June than at any other time of the year. It was the reason for an average of 11 per cent and EPH-gestosis plus essential hypertension for about 13 per cent of the admissions in 1965–1968.

Results

The effect of the daily mean temperature on admissions appears on Tab. 3. The mean temperatures are tabulated at intervals of 10° and in the following column are entered the number and per cent of days belonging to the corresponding temperature

Tab. 3. Effect of daily mean temperature on the admission of patients to hospital.

Daily temperature	Days		Patients of the material		
C°	No.	%	No.	%	Per day
≤ - 30	7	0.5	5	0.4	0.71
- 29 – - 20	79	5.4	68	5.0	0.81
- 19 – - 10	163	11.0	161	11.8	0.99
- 9 – 0	345	23.7	295	21.7	0.86
0 – + 9	458	31.4	409	30.1	0.89
+ 10 – + 19	394	27.0	404	29.7	1.02
≥ + 20	15	1.0	19	1.4	1.26

groups. In the next column are the number of admissions in each temperature interval and the corresponding per cent distribution. The last column shows the calculated daily frequency of admissions. Fig. 3 shows graphically the ratio between the mean

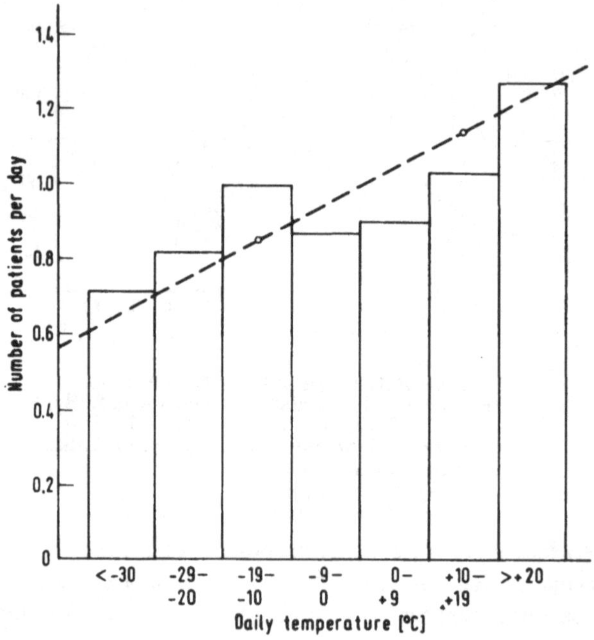

Fig. 3. Daily number of patients in the material in the mean temperature groups

temperature and the daily distribution. When the temperature is over 0°C, the number of admissions rises with the temperature. A minor decrease in the admission frequency occurs in the temperature range - 10° – + 10°C; otherwise, the admission frequency correlates well with the temperature on the day of admission (equation of the regression line $y = 0.0096 X + 0.99$, correlation coefficient $r = +0.855$). Analysing the same point by diagnostic groups (Fig. 4), the incidence of eclampsia is highly significantly ($p < 0.001$) greater at higher and lower temperatures than in the middle range. The change is similar to that in the total EPH-gestosis material, but is more accentuated. Gradual elevation was seen in the daily readings on moving from - 20° to + 20°C ($p < 0.05$) in the groups with superimposed EPH-gestosis and essential hypertension. No significant differences were seen in the other diagnostic groups. The incidence of the different individual symptoms of EPH-gestosis, such as edema, proteinuria and hypertension, on the day of admission increased on moving from colder to warmer temperatures, but there was a decrease in the temperature range from

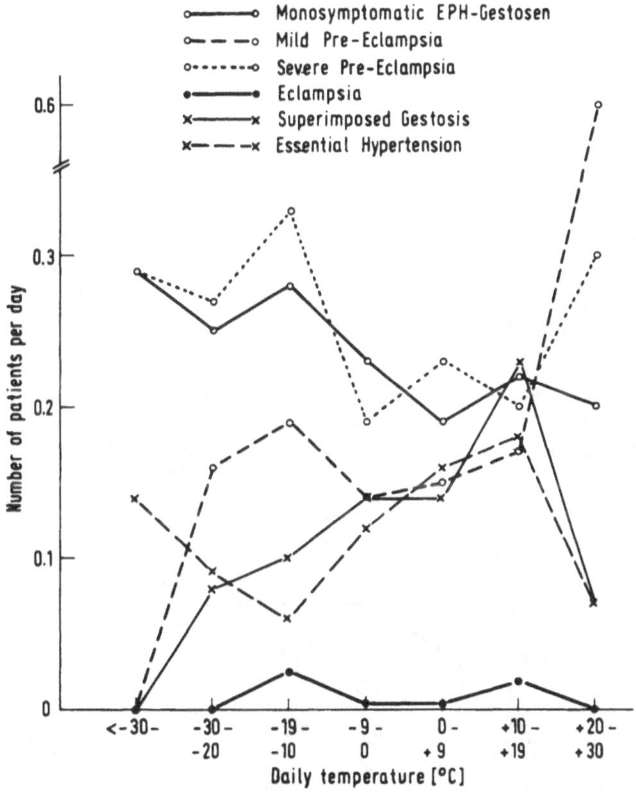

Fig. 4. Distribution of the daily number of patients in the material according to the diagnostic and mean temperature groups

- 10°– + 10°C (Fig. 5). No definite differences were observed between the temperature intervals in the subjective symptoms on the day of admission, i.e. headache, visual disturbances.

The effect of temperature change on the admission rate on both the 1st and 2nd day was examined. The result obtained was expressed in so-called daily readings. The daily readings were obtained by dividing the number of admissions in the different temperature change groups by the number of corresponding days. The daily reading is entered in the graph as the ordinate and the temperature change groups as the abscissa (Fig. 6). No significant differences were noted. The result is similar for the effect of temperature changes during the coldest months, January–February, and the warmest, July–August (Fig. 7).

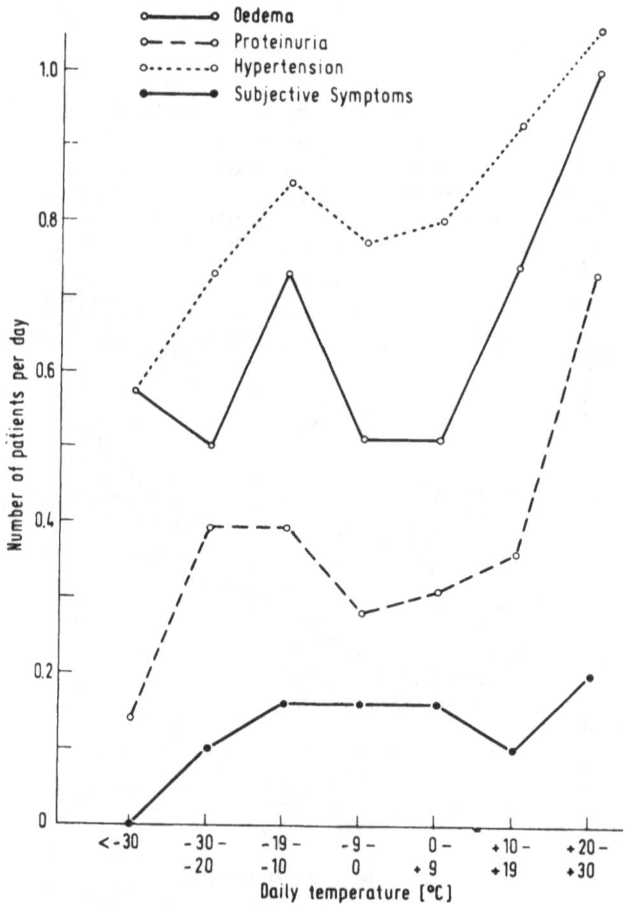

Fig. 5. Occurrence of the various symptoms of EPH-Gestosis daily in the different temperature groups

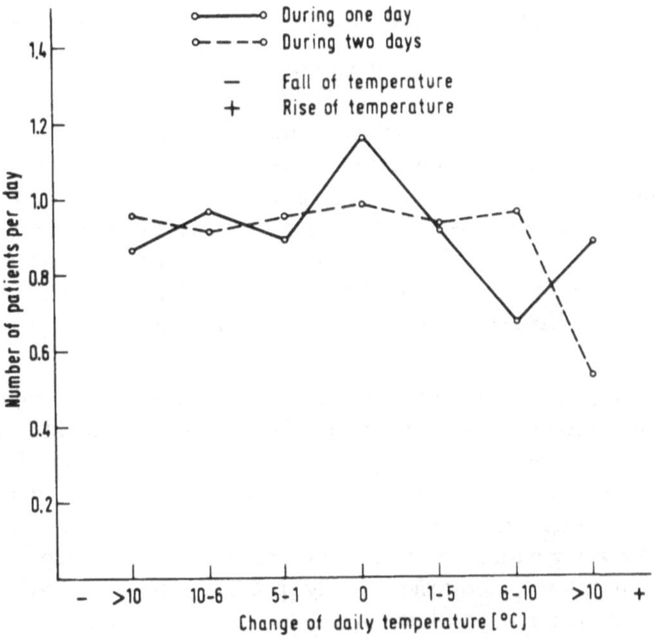

Fig. 6. The daily number of patients in the material in the temperature change groups. The change of temperature was calculated for 1 day and 2 days before the day of admission

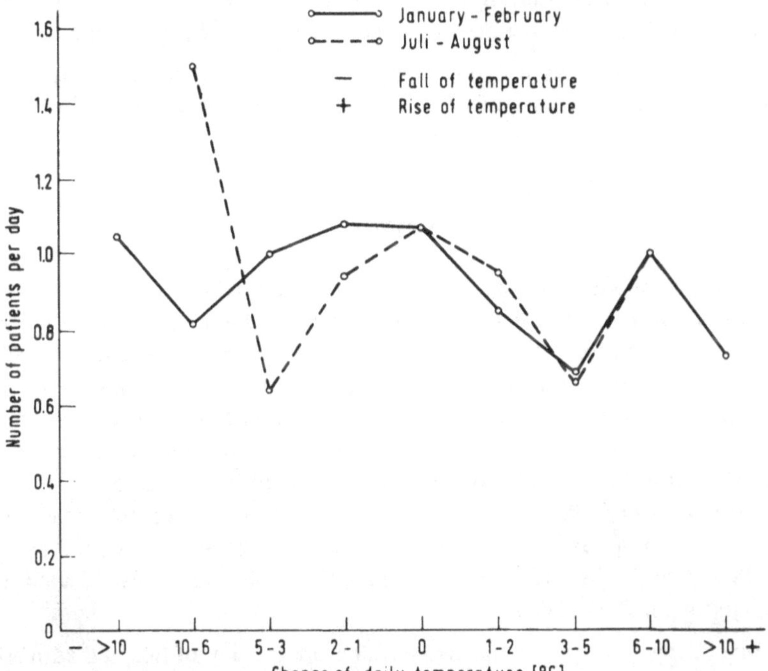

Fig. 7. The daily number of patients in the material in the temperature change groups, during January–February and during July–August, calculated for 2 days before the day of admission

Conclusions

The environmental temperature in a subarctic area is correlated with the admissions of toxemic patients. The higher the temperature, the greater is the number of admissions. The proportion of admissions was higher in April–May–June than at any other time of the year. A minor drop was seen in the rate of admissions of toxemic patients in the temperature range - 10° – + 10°C, and the same phenomenon was observed in the frequency of the individual symptoms of EPH-gestosis: edema, proteinuria and hypertension. On the other hand, no such decrease was seen in the occurrence of subjective symptoms.

Application of the x^2-test to compare the distribution of the diagnostic groups according to temperature groups and to the number of corresponding days in 1965–1968 showed a highly significant difference ($p < 0.001$) in the incidence of eclampsia. It was higher in the temperature ranges - 10° – - 19°C and + 10° – + 19°C and lower in the 10° – - 10°C range, that is the change established in the total EPH-gestosis material accentuated. The group with superimposed EPH-gestosis and the group with essential hypertension also differed almost significantly ($p < 0.05$) from the distribution of days into temperature groups, with the incidence rising fairly evenly in the range - 20° – + 20°C as the temperature rose. No significant differences were seen in the other distributions of the diagnostic groups.

Temperature change during the 1st and 2nd day before the day of hospital admission was not found to exert a distinct effect on the frequency of hospital admission.

The most favourable temperature range for pregnancy in a subarctic area is - 10° – + 10°C if the occurrence of EPH-gestosis is taken into consideration.

Summary

A study has been conducted on the effect of environmental temperature and its variations on the admission of patients with EPH-gestosis in a subarctic area. EPH-gestosis was the reason for 1,152 admissions in 1965–1968, and essential hypertension was the reason for 209 admissions. The environmental temperature was correlated with the admissions: the higher the temperature, the greater was the number of admissions. A minor drop was seen in the rate of admissions in the temperature range - 10° – + 10°C, and the same phenomenon was observed in the frequency of the individual symptoms of EPH-gestosis: edema, proteinuria and hypertension. The incidence of eclampsia was higher in the temperature ranges - 10° – - 19°C and + 10° – + 19°C than in the - 10° – + 10°C range, that is the change established in the total EPH-gestosis material accentuated.

Temperature change during one and two days before the day of hospital admission was not found to exert a distinct effect on the frequency of hospital admission.

A Proposed New Gestosis Index

L. Tervilä, C. Goecke, S. Timonen

Geburtshilfl.-gynäkol. Abteilung, Stadtkrankenhaus Lahti, Finnland,
und Universitäts-Frauenklinik, Würzburg, BRD

At the meeting of the Gestosis Association in Paris last year certain studies were presented in which the so-called Gestosis Index was applied. The results were not very encouraging. This is understandable, considering that the index was far from precise, being constructed on the basis of common sense more than facts. The use of the index is moreover both time-consuming and rather difficult. An attempt has therefore been made to determine the prognosis for the newborn on the basis of symptoms of gestosis and to construct an index of a better model. For this purpose Dr. *Goecke* collected 2077 consecutive cases of gestosis in Würzburg from the last 10 years, and Prof. *Timonen* and I collected 2327 cases from Helsinki University Central Hospital from a period of five years. On admission these 4404 patients were all examined for the classic symptoms of gestosis. Moreover, a large number of criteria relating to the newborn were collected from the hospital records. To begin with the symptoms of gestosis were correlated one by one to the criteria for the infant. The results appear on the slides. First, the *systolic blood pressure.* Below you see the blood pressure in millimetres, to the left the frequency percentage. The curve at the bottom shows perinatal mortality, the next curve represents the infants given 6 or less Apgar scores at one minute, the third curve shows the incidence of infants with a birth-weight under 2500 g, and the uppermost curve shows the rate of infants small for date. This percentage was obtained from the birth-weight figures and gestation times taking into account that in the general population 10% of the newborn are small for date, according to a probability table previously made. As you will notice, the incidence of infants in poor condition shows a relatively slow rise. The curve rises more abruptly only when the blood pressure axceeds 180 mm.

Tab. 2 shows the curves related to the *diastolic blood pressure.* Again, the incidence of infants in poor condition increases slowly up to 115 mm, after which a steeper rise is seen.

The corresponding correlations for *proteinuria* are shown on Tab. 3. The rise is somewhat steeper from the beginning than in connection with the blood pressures. The most abrupt rise begins when protein increases to 2 per thousand.

The diagram for *oedema* is a bit more complicated. The Finish and German results are presented separately. In regard to the foregoing parameters the correlations

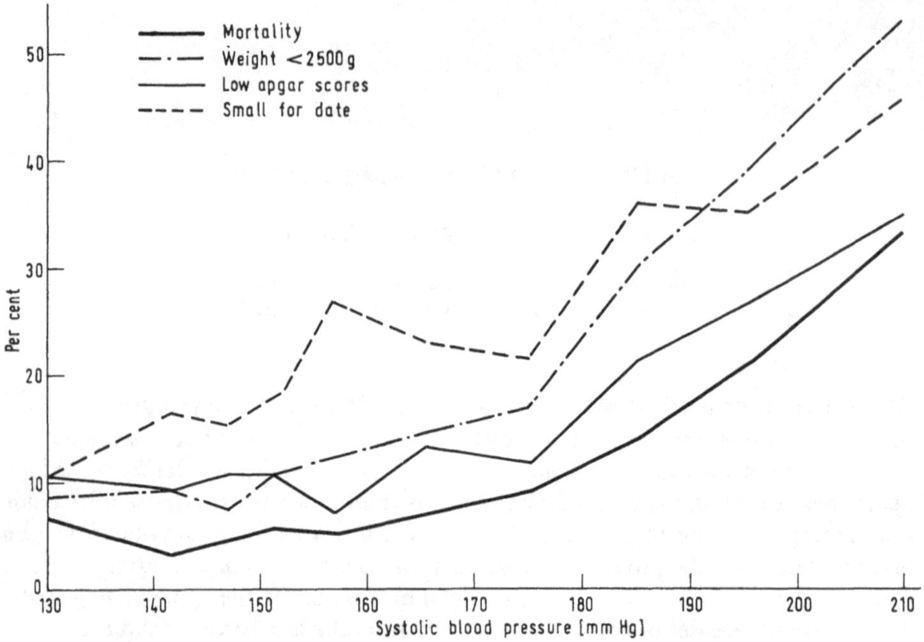

Mortality
Weight <2500g
Low apgar scores
Small for date
Per cent
0
10
20
30
40
50
130
140
150
160
170
180
190
200
210
Systolic blood pressure [mm Hg]

Tab. 1.

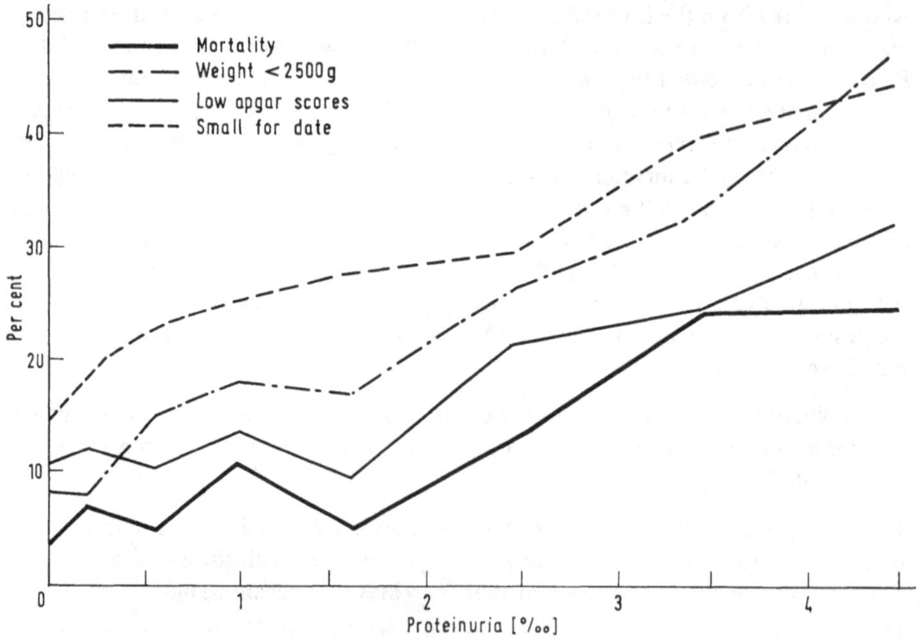

Mortality
Weight <2500g
Low apgar scores
Small for date
Per cent
0
10
20
30
40
50
1
2
3
4
Proteinuria [°/₀₀]

Tab. 2.

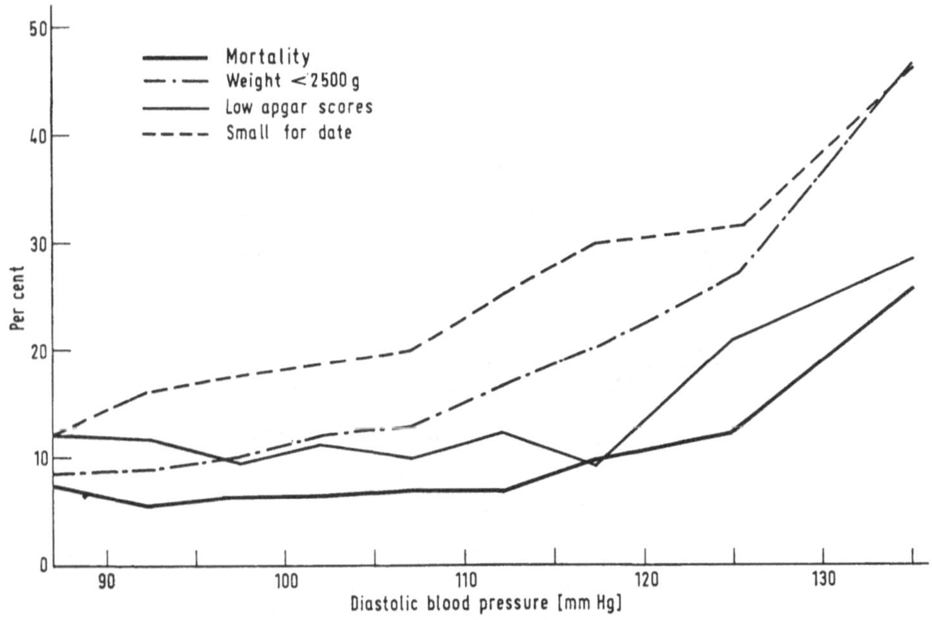

Tab. 3.

obtained were very much alike in the two series, which therefore were pooled. For oedema, the results differed considerably. In the Finish series the prognosis improved with an increase of oedema. In the German series an improvement of prognosis was observed with a shift from the *non-oedematous* group to the group with slight oedema, but abundant oedema was associated with a clearly poorer prognosis. Obviously oedema is differently assessed in the two countries, as appears from this table showing the frequency of the symptom in Germany and in Finland. The inconvenience caused by the deplorably subjective assessment of oedema is again illustrated.

Using these results the correlation coefficients for the relationship between the different symptoms and the condition of the infant were calculated. The calculations were made at the Computing Centre of Helsinki University, and my knowledge of statistical mathematics unfortunately is not thorough enough to permit presentation of the figures in greater detail.

Anyhow the results showed that oedema is negatively correlated with smallness for date. The same is true for prematurity, though to a lesser degree. However as oedema correlates with the other symptoms, no important additional information is thus obtained.

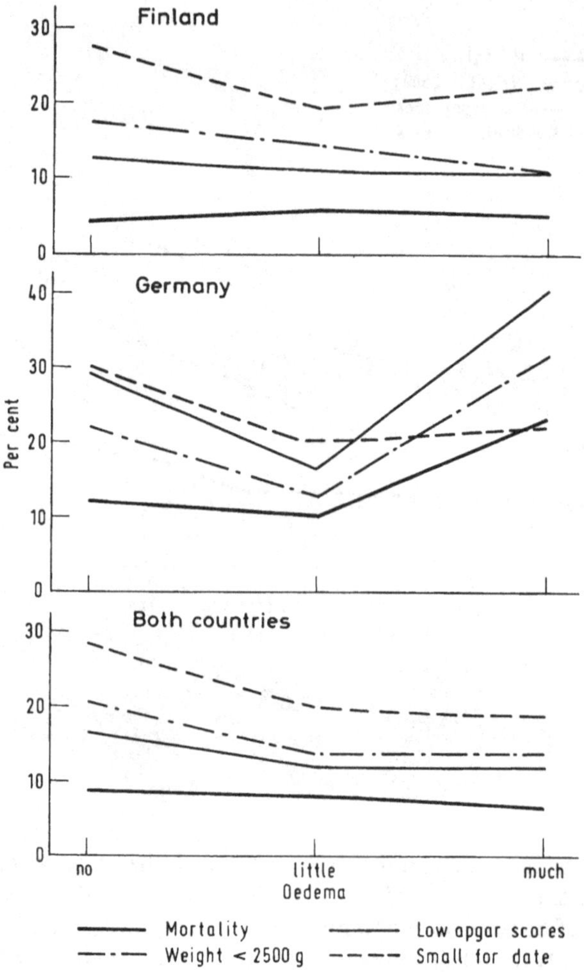

Tab. 4.

Tab. 5. Frequency of oedema.

	–	+	++	n
Helsinki	13.4%	50.9%	35.7%	2327
Würzburg	18.1%	76.9%	5.0%	2077

Tab. 6. Correlation coefficients for the relationship between various symptoms and the criterion for the newborn.

	mortality	prematurity	low Apgar scores	small for date	duration of pregnancy
Oedema (Helsinki)	+ 0.01	– 0.04	– 0.02	– 0.07	– 0.02
Oedema (Würzburg)	– 0.02	– 0.09	–	– 0.09	– 0.08
Proteinuria (pooled)	+ 0.198	+ 0.253	+ 0.112	+ 0.192	+ 0.159
syst. RR (pooled)	+ 0.155	+ 0.228	+ 0.097	+ 0.176	+ 0.144
diast. RR (pooled)	+ 0.093	+ 0.186	+ 0.046	+ 0.155	+ 0.107
Significance levels:	0.030 – p < 0.05, 0.040 – p < 0.01, 0.050 – p < 0.001				

Tab. 7. Partial correlation coefficients obtained by omitting the effect of other symptoms.

	mortality	prematurity	low Apgar scores	small for date
systolic blood pressure	0.11	0.13	0.07	0.09
diastolic blood pressure	0.00	0.07	0.01	0.07

Significance levels for the correlation coefficients:
0.030 – p < 0.05, 0.040 – p < 0.01, 0.050 – p < 0.001

The other symptoms showed a highly significant positive correlation with the variables for the condition of the infant. Proteinuria proved to be the most significant factor. In order to test the importance of the systolic and diastolic blood pressures, partial correlations with the variables for the condition of the infant were calculated by eliminating in turn the effect of protein and of systolic and diastolic blood pressure. The results are shown on this slide.

The systolic blood pressure was found to be a factor of significance for the prognosis also when the effect of the other symptoms had been eliminated.

The diastolic blood pressure proved to be a clearly less important factor, although it has a significant effect on the size of the child.

The next step was to construct a table of scores. Since the effect of oedema and diastolic blood pressure on the prognosis for the infant had proved to be so slight, it was decided to omit these variables. In this way the table gained considerably in simplicity, and the subjective factor relating to the estimation of oedema was eliminated.

Then, an entirely subjective estimate was made, the only one in the whole system, we decided that the prognosis for the infant was best illustrated by a totality in which 50 per cent of the weight was allotted to infant mortality. The remaining 50 per cent was divided between prematurity, low Apgar scores and smallness for date. Consequently, a dead child was given a score of 50 and the other three criteria were given scores of 17 each. The mean values for the scores given in the individual cases were calculated and plotted against proteinuria and systolic blood pressure of four degrees. The table seen on this slide was thus obtained, and the figures are mean values.

Tab. 8. Mean scores and number of cases in the various groups.

	Systolic blood pressure mm			
Proteinuria in %	−149	150−169	170−189	190−
0	6.10 672	7.40 901	8.45 321	17.86 59
0.1−0.7	6.58 338	9.71 464	13.09 172	24.81 47
0.8−2.9	11.40 368	12.66 407	19.06 146	30.00 49
3.0	15.67 101	24.90 153	32.36 107	41.53 92

Results of two-way variance analysis:
Effect of proteinuria $F = 112.27^{xxx}$, $p < 0.1\%$
Effect of syst. blood pressure $F = 65.60^{xxx}$, $p < 0.1\%$
Interaction $F = 3.79^{xxx}$, $p < 0.1\%$

Of the variance, protein accounted for about 60 per cent and systolic blood pressure about 35 per cent. Although the combined effect accounted for only 5 per cent, we decided to make a two-dimensional table, because the highest mean scores were obtained in groups with a small number of cases. Consequently their share in the variance is slight, as compared to the total material. The scores for these groups would have been too low if the two symptoms had been rated separately.

When the mean values were compared by the t-test, the difference between a minimum of two steps in the table was found to be highly significant ($p < 0.001$). Adjacent steps in the horizontal and vertical directions did not always differ significantly from each other.

Tab. 9. Proposed Gestosis Index.

	Systolic blood pressure mm			
Proteinuria ‰	−149	−169	−189	190−
0	0	1	2	9
0.1−0.7	0	3	5	14
0.8−2.9	4	5	10	18
3.0−	7	14	20	27

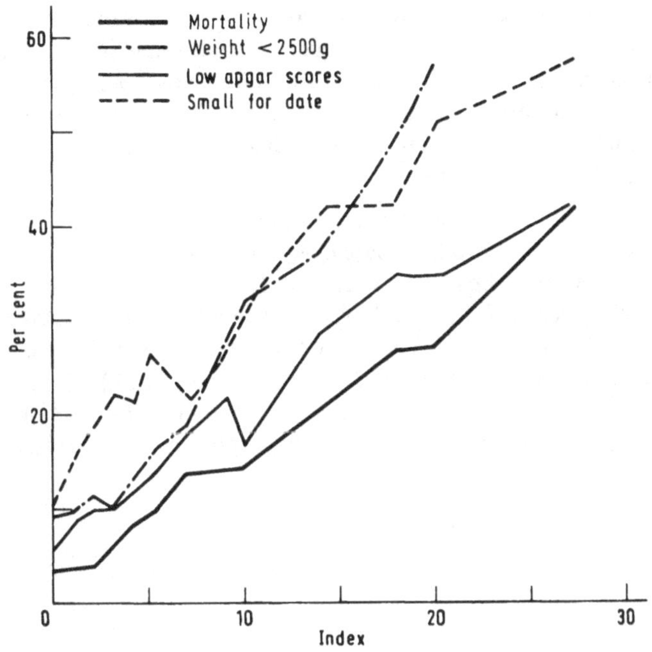
Mortality
Weight <2500g
Low apgar scores
Small for date
60
40
20
Per cent
0
10
20
30
Index

Tab. 10.

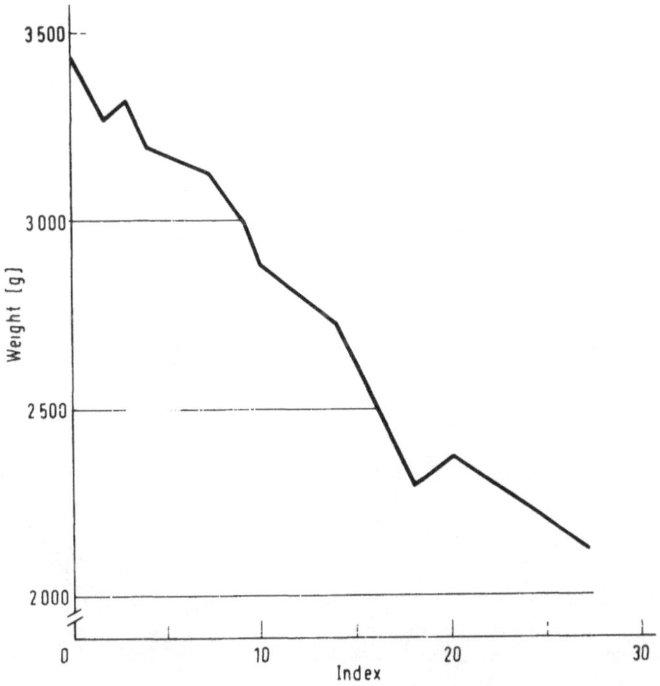
3500
3000
2500
2000
Weight [g]
0
10
20
30
Index

Tab. 11.

The figures were then reduced and rounded off, and this gave the table seen on this slide. There are 13 classes, the weight of which was calculated using the same material for all. On the next slide you will see the scores used below, and to the left the ratios of perinatal deaths, infants weighing under 2500 g, infants given less than 7 Apgar scores and infants small for date. On the next slide, which is my last, you see the weight changes of the newborn in scores.

Finally, it may be stated that the corralation is not too bad. For example, if a woman is admitted with a systolic blood pressure of 175 mm and proteinuria of 0.5 per thousand, we can say that the mortality risk for her child is about 9 per cent, because there is a risk of 15 per cent that it will have a birth-weight under 2500 g, a 13 per cent risk that the Apgar scores will be 6 or under, and a 25 per cent risk that it will be small for date when the average risk is 10 per cent. And if the child is not prematurely born, it is supposed to weigh 3165 g and measure 49.5 cm. The supposed weight of the placenta is 596 g, and the supposed duration of pregnancy is 274 days.

Changes of Selected Serum–Factors in Pregnancy and EPH-Gestosis

Immunoelektrophoretische Untersuchungen der Proteine im Blutserum und Harn in der EPH-Gestose

K. Bernacka, A. Cretti, S. Jaworski

Klinik für innere Krankheiten und II. Frauenklinik der Medizinischen Akademie, Bialystok, Polen

Bis jetzt wurden keine gleichzeitige, vergleichende immunoelektrophoretische (IE) Untersuchungen der Proteine im Blutserum und Harn in der EPH-Gestose beschrieben. Die vorliegende Mitteilung spricht von solchen Untersuchungen, die 23 Patientinnen mit EPH-Gestosen umfassen.

Die IE-Untersuchungen wurden nach *Scheidegger* [5] durchgeführt, wobei wir uns des polyvalenten, resistenten Pferdeserums der Pharmazeutischen Werke – Krakowska Wytwórnia Surowic i Szczepionek – bedienten. Die Objektträger wurden mit einem im eigenen Labor hergestellten Agar bedeckt. Die Ergebnisse wurden laufend mit dem IE-Bild gesunder Menschen verglichen. Die Untersuchungen wurden mit Vollserum und konzentriertem Harn, und in der Verdünnung mit physiologischer Kochsalzlösung in den Verhältnissen 1:2 und 1:8 durchgeführt. Der Harn wurde in einer 50%igen Gummi-Arabicum-Lösung in zur Eiweißkonzentration dienenden Zellophanbeuteln bis zum Werte der Eiweißkonzentration des untersuchten Serums konzentriert.

Die Untersuchungsergebnisse zeigt Tab. 1; die klinischen Daten Tab. 2. In beiden Tabellen wurden die Daten gleichartig nach der Schwere des klinischen Bildes zusammengestellt, das mit Hilfe des Gestose-Indexes nach *Goecke* u. Mit. [2] in eigener Modifikation [1] beurteilt wurde (Tab. 3).

Die vergleichende Analyse der IE-Untersuchungen im Blutserum und Harn zeigt, daß der Übertritt immer zahlreicherer Eiweißfraktionen sich parallel zur Verschlechterung des klinischen Zustandes steigert.

Interessant ist auch die Anwesenheit des IgG-Globulins im Harn bei 21 Fällen; gleichzeitig wurde eine Senkung des Spiegels dieser Fraktion im Blutserum bei 18 von 23 untersuchten Fällen beobachtet (Tab. 1 u. 2). Unabhängig von den Erwägungen, ob der Übertritt so großer Moleküle, wie das IgG-Globulin, eine Folge der „essentiellen" Gestose oder Pfropfgestose sei, spricht dieses für eine bedeutende, bleibende oder vorübergehende Beschädigung der Nieren.

Der Übertritt des IgA-Globulins in den Harn wurde bei 16 von 23 Fällen festgestellt. Dieses könnte durch die Steigerung der immunologischen Störungen erklärt werden; nach *Jones* u. Mit. [3] gehören die IgA-Globuline zu den frühen Antikörpern.

Tab. 1. Die Ergebnisse der immunoelektrophoretischen Untersuchung der Proteine im Blutserum und im Harn in 23 EPH-Gestose-Fällen.

Fall Nr.		Gesamt Eiweiß	Präalbumine	Präalbumine	Albumine	Orosomuk.	$Alpha_1$ L	$Alpha_1$ Glyk.	Haptoglobin	$Alpha_2$ M	Coerulopl.	$Alpha_2$ Lip.	$Beta_1$ Glyk.	$Beta_1$ B Glob.	Transferrin	$Beta_1$ C Glob.	$Beta_1$ L	IgM	IgA	IgG	Alpha-Beta Bogen
1	Serum	6,0				+↑		+↑	+↑	+↑	+↑									+↓	
	Harn	4,9			+				+	+					+	+		+	+	+	
2	Serum	6,0							+↑	+↑	+↑									+↑	
	Harn	1,65			+				+											+	+
3	Serum	6,5	+		+↓	+↑		+↑												+↓	
	Harn	1,65			+				+		+									+	+
4	Serum	7,0							+↑		+↑							+↑		+↓	
	Harn	1,32			+										+				+	+	+
5	Serum	6,5						+↑	+↑	+↑	+↑								+↑	+↑	
	Harn	1,65			+				+						+				+	+	
6	Serum	6,5			+↓			+↑	+↑	+↑	+↑	+↑							+↓	+↓	
	Harn	0,66			+				+		+				+				+	+	
7	Serum	6,25			+↓	+↑				+↑	+↑		+↓		+↓		+↓		+↓	+↓	
	Harn	0,66			+				+	+	+										
8	Serum	6,0			+↓	+↑	+↑	+↑		+↑					+↑			+↑	+↓	+↓	
	Harn	3,3			+				+										+	+	+
9	Serum	5,5			+↓				+↑	+↑	+↑								+	+↓	
	Harn	3,3			+	+			+										+	+	+
10	Serum	6,25			+↓		+	+	+↓		+↓								+↓	+↓	
	Harn	6,6			+				+		+								+	+	+
11	Serum	6,25			+↓			+↑		+↑		+↑			+↑					+↓	
	Harn	1,65			+			+	+		+					+			+	+	+
12	Serum	6,6			+		+↑	+↑							+↑			+↑	+↓	+↓	
	Harn	3,3			+				+		+								+	+	+
13	Serum	6,25			+↓				+↑	+↑				+↑	+↑			+↑		+↓	
	Harn	6,6			+					+				+	+					+	
14	Serum	4,9			+↓			+↑							+↓					+↓	
	Harn	3,3			+				+		+								+	+	+
15	Serum	4,5			+↓		+↑		+↑	+↑	+↑				+↓			+↑	+↓	+↓	
	Harn	3,3			+										+				+	+	
16	Serum	5,8			+↓			+↑	+↑	+↑		+↑							+↓	+↓	
	Harn	3,3			+	+		+	+		+	+							+	+	+
17	Serum	5,6			+↓				+↑	+↑	+↑							+↓		+↑	
	Harn	16,5			+				+		+				+					+	+
18	Serum	6,0			+	+↓			+↓		+↓				+↑			+⇈		+⇈	
	Harn	3,3			+				+											+	+
19	Serum	7,8		+↑							+↑	+↑							+↓	+↓	
	Harn	3,3			+				+			+			+				+	+	
20	Serum	6,6			+↓			+↑			+↑									+↓	
	Harn	3,3			+	+			+	+			+	+		+			+	+	+
21	Serum	6,25		+				+↑	+⇈	+⇈					+↓				+↑	+↓	
	Harn	9,9		+				+	+	+					+				+	+	+
22	Serum	6,6			+↓	+↑		+↑	+↑		+↑	+↑							+↓	+↓	
	Harn	3,3			+			+	+		+				+				+	+	+
23	Serum	6,25						+↑			+↑	+↑							+↑	+↑	
	Harn	6,6			+										+						+

↓ erniedrigt ↑ erhöht ⇈ erheblich erhöht

Tab. 2. Klinische Daten der EPH-Gestose-Fälle, deren Ergebnisse der immunoelektrophoretischen Untersuchung der Proteine im Blutserum und Harn auf Tab. 1 abgegeben sind.

Fall Nr.	Alter	Geburt	Schw.-Woche	Gestose Index	Komponente des Gestose Indexes	Kind		Bemerkungen
						Gewicht	Apgar	
1	23	1	40	3	$E_1 P_2$	3480	7	
2	27	2	40	3	$E_1 P_2$	Schwangere		
3	24	1	38	6	$E_1 P_1 H_4$ (2 + 2)	3470	8	
4	17	1	35	7	$E_2 P_1 H_4$ (1 + 3)	1250	2	Kind gestorben 7 Tage nach Geburt
5	24	1	40	7	$E_1 P_1 H_5$ (2 + 3)	2750	8	
6	19	1	40	7	$E_1 P_1 H_5$ (2 + 3)	3570	10	
7	28	1	35	8	$E_2 P_1 H_5$ (2 + 3)	2070	3	Asphyxie, Kaiserschnitt
8	35	3	40	8	$E_1 P_2 H_5$ (3 + 2)	3180	8	
9	23	4	28	8	$E_2 P_2 H_4$ (2 + 2)	Schwangere		
10	23	1	40	8	$E_1 P_3 H_4$ (2 + 2)	3700	10	Asphyxie, Kaiserschnitt
11	26	1	38	8	$E_2 P_1 H_5$ (2 + 3)	I: 2400 II: 1850	5 5	
12	26	2	40	8	$E_2 P_2 H_4$ (2 + 2)	3850	10	
13	22	1	40	9	$E_1 P_3 H_5$ (2 + 2)	2180	1	
14	27	2	31	9	$E_2 P_3 H_4$ (2 + 2)	900	–	Intrauterin abgestorben
15	27	3	40	9	$E_2 P_2 H_5$ (2 + 3)	3100	1	Asphyxie Kaiserschnitt
16	33	2	40	9	$E_2 P_2 H_5$ (2 + 3)	2800	7	Asphyxie Kaiserschnitt
17	40	3	40	9	$E_2 P_3 H_4$ (2 + 2)	920	–	Intrauterin abgestorben
18	26	1	40	9	$E_1 P_2 H_6$ (3 + 3)	3050	3	Asphyxie Kaiserschnitt
19	28	4	32	10	$E_2 P_2 H_6$ (3 + 3)	1750	3	Pfropfgestose bei Nephrosonephritis. Asphyxie, Kaiserschnitt
20	22	1	36	10	$E_2 P_2 H_6$ (3 + 3)	2000	5	Asphyxie, Kaiserschnitt
21	18	1	36	11	$E_2 P_3 H_6$ (3 + 3)	3000	10	Asphyxie Kaiserschnitt
22	37	1	24	11	$E_2 P_3 H_6$ (3 + 3)	600	–	Intrauterin abgestorben. Pfropfgestose bei essentieller Hypertension
23	25	2	35	11	$E_2 P_3 H_6$ (3 + 3)	900	3	Eklampsie, Asphyxie Kaiserschnitt

Tab. 3. Gestose Index nach *Goecke* u. Mit. in eigener Modifikation.

		0	1	2	3	Dat.	Dat.	Dat.
E	Oedeme trotz Bettruhe	keine	tibiale	generalisierte	–			
P	Proteinurie in ‰	weniger als 0,1	0,1–1,99	2–4,99	5 und mehr			
H	Blutdruck systol.	niedriger als 140	140–159	160–179	180 und höher			
	Blutdruck diastol.	niedriger als 90	90–99	100–109	11 und höher			
					Gestose Index			

Die Alpha$_2$M-Fraktion wurde im Harn der 5 Kranken nachgewiesen; unter diesen 5 Fällen wurden bei den 4 Neugeborenen Schäden beobachtet, deren Ursache eine chronische oder akute Asphyxie gewesen war. Dieses stimmt überein mit den Beobachtungen von *McEwan* [4], welche der Ansicht ist, daß das Auftreten dieser Fraktion ein Faktor sei, der eine ungünstige Prognose für die Frucht voraussagen läßt.

Zusammenfassung

Bei 23 EPH-Gestosefällen wurden gleichzeitige, vergleichende immunoelektrophoretische Untersuchungen der Proteine im Blutserum und Harn durchgeführt. Die Daten wurden mit dem klinischen Bild verglichen. Es wurde festgestellt, daß das Übertreten zahlreicher Eiweißfraktionen sich parallel zur Verschlechterung des klinischen Bildes steigert. Von einer bedeutenden Beschädigung der Nieren zeugt das Übertreten der IgG-Globuline in den Harn bei gleichzeitigem Sinken der Werte im Blutserum. Diese Erscheinung wurde bei der Mehrzahl der Fälle beobachtet. Das Übertreten des IgA-Globulins, das bei 16 auf 23 Fälle beobachtet wurde, könnte durch eine Steigerung der immunologischen Störungen in der Gestose erklärt werden. Die Alpha$_2$M-Fraktion wurde im Harn von 5 Kranken beobachtet; 4 davon gebaren Kinder mit Schäden, die durch eine Asphyxie bedingt waren.

Literatur

[1] *Cretti, A.:* Ginek. Pol. 42 (1971) S. 247.
[2] *Goecke, C.* u. *G. Schwabe:* Zbl. Gynäk. 87 (1965) S. 1439
[3] *Jones, B. M.* u. *R. B. Kemp:* Nature 221 (1969) S. 829.
[4] *McEwan, H. P.:* J. Obst. Gyn. Brit. Cwth. 76 (1969) S. 809.
[5] *Scheidegger, J. J.:* Int. Arch. Allergy 7 (1955) S. 103.

Die Serum-Elektrolytveränderungen während der physiologischen Schwangerschaft

M. Bletka

II. Universitäts-Frauenklinik der Karls Universität, Prag, CSSR

Eine kurze Zusammenfassung unserer Arbeit:

1. In unserem Forschungsplan widmen wir jetzt unsere Aufmerksamkeit den Konzentrationsveränderungen einiger Serum-Elektrolyte während der Schwangerschaft.
2. Wir benützen zur Untersuchung „flame atomic spectrometry".
3. Wir studieren die Serum-Konzentrationsveränderungen folgender Electrolyte: Natrium, Calcium, Magnesium, Cuprum, Ferrum, Zincum.
4. Wir verfolgen die Veränderungen im Laufe der physiologischen Schwangerschaft vom 2. bis 10. Monat und vergleichen die Resultate mit den Befunden bei gesunder Nichtschwangeren (NeT: G_2–G_{10}).
5. Die Ergebnisse wurden statistisch gesichert (95% Wahrscheinlichkeit) und sind ad a / in der Tab. 1 zusammengestellt (mg %)
   ad b / graphisch dargestellt (mE/L).
6. Diese Veränderungen sind statistisch signifikant:
   Natrium – Die Senkung der Serumkonzentration im 7. Monate. Die Erhöhung der Serumkonzentration im 8. Monate.
   Calcium und Magnesium – die Erniedrigung der Serumkonzentration im Laufe der Schwangerschaft gegen den Nichtschwangeren.
   Kupfer – Der Anstieg der Serumkonzentration im Laufe der Schwangerschaft.
7. Die Ursachen dieser Veränderungen sind sehr kompliziert; sie resultieren aus manigfaltigen Schwangerschaftseinflüssen.
8. Sie stellen den Ausgangspunkt für unsere weitere Forschungsarbeit dar.

Tab. 1. The changes of the concentration of some serum-electrolytes in the course of pregnancy.

Group	Number of investigations	Natrium mg %	Calcium mg %	Magnesium mg %	Cuprum mg %	Ferrum mg %	Zincum mg %
Non-gravidae	7	307.1 ± 14.6	12.29 ± 0.33	2.50 ± 0.17	0.127 ± 0.011	0.089 ± 0.024	0.170 ± 0.055
Grav. m. II.	25	296.1 ± 4.35	10.09 ± 0.30	2.09 ± 0.09	0.156 ± 0.019	0.146 ± 0.016	0.182 ± 0.029
Grav. m. III.	46	301.5 ± 5.32	10.13 ± 0.30	2.07 ± 0.04	0.205 ± 0.017	0.194 ± 0.023	0.209 ± 0.025
Grav. m. IV.	11	300.6 ± 11.8	10.37 ± 0.46	2.14 ± 0.15	0.235 ± 0.022	0.149 ± 0.062	0.135 ± 0.040
Grav. m. V.	12	304.7 ± 5.6	9.93 ± 0.30	2.05 ± 0.10	0.221 ± 0.025	0.181 ± 0.093	0.185 ± 0.064
Grav. m. VI.	9	291.6 ± 8.9	10.14 ± 0.15	2.12 ± 0.12	0.273 ± 0.025	0.139 ± 0.056	0.131 ± 0.018
Grav. m. VII.	12	293.5 ± 6.2	9.90 ± 0.64	2.13 ± 0.12	0.254 ± 0.033	0.130 ± 0.041	0.145 ± 0.044
Grav. m. VIII.	21	305.2 ± 5.1	10.29 ± 0.54	2.11 ± 0.07	0.269 ± 0.023	0.115 ± 0.020	0.120 ± 0.019
Grav. m. IX.	30	302.2 ± 4.5	10.60 ± 0.39	2.10 ± 0.07	0.260 ± 0.022	0.087 ± 0.016	0.132 ± 0.028
Grav. m. X.	14	300.3 ± 8.3	10.47 ± 0.69	2.11 ± 0.08	0.266 ± 0.014	0.106 ± 0.027	0.144 ± 0.034
Oedema of pregnancy							
Grav. m. VIII.	8	309.3 ± 5.3	11.83 ± 0.38	2.30 ± 0.18	0.268 ± 0.026	0.097 ± 0.023	0.132 ± 0.015
Grav. m. IX.	11	300.2 ± 6.7	10.80 ± 0.78	2.15 ± 0.21	0.265 ± 0.045	0.098 ± 0.036	0.151 ± 0.055
Grav. m. X.	25	301.2 ± 6.3	10.70 ± 0.59	2.18 ± 0.10	0.274 ± 0.023	0.099 ± 9.016	0.137 ± 0.030

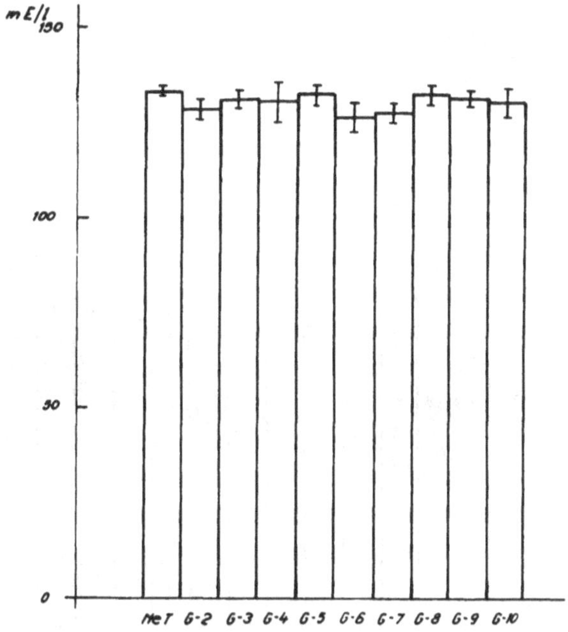

Abb. 1. [Na^+]

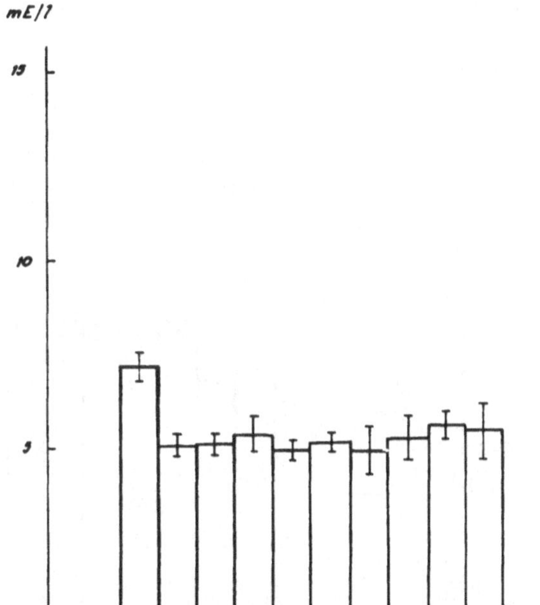

Abb. 2. [Ca^{++}]

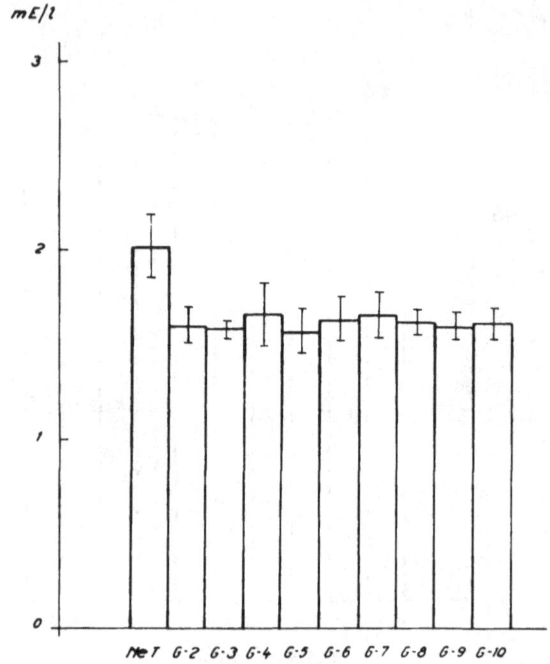

Abb. 3. [Mg^{++}]

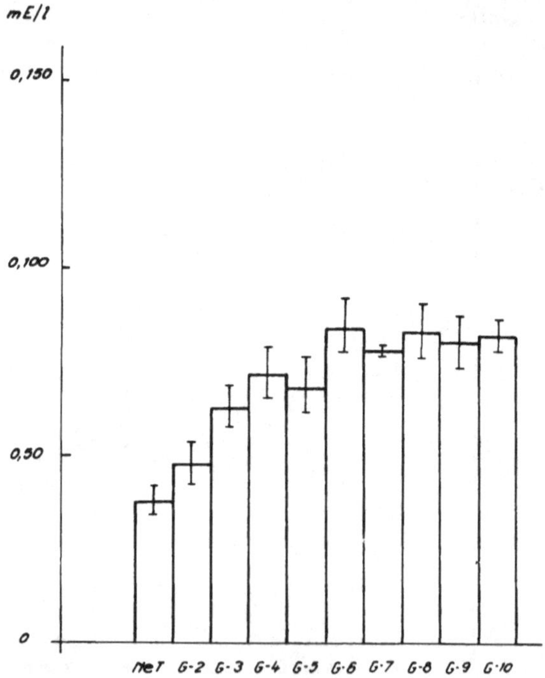

Abb. 4. [Cu^{++}]

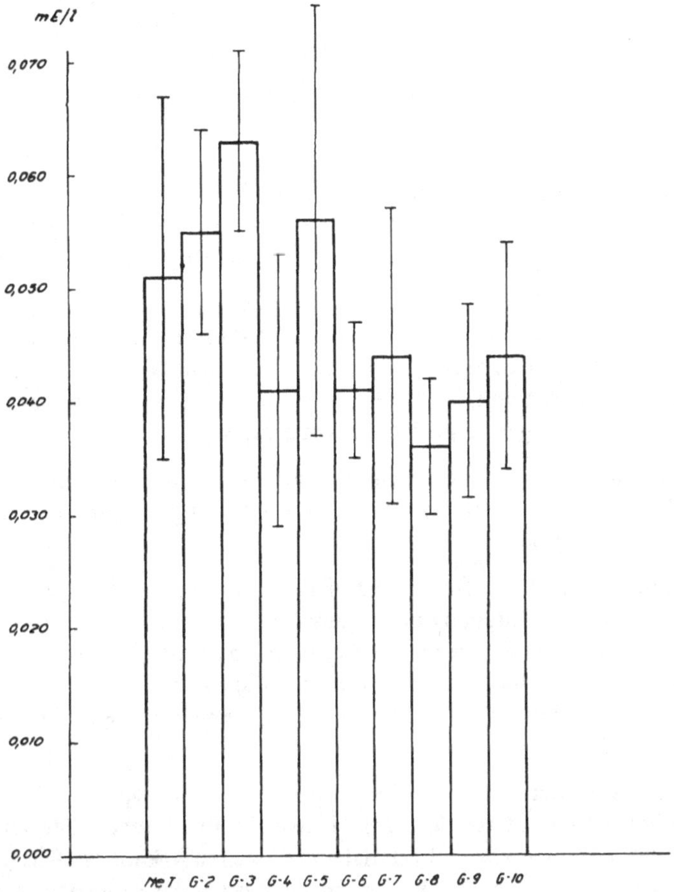
mE/l
0,070
0,060
0,050
0,040
0,030
0,020
0,010
0,000
MeT
G·2
G·3
G·4
G·5
G·6
G·7
G·8
G·9
G·10

Abb. 5. [Zn^{++}]

Arteriovenous Kininogen in Toxemic Pregnancies

P. Periti, V. Levi D'Ancona and *S. Severi*

Clinica Ostetrica e Ginecologica dell' Università, Firenze, Italia

In a previous communication (*Periti* and *Gasparri,* 1965) we reported that the blood of a pregnant woman in her third trimester shows a significant difference between the kininogen contents of the arterial and venous plasma. The mean of this difference is 1000 μg/ml, in favour of the former.

We later reported (*Gasparri* and *Periti,* 1969) the data referring to a small number of cases of late pregnancy toxemias, in which the mean values of the arterial and venous kininogen did not differ significantly. We have controlled the behaviour of arterio-venous kininogen in a larger number of toxemia cases.

We know that when *in vitro* blood is cooled there is a decrease in kininogen (*Armstrong,* 1965). A decrease of barely 10°C gives rise to a significant depletion of kininogen (*Melmon,* 1968).

Since the methods used by us from 1962 to 1968 for plasma kininogen assay (*Diniz,* 1963) did not foresee maintaining blood samples at body temperature from the moment the blood was drawn until it was used in laboratory, we decided to carry out controls. The blood was drawn with a warmed syringe and immediately transferred to test tubes placed in a bath at 38°C. Samples of the same blood were kept as controls at room temperature.

In Fig. 1.33 cases of normal or pathological pregnancies are reported. The women were hospitalized in the Clinica Ostetrica of the University of Florence. The values of kininogen in 86 blood samples (33 arterial and 53 venous), kept at 38°C (the mean value is 6.9 μg/ml) are shown on the left. On the right is the kininogen of a few of the same samples of blood (20 arterial and 44 venous), kept at room temperature (the mean value this time is 5.2 μg/ml). The time lag between the moment the blood was drawn and the time it was used for kininogen assay ranges from a minimum of 15 to a maximum of 120 minutes. The difference between the two mean kininogen values, directly related to the different storage temperature, is significant (P was calculated according to Student's t). The kininogen depletion, caused by the cooling of the blood samples at room temperature, is the same in arterial and in venous blood and mostly occurs during the first 15 minutes after drawing the blood.

A period of 15 minutes (which is often the time needed for taking the blood to the laboratory, centrifugating it and waiting for the separation of plasma) at room tempe-

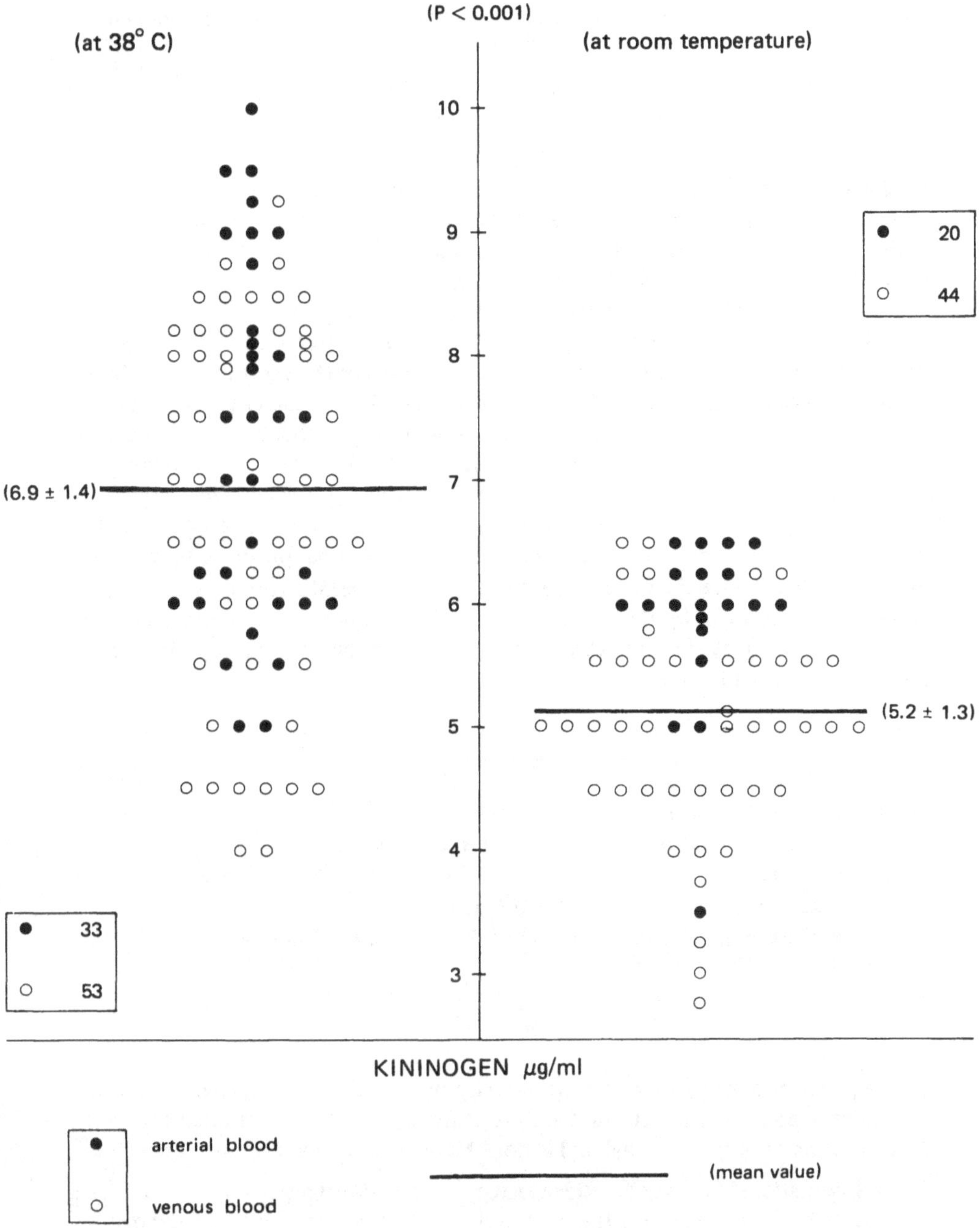

normal and toxemic pregnancies during the 3rd. trimester

Fig. 1

rature (and in any case below 38°C) is enough to cause a depletion of kininogen of about 30%.

The conclusion we have reached is that for plasma kininogen assay the blood should be drawn and kept at a temperature of 38°C until the plasma is used.

Fig. 2 refers to 20 cases of toxemia, characterized by edema, proteinuria and hypertension (EPH-Gestosis), and 12 healthy women in their third trimester of pregnancy with a normal course. On the average, the two groups of cases do not show differences in the arterial plasma kininogen level (7.3 for the toxemic cases, 7.1 for the normal ones). The kininogen contents in the venous blood are, instead, different (6.6 and 5.5 respectively). The arteriovenous ratio is therefore much higher in the cases of normal pregnancy (7.1/5.5). In other words, the difference between the mean kininogen value in the arterial blood and in the venous blood is significant (P according to Student's t) for the cases of normal pregnancies, but not for toxemic pregnancies. Presuming that the blood is subjected to kininogenase activation in the peripheral vascular walls and that this activation is reflected by the kininogen depletion, we could therefore reach the conclusion that in the case of toxemia this activation is reduced. We cannot as yet explain the significant difference between the mean values of the arterial and of the venous plasma kininogen during the third trimester of normal pregnancies. We can therefore only advance the simple hypothesis that in cases of toxemia the condition of the tissues expressed by the edema and the microcirculatory pathology characterizing the syndrome may, in some way, be tied to the missing or reduced peripheral depletion of plasma kininogen.

References

Armstrong, D. and *G. L. Mills:* Physiol. 170 (1065) p. 89 P.

Diniz, C. R. and *I. F. Carvalho:* Ann. N.Y. Acad. Sci. 104 (1963) p. 77.

Gasparri F., P. Periti: in „Die Spätgestose", S. 119. Schwabe & Co, Basel, Stuttgart (1969).

Melmon, K. L. et al.: J. Clin. Invest. 47 (1968) p. 1295.

Periti, P., F. Gasparri: in „Hypotensive Peptides", S. 536. Springer-Verlag, New York Inc. (1966).

Summary

During pregnancy the plasma kininogen level progressively increases, reaching levels which rise to above normal during the third trimester. At the end of pregnancy a difference can be seen in arterial and venous kininogen, with a ratio over one.

At the International Meeting on EPH-Gestosis (Basle, 1969) we reported that during serious late pregnancy toxemia the ratio between the two types of blood decreases, reaching a non-significant value; the difference, that is, between arterial and venous kininogen is annulled.

We had recently observed that the values obtained for plasma kininogen were considerably higher if blood was drawn with a warm syringe and kept at 38°C until

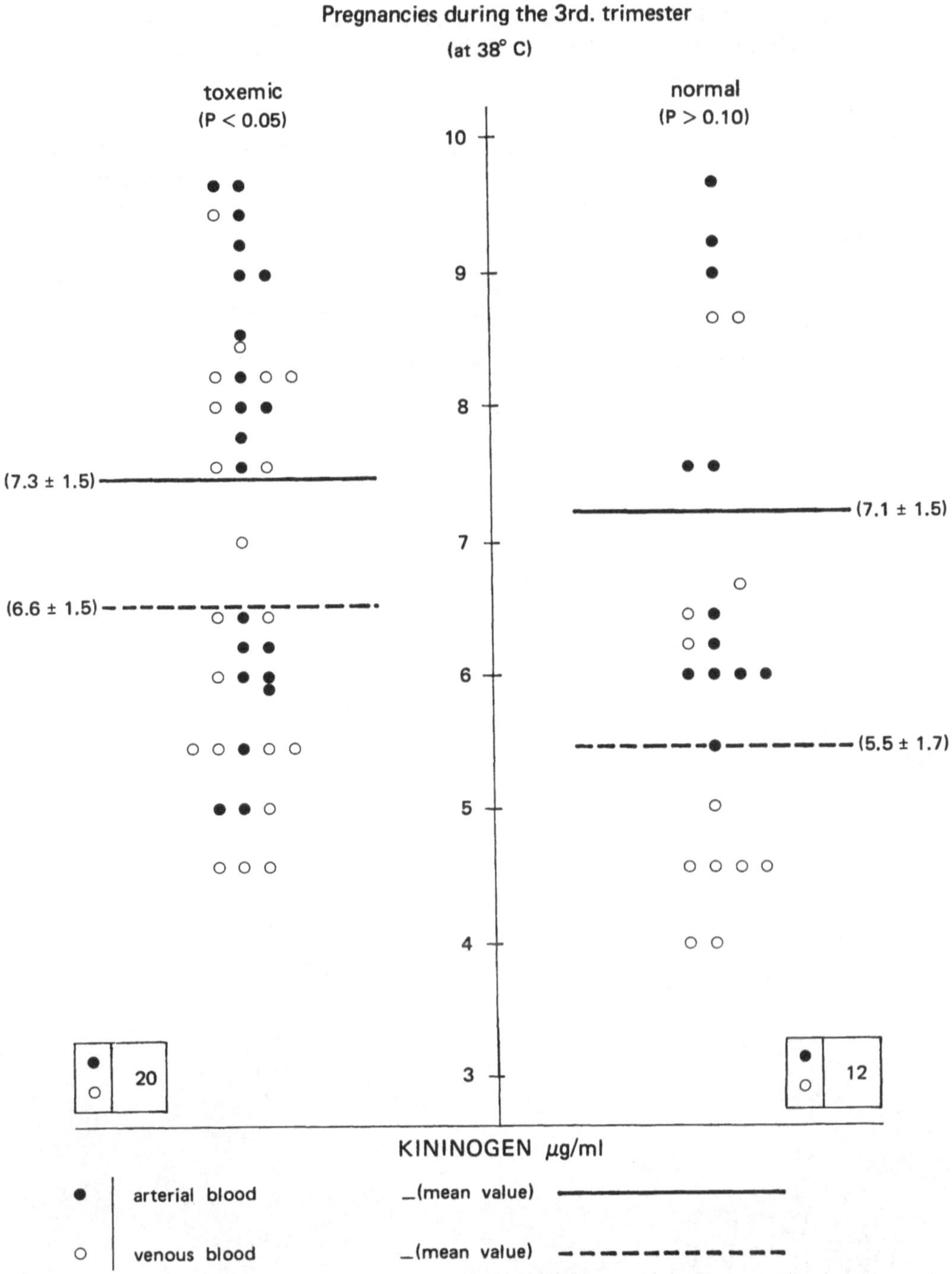
Pregnancies during the 3rd. trimester
(at 38° C)
toxemic
(P < 0.05)
normal
(P > 0.10)
10
9
8
7
6
5
4
3
(7.3 ± 1.5)
(6.6 ± 1.5)
(7.1 ± 1.5)
(5.5 ± 1.7)
20
12
KININOGEN µg/ml
arterial blood
venous blood
(mean value)
(mean value)

Fig. 2

use, rather than if the procedure was carried out at room temperature (14–22°C). We therefore reached the conclusion that the cooling of blood samples is to be considered an error which may lead to variations of over a third of the true value of plasma kininogen.

Further assays of arterial and venous kininogen have now been carried out, withdrawing blood and keeping it at 38°C until laboratory use. The results previously reported can be confirmed (the values obtained with this procedure being double those obtained with the room temperature procedure):

Arterial and venous kininogen (μg/ml) in pregnancies during the 3rd trimester.

Pregnancies	arterial blood	venous blood	P
Normal	7.1 ± 1.5	5.5 ± 1.7	> 0.10
Toxemic	7.3 ± 1.5	6.6 ± 1.5	< 0.05

Immunoglobulins in Normal Pregnancy and EPH-Gestosis

J. W. W. Studd, M.D., M.R.C.O.G.

Birmingham Maternity Hospital, England

The concentration of albumin and individual $alpha_1$, $alpha_2$ and beta globulins in the serum of patients with normal pregnancy and EPH-gestosis has previously been reported using the technique of Laurell immunoelectrophoresis (*Studd* et al., 1970 A, 1970 B). They claim that the depression of albumin and transferrin and elevation of the larger proteins $alpha_2$ macroglobulin and beta lipoprotein are identical to the changes in serum protein concentration in patients with nephrotic syndrome. There is little information about the immunoglobulins in normal and abnormal pregnancy and the purpose of this study was to establish normal values for the serum concentrations of these proteins and to investigate the effect that heavy proteinuria has upon these values.

Patients and methods

Ten normotensive patients with normal single pregnancies were investigated serially through pregnancy, blood being taken by venepuncture at 8 weeks and 30 weeks gestation, at term and also at three months postpartum.

Four patients with confirmed nephrotic syndrome with a urinary protein loss of 6 to 13 g per day were studied towards the end of their pregnancy.

Eighteen patients with severe pre-eclampsia who had a blood pressure of 160/110 mm/Hg or more and heavy proteinuria were also studied. The majority of these patients had a urinary protein loss in excess of 5 g per 24 hours.

The immunoglobulins IgG, IgA, IgM and IgD were estimated by the *Mancini* method of immunodiffusion using a specific anti-serum obtained from the Department of Experimental Pathology, University of Birmingham.

Results

The mean concentration and standard deviations of immunoglobulins and the serial study of normal pregnancy is shown in Tab. 1. The mean of the normal term pregnancies and the mean concentration from the 18 patients with pre-eclampsia and the four with nephrotic syndrome are shown in Tab. 2. The statistical significance of these differences is given in Tab. 3.

Tab. 1. Mean concentration and standard deviation of serum IgG, IgA, IgM, IgD, in normal pregnancy (mg per 100 ml).

	8 weeks	20 weeks	30 weeks	40 weeks	3 months postpartum
IgG	1100	972	948	826	1304
S.D.	430	381	385	269	369
IgA	257	256	272	254	322
S.D.	109	80	109	82	125
IgM	100.2	134.7	120	85	106
S.D.	64.7	101	89	38	63
IgD	11	11.2	11.25	15.2	8.6
S.D.	8.5	9.9	10.2	10.6	12

Tab. 2. Mean and standard deviation of concentration of serum immunoglobulins in normal pregnancy at term, pre-eclampsia and pregnancy complicated by nephrotic syndrome (mg per 100 ml).

	Normal pregnancy at term	Pre-eclampsia	Nephrotic syndrome
n	10	18	4
IgG	826	559	580
S.D.	262	202	155
IgA	254	292	241
S.D.	82	146	88
IgM	85	115	123
S.D.	38	76	51.7
IgD	15.2	6.62	5.7
S.D.	10.6	6.82	6.5

Tab. 3. Significance of differences of serum immunoglobulin concentration in normal pregnancy, pre-eclampsia and pregnancy complicated by nephrotic syndrome.

	Non-pregnant X late pregnancy	Late pregnancy X pre-eclampsia	Pre-eclampsia X nephrotic syndrome
IgG	$p < 0.001$	$p < 0.01$	N.S.
IgA	$p < 0.05$	N.S.	N.S.
IgM	N.S.	N.S.	N.S.
IgD	$p < 0.01$	$p < 0.01$	N.S.

It can be seen that in normal pregnancy there is a depression in the serum concentration of IgG and an elevation in the serum concentration of IgD. The concentrations of IgA and IgM are unaltered throughout pregnancy. When proteinuria complicates pregnancy there is a further depression in serum IgG and the serum IgD falls to below non-pregnant values. Both proteins have a molecular weight of 160 000 and would be expected to be lost in the urine. Certainly IgG is invariably found in the urine in EPH-Gestosis. The serum immunoglobulin concentration changes in pre-eclampsia are all similar to those found in nephrotic syndrome which again draws attention to the biochemical similarities in these two conditions. The depression of IgG is notable and may pre-dispose to infection during pregnancy as is the case when pregnancy is complicated by nephrotic syndrome (*Studd* and *Blainey*, 1969).

These identical serum protein changes in nephrotic syndrome and pre-eclampsia suggest a comparable mechanism of protein loss from the serum into the urine. The proteinuria of pre-eclampsia results from a glomerular loss of protein rather than an inability of the tubules to re-absorb proteins of low molecular weight from the glomerular filtrate and immunoclearance studies of this glomerular proteinuria show a very poorly selective proteinuria similar to that found in membranous glomerulonephritis and renal vein thrombosis (*Studd*, 1971). A striking pathological feature of pre-eclamptic nephropathy is the massive deposition of fibrin within the basement membrane and endothelial cells and it is considered to be significant that this "intrarenal thrombosis" produces by molecular sieving of proteins the same character of proteinuria as is found in renal vein thrombosis.

References

Studd, J. W. W. and *J. D. Blainey:* "Pregnancy and the Nephrotic Syndrome". Brit. Med. J. 1 (1969) p. 276.

Studd, J. W. W., J. D. Blainey and *D. E. Bailey* (1970A): "A Study of Serum Protein changes in late Pregnancy and identification of the Pregnancy Zone Protein using Antigen Antibody crossed Immunoelectrophoresis". J. Obs. Gynae. of the British Commonwealth 77 (1970A) p. 42.

Studd, J. W. W., J. D. Blainey and *D. E. Bailey* (1970B): "Serum Protein changes in the Pre-eclampsia-Eclampsia Syndrome". J. Obs. Gynae. of the British Commonwealth 77 (1970B) p. 796.

Studd, J. W. W., M. D. Thesis: University of Birmingham. "Serum Proteins in Pregnancy" (1971).

Hormone–Findings in Gestosis

Vergleichende Untersuchungen über den Aussagewert der Oestriolausscheidung im 24/h-Urin und des Dehydroepiandosteronsulfat-Belastungstests mit Hinzuziehung der histologischen Placentabefunde

H. von der Crabben, Ch. Werner

Universitätsfrauenklinik, Düsseldorf, BRD

Die Placenta ist nicht in der Lage, Östrogene de novo zu synthetisieren, da ihr die hierfür erforderlichen Enzymsysteme fehlen. Sie ist vielmehr auf die zu 80% vom Feten und zu 20% von der Mutter gebildeten Precursoren, vor allem des DHEA-S, angewiesen. *Lauritzen* entwickelte folgenden Belastungstest: Er ließ die Patientin einen 24/h-Urin sammeln, injizierte ihr dann 30 mg DHEA-S i.v. und bestimmte sowohl in der ersten, als auch in einer darauf folgenden zweiten 24/h-Urinportion die Östriolausscheidung. Wir modifizierten diesen Test, so daß er sich jetzt als klinischer Test bei Verdacht auf Vorliegen einer Placentainsuffizienz bewährt hat.

Nach Sammlung einer 2-Stunden-Urinportion zur Bestimmung der Östriolausgangslage erfolgt die Applikation von 50 mg DHEA-S i.v. In vier anschließend gesammelten Zweistunden-Urin-Portionen wird die Östriolausscheidung bestimmt. Handelt es sich um eine normal verlaufende Schwangerschaft, so findet eine optimale Metabolisierung des Precursors zu Östriol – ca. 25%–40% – in den ersten zwei Stunden nach Applikation des DHEA-S statt. Besteht dagegen eine leicht eingeschränkte bzw. pathologische Funktion der feto-placentaren Einheit, so wird das Maximum der Östriolausscheidung erst 4 h bzw. 6 h nach Applikation des Precursors beobachtet, und man spricht von verzögertem bzw. pathologischem Belastungstest.

Die Brauchbarkeit des Funktionstests zeigen unsere Untersuchungen mit markiertem DHEA-S. Wir verabreichten 0,5 mc Tritium markiertes DHEA-S mit einer Aktivität von 311 mC/mM einer gesunden Schwangeren und einer Patientin mit allen Zeichen einer hochgradigen Placentainsuffizienz, die auch histologisch verifiziert werden konnte.

Die Meßdaten zeigen – es wurde Östriol H^3 bestimmt – daß bei einer normalen Funktion der feto-placentaren Einheit, histologisch post partum gesichert, die maximale Umwandlung des Östrogen-precursors innerhalb der ersten beiden Stunden stattfindet, dagegen bei Vorliegen einer Placentainsuffizienz diese Umwandlung deutlich verzögert ist.

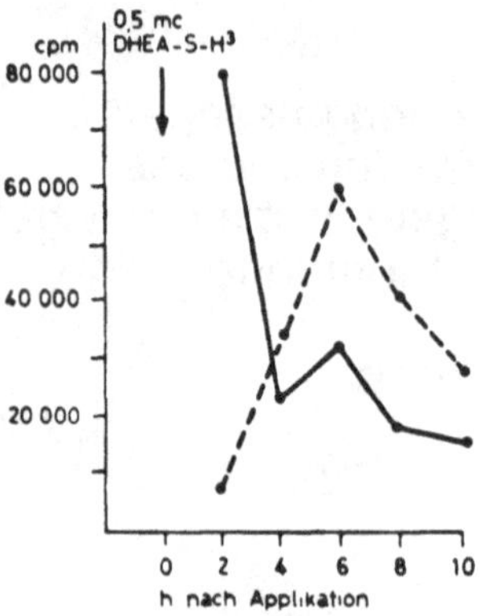

Abb. 1

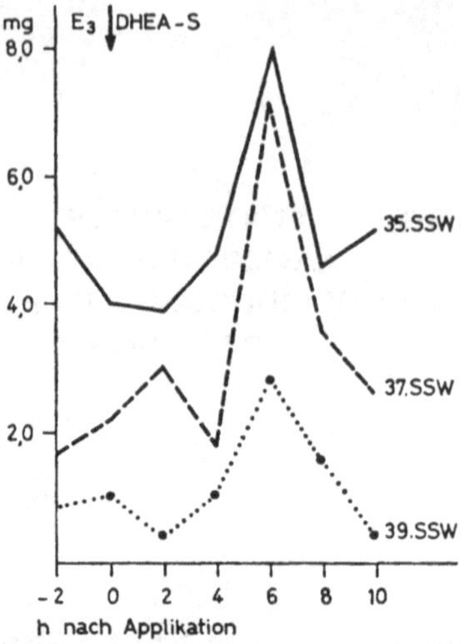

Abb. 2

Damit ist die Aussagekraft des Belastungstests keinesfalls schon erschöpft. Besteht nämlich eine fortschreitende, hochgradige Placentainsuffizienz, z. B. bei schwerer EPH-Gestose, so findet sich nicht nur eine Verzögerung der Metabolisierung in der Zeiteinheit, sondern sogar eine Verringerung der Östriolausscheidung, aus der auf den Grad der fetalen Gefährdung geschlossen werden kann, wenn man diesen Test in mehrtägigen Intervallen durchführt.

DHEA-S-Test Gruppe	N	Morphologisch nachgewiesene Placentainsuffizienz Klasse 1	Klasse 2	Klasse 3
1	66	42	23	1
2	69	21	42	6
3	66	16	32	18
Summe	201	79	97	25

Abb. 3. DHEA-S-Test Ergebnisse und morphologische Placentabefunde

Bei der Auswertung von 200 durchgeführten DHEA-S-Belastungstests sahen wir bei 66 der Fälle mit pathologischem Ausfall (DHEA-S-Testgruppe 3) in 50 d. h. in 75,8% ($p < 0{,}001$) eine mittelgradige bis hochgradige histologisch von *Werner* nachgewiesene Placentainsuffizienz in Form von Reifungsretardierung (Placentaklasse 2 und 3); in

16 d. h. 24,2% war eine reife Placenta nachzuweisen (Placentaklasse 1). Bei normalem Ausfall des DHEA-S-Belastungstests waren in 42 Fällen d. h. in 63,6% ($p < 0{,}001$) reife Placenten histologisch nachzuweisen, aber in 24 Fällen d. h. 36,4% waren morphologische Veränderungen vorhanden. Bei histologisch nachgewiesener hochgradiger Reifungsretardierung der Placenta fanden wir in 72% einen pathologischen DHEA-S-Test. Das bedeutet, daß wir mit diesem Test in der Mehrzahl der Fälle schon frühzeitig eine Placentainsuffizienz erkennen können.

Bei 35 Patientinnen wurden gleichzeitig Östriolbestimmungen im 24/h-Urin und DHEA-S-Belastungstests ab 30. Woche durchgeführt. Alle Placenten wurden post partum histologisch untersucht. Von den 35 Patientinnen hatten 26 eine EPH-Gestose.

Placenta-histologie	DHEA-S-Test norm.	DHEA-S-Test pathol.	Östriol-norm	24 h pathol.
reif	16	5	21	1
reifungsretard.	0	14	12	1

Abb. 4. Ergebnisse des DHEA-S-Tests und der Östriolbestimmung im 24/h-Urin im Vergleich zur Plazentahistologie

Aus der Abbildung geht hervor, daß bei normalem DHEA-S-Belastungstest in 16 Fällen histologisch eine reife und in keinem Fall eine reifungsretardierte Placenta diagnostiziert wurde. Bei pathologischem Ausfall des DHEA-S-Tests fanden wir in 5 Fällen eine unauffällige und in 14 Fällen eine reifungsretardierte Placenta. Die Östriolausscheidung dagegen zeigte bei normalen Werten 21 mal eine reife und 8 mal eine reifungsretardierte Placenta. Nur in 2 Fällen sahen wir pathologische Ausscheidungswerte, in 1 Fall handelte es sich um einen intrauterinen Fruchttod.

Von den 5 pathologischen DHEA-S-Tests mit reifer Placenta waren 3 Kinder dystroph. Hier scheint eine fetale Störung vorgelegen zu haben. Es zeigt sich, daß man mit dem DHEA-S-Test eine Placentainsuffizienz schon dann erkennen kann, wenn die Östriolausscheidungswerte noch im Bereich der Norm liegen. Ein verzögerter Belastungstest wird sich klinisch selten einmal negativ auswirken, da die feto-placentare Einheit imstande ist, Störungen kompensatorisch voll auszugleichen, so daß unter Normalbedingungen keine Gefahr für das Kind zu erwarten ist. Bei Vorliegen eines pathologischen Belastungstests kann durchaus noch mit kompensatorischen Maßnahmen der feto-placentaren Einheit gerechnet werden, doch kann bei einer schon geringen Stressreaktion es zu einer Dekompensation des kindlichen Kreislaufs und damit zum intrauterinen Fruchttod kommen.

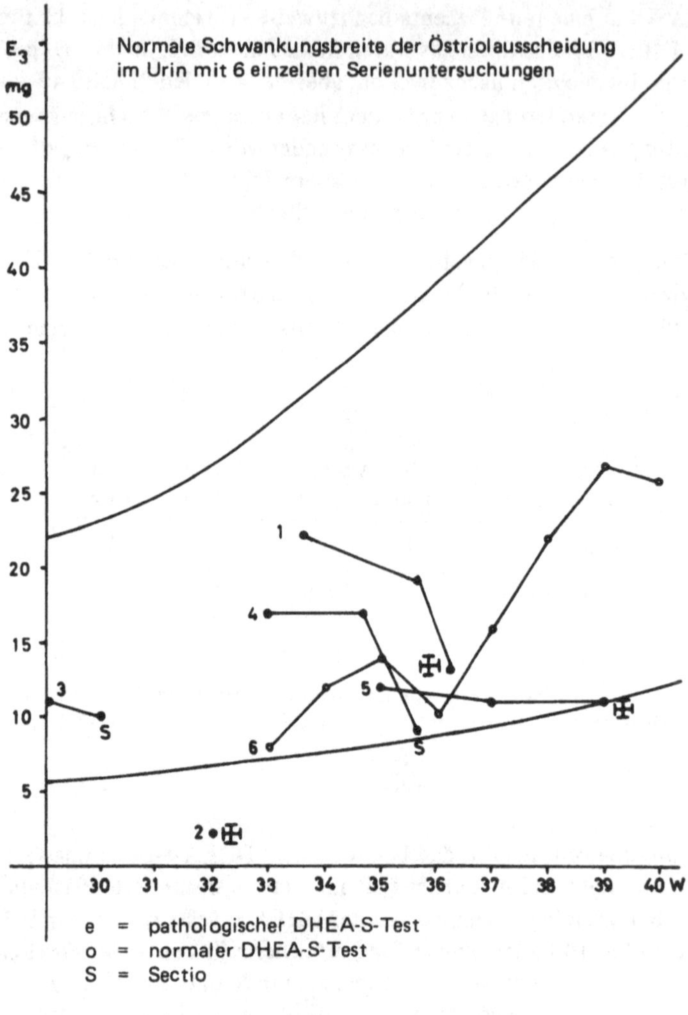

Abb. 5. Normale Schwankungsbreite der Östriolausscheidung im Urin mit 6 einzelnen Serienuntersuchungen

Auf diesem Dia sind einige typische Verlaufskurven dargestellt. Die einzelnen Punkte stellen die Östriolausscheidungswerte im 24/h-Urin dar, wobei ein schwarzer Punkt einen pathologischen Ausfall und ein Kreis einen normalen Ausfall des gleichzeitig durchgeführten DHEA-S-Tests darstellt. Wir sehen, daß bei pathologischen Verlaufskurven der 24/h Östriolausscheidung der DHEA-S-Test schon pathologisch ausfällt, wenn sich die Östriolausscheidungswerte noch im Bereich der Norm befinden. Wir erhalten damit schon 3 Wochen eher einen Hinweis auf eine bestehende Placentainsuffizienz.

Beim Vergleich des DHEA-S-Tests mit der 24/h-Östriolausscheidung können wir feststellen, daß der DHEA-S-Test mit einer Bestimmung schon frühzeitig eine beginnende Placentainsuffizienz anzeigt. Die normalen Östriolausscheidungswerte im 24/h-Urin bei pathologischem DHEA-S-Test können bedeuten, daß es sich hier um eine noch kompensierte Placentainsuffizienz handelt. Diese Fälle überwachen wir mit der Cardiotokographie intensiv. Die Bestimmung der 24/h Östriolausscheidung im Urin alleine hat den Nachteil, daß sich erst bei Zusammenbruch der Placentafunktion ein Abfall der Ausscheidungswerte zeigt, in einem Moment also, wo das Kind schon einer erhöhten Gefährdung ausgesetzt ist. Außerdem kann mit einem Wert keine Aussage gemacht werden, man muß also einen weiteren Wert abwarten und verliert dadurch kostbare Zeit. Eine Kombination beider Methoden ist daher sinnvoll, denn man kann bei pathologischem Ausfall des DHEA-S-Tests kombiniert mit einem Abfall der Östriolausscheidung und unter Hinzuziehen der Cardiotokographie eine erhöhte Gefährdung des Feten sicherer erkennen.

Actions of Prolactin on Human Renal Function

D. F. Horrobin

University College Nairobi, Dept. of Medical Physiology, Nairobi, Kenya

Prolactin is a hormone of major importance in the regulation of fluid and electrolyte balance in fishes, amphibians and birds but its role in this area has received little attention from those concerned with mammalian and human function. *Lockett* and co-workers demonstrated some years ago that in the perfused cat kidney and in the conscious intact rat growth hormones and prolactins from several sources could produce renal retention of water, sodium and potassium.

These findings are of potential human clinical importance. Prolactin has a role in lactation, it is secreted at the end of the human menstrual cycle and large amounts of prolactin-like material of placental origin are produced during pregnancy. *Becks* group in Montreal have recently shown that pituitary prolactin output also rises several fold during human pregnancy. We therefore decided to investigate the action of prolactin on human renal function. We used sheep pituitary prolactin which in unpublished work *Becks* group has shown to be very closely related to both placental lactogen and human pituitary prolactin.

Five male Europeans took part in the experiments. With each experiment no food was taken after 22 h the previous night. Between 6 and 6.30 in the morning each subject drank a litre of fluid. At 7 and every half hour thereafter the bladder was emptied, the volume of urine measured and an equivalent amount of water drunk back. Within about two hours a steady state was reached with the half hourly urine volumes remaining approximately constant. The sodium and potassium concentrations and pH of each urine sample were estimated. At 11 a.m. each subject was given an intramuscular injection of prolactin or distilled water which caused pain similar to that caused by the prolactin. Half hourly urine collections were continued until 18 h. Between 18 and 20 h each subject ate a standardised meal. The bladder was emptied at 23 h and again the following morning at 8 h. The urine was analysed and mean half hourly overnight excretion rates for water sodium and potassium were estimated.

Experiments were run on four separate days at least 72 hours apart. Each subject received two control and two prolactin injections. On one control day and on one prolactin day blood samples were taken from each subject immediately before the injection and 2 and 6 hours later. Plasma sodium, potassium and osmolality were measured.

The dose of prolactin used was 8 mg. If this had been injected intravenously and diluted only by the plasma volume the peak concentration would have been about 3 microg/ml (μg/ml) as compared to a placental lactogen concentration near term of around 8–10 microg/ml.

The prolactin caused retention of water, sodium, and potassium, a rise in plasma sodium and a rise in plasma osmolality in all subjects. The changes in water excretion are shown in Fig. 1. The control experiments showed a steady decline presumably due to water loss from extra-renal sources. Prolactin caused a very sharp drop in water excretion during the first hour. After this water excretion rose to a plateau which was nevertheless significantly below control values. The initial sharp drop was similar to the action of ADH but the manufacturers (*Ferring, Sweden*) claimed that the preparation was ADH-free and we have not been able to find any evidence of its presence using paper chromatography. The prolactin itself may have ADH-like action or it may stimulate ADH release from the pituitary.

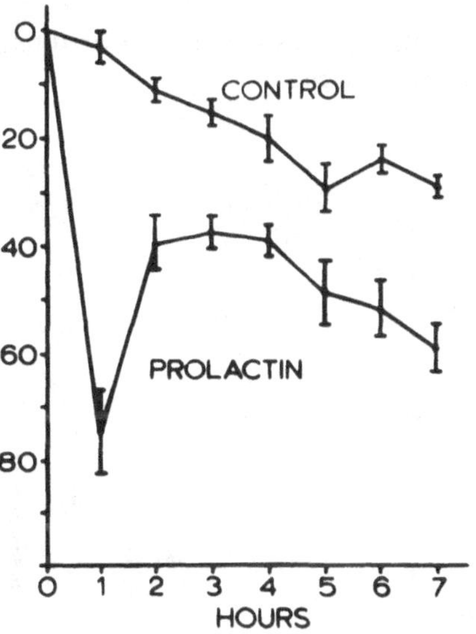

Fig. 1. Percentage change in water excretion

The control sodium excretion rate (Fig. 2) showed an initial steady decline followed by a rise in the late afternoon. This pattern may be accounted for by the normal diurnal variation in adrenal steroid secretion rates which are at their lowest in the afternoon. After prolactin treatment sodium excretion was consistently lower and failed to show the late afternoon rise.

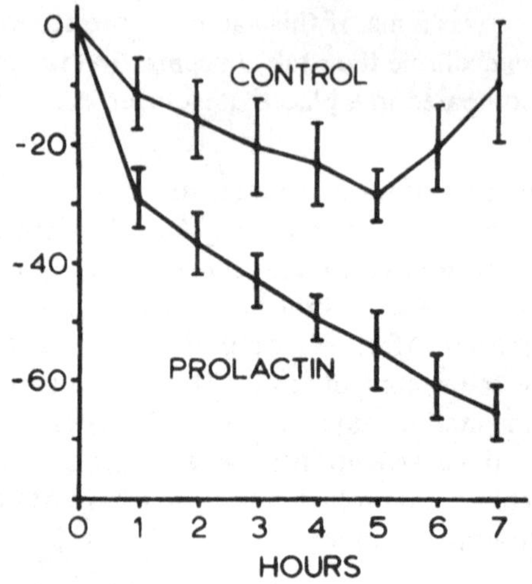

Fig. 2. Percentage change in sodium excretion

Prolactin also caused retention of potassium as compared to control (Fig. 3) although in this case the effect was less striking.

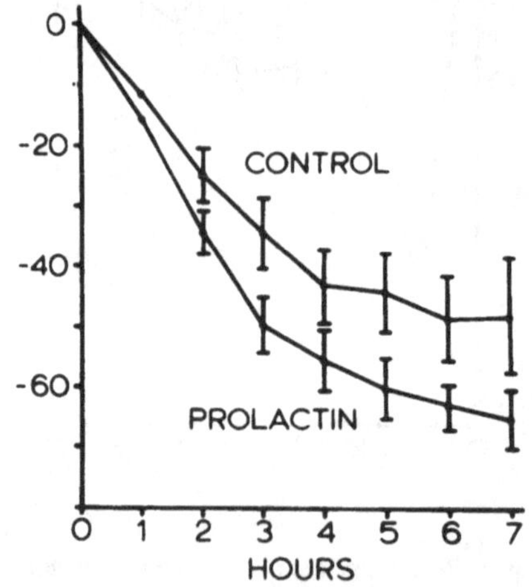

Fig. 3. Percentage change in potassium excretion

During the six hours after prolactin injection the mean plasma sodium concentration rose from 140.20 to 147.00 mEq/L. During the same period the mean plasma osmolality rose from 351.40 to 360.80 mosmoles/L. During the same period, although they were well hydrated with hourly urine volumes of over half a litre, most subjects had strong subjective sensations of thirst. Those changes could not be accounted for by a relatively greater renal retention of sodium than of water. They could be accounted for if prolactin caused a movement of water into cells. The sodium, potassium and water retention persisted for 12–18 hours.

It seems possible therefore that prolactin and placental lactogen may have profound effects on fluid and electrolyte balance in pregnancy. There is no need to stress the possible importance of this finding for our understanding of gestosis.

Determination of Newer Oestrogens – Physiopathological Importance, Diagnostic and Prognostic Value and Methodological Limits

J. Stastny, L. Dubey

Clinique Universitaire de Gynécologie et d'Obstétrique, Laboratoire d'Hormonologie, Genève, Suisse

During the past decade a considerable amount of informations on the biosynthesis, catabolism, conjugation and transport of oestrogens during pregnancy has been accumulated and the concept of the placenta and foetus as two specialized compartments of an integrated functional foetoplacental unit has been established by the group associated with *Egon Diczfalusy*.

The gradual increase of urinary oestrogens during pregnancy is accompanied by elevated oestrogen levels in maternal blood, in amniotic fluid and cord blood as well as by an elevated oestriol excretion in the urine and meconium of the newborn. The oestrogen pattern of all these biological materials is dominated by oestriol.

From late pregnancy urine some 20 oestrogens have been isolated and at least 10 have been detected. (For reviews see *Diczfalusy* and *Lauritzen,* 1961; *Breuer,* 1964, 1968; *Diczfalusy* and *Mancuso,* 1969; *Klopper,* 1969; *Oakey,* 1970; *Adlercreutz* and *Luukkainen,* 1968, 1970.)

A small number of reports giving quantitative data on these oestrogens in pregnancy urine as well as on oestrogen levels in maternal plasma, cord plasma and amniotic fluid has recently been summarized by *Adlercreutz* and *Luukkainen* from methological as well as pathophysiological point of view.

Gas chromatographic determinations of 13 oestrogens in all four biological fluids and mass spectrometric identification of these compounds in maternal urine in normal, twin and anencephalic pregnancies as well as in a pregnant woman with Addison desease have recently been published by *Adlercreutz* and *Luukkainen* and made it possible to obtain a view of the origin of these oestrogen metabolites. Some of their results are listed in Tab. 1.

Comparing the oestrogen levels in the four biological fluids, the authors concluded that following oestrogens are mainly of foetal origin: oestriol, 17-epioestriol, 16α-hydroxyoestrone, 16β-hydroxyoestrone, 16-oxo-oestradiol-17β, and especialy 15α-hydroxyoestriol, which is a specific metabolite of the foetal liver and 11-dehydro-oestradiol-17α which seems to be the most specific indicator of foetal adrenal function. However, about half of the oestrone and oestradiol-17β as well as the main part of 16-epioestriol and 2-methoxyestrone are of maternal origine.

Tab. 1. Trivial names and systematic names of the steroids mentioned in this paper.

Abbreviation	Trivial name	Systematic name
E_1	Oestrone	3-Hydroxyoestra-1,3,5/10/-trien-17-one
$2\text{-}CH_3\text{-}O\text{-}E_1$	2-Methoxy-oestrone	2-Methoxy-3-hydroxyoestra-1,3,5/10/-trien-17-one
$15\alpha\text{-}OH\text{-}E_1$	15α-Hydroxy-oestrone	3,15α-Dihydroxyoestra-1,3,5/10/-trien-17-one
$16\alpha\text{-}OH\text{-}E_1$	16α-Hydroxy-oestrone	3,16α-Dihydroxyoestra-1,3,5/10/-trien-17-one
$16\beta\text{-}OH\text{-}E_1$	16β-Hydroxy-oestrone	3,16β-Dihydroxyoestra-1,3,5/10/-trien-17-one
$16\text{-}oxo\text{-}E_1$	16-Oxo-oestrone	3-Hydroxyoestra-1,3,5/10/-triene-16,17-dione
E_2	17β-Oestradiol	Oestra-1,3,5/10/-triene-3,17β-diol
$2\text{-}CH_3O\text{-}E_2$	2-Methoxy-17β-oestradiol	2-Methoxyoestra-1,3,5/10/-triene-3,17β-diol
$6\alpha\text{-}OH\text{-}E_2$	6α-Hydroxy-17β-oestradiol	Oestra-1,3,5/10/-triene-3,6α,17β-triol
$16\text{-}oxo\text{-}E_2$	16-Oxo-17β-oestradiol	3,17β-Dihydroxyoestra-1,3,5/10/-trien-16-one
$^{11}\text{-}E_2\text{-}17\alpha$	11-Dehydro-17α-oestradiol	Oestra-1,3,5/10/,11-tetraene-3,17α-diol
E_3	Oestriol	Oestra-1,3,5/10/-triene-3,16α,17β-triol
$2\text{-}MeO\text{-}E_3$	2-Methoxy-oestriol	2-Methoxyoestra-1,3,5/10/-triene-3,16α, 17β-triol
$6\text{-}OH\text{-}E_3$	6α-Hydroxy-oestriol	Oestra-1,3,5/10/-triene-3,6α,16α,17β-tetrol
$E\text{-}5\alpha\text{-}OH\text{-}E_3$	15α-Hydroxy-oestriol	Oestra-1,3,5/10/-triene-3,15α,16α,17β-tetrol
$16\text{-}Epi\text{-}E_3$	16-Epi-oestriol	Oestra-1,3,5/10/-triene-3,16β,17β-triol
$17\text{-}Epi\text{-}E_3$	17-Epi-oestriol	Oestra-1,3,5/10/-triene-3,16α,17α-triol
$16,17\text{-}Epi\text{-}E^3$	16,17-Epi-oestriol	Oestra-1,3,5/10/-triene-3,16β,17α-triol
Δ16	Oestratetrenol	Oestra-1,3,5/10/,16-tetran-3-ol
6-OH-Equilenin 3,6-ME	6-Hydroxyequilenin-3,6-dimethylether	3,6-Dihydroxyoestra-1,3,5/10/,6,8/9/-pentaen-17-one 3,6-dimethylether

The data of *Adlercreutz* and *Luukkainen* represent the recent progress in methodology and demonstrate the physiopathological as well as clinical importance of serial determinations of the newer oestrogens in clinical research. The latest development in oestrogen methodology, the combination of gas chromatography and mass spectrometry, providing the maximum of specificity, remains nevertheless reserved for basic research.

During the past decade only a few serious attempts have been made to develop suitable methods for the determination of newer oestrogens by means of classical chemical methods. Detailed studies of the experimental conditions required for the hydrolysis, extraction, purification, separation of ketonic and non-ketonic oestrogens by means of the *Girard* reaction, separation of the individual oestrogens by means of chromatography on columns, paper and thin layers as well as for the quantitative determination

Tab. 2. Oestrogens in urine, maternal plasma, cord plasma and amniotic fluid in late pregnancy and at term. (After *Adlercreutz* and *Luukkainen*, 1970).

Oestrogen	Urine /24/	Maternal Plasma /3/		Cord Plasma /5/		Amniotic Fluid /7/	
	mg/24h	μg / 1				μg / 1	
	Conjug.	Free	Conjug.	Free	Conjug.	Free	Conjug.
E_1	0.67	11.1	79.2	24.3	26.2	5.6	8.0
E_2	0.17	19.0	4.4	7.4	3.4	+	1.4
E_2-17α	0.03	–	0.9	–	+	–	–
Δ^{11}-E_2-17α	0.14	–	1.4	–	2.2	–	2.0
E_3	25.90	6.5	124.0	137.0	1260.0	56.2	932.0
17-epi-E_3	0.19	–	–	+	1.0	+	1.9
16-epi-E_3	1.14	+	6.3	1.7	5.4	–	5.7
16α-OH-E_1	2.67	0.8	27.8	2.6	46.0	2.7	24.7
16β-OH-E_1	0.72	–	4.1	1.4	9.3	–	17.8
16-oxo-E_2	1.87	0.9	15.5	3.4	60.7	3.6	26.5
2-MeO-E_1	0.07	2.2	2.1	1.4	2.8	+	+
15α-OH-E_1	0.24	+	3.4	2.7	5.5	1.0	5.5
15α-OH-E_3	2.28	–	–	–	–	–	–

/ / Values in brackets indicate numbers of determinations /pools/.
\+ Compound present, number of pools not sufficient for mean calculation.
– Compound not present in detectable amounts.

have been undertaken in order to obtain a maximum of specificity with a reasonable degree of experimental losses and other factors limiting the practical use. (For critical reviews see *Breuer*, 1964, 1968; *Nocke*, 1968; *Lisboa*, 1966; *Stoa*, 1968; *Scholler* and coll., 1966; *Preedy*, 1962.)

As far as the final detection is concerned, the *Kober* reàction of oestrogens has been extensively studied in its *colorimetric* form and optimal conditions have been established for the majority of the newer oestrogens (*Nocke*, 1961, 1964). The *fluorometrical* version of the *Kober* reaction combined with the *Ittrich* extraction of the fluorescent complex by organic solvents (*Ittrich*, 1958, 1960) has been investigated by *Scholler* and coll. Several phenolic steroids have been carefuly investigated under constant conditions of the *Kober-Ittrich* reaction. No attempt was made to find optimum reaction conditions. *Bauld* and coll., 1960 described these conditions without *Ittrich* extraction.

Tab. 3/I. Optimal conditions of the *Kober-Ittrich-Brown*-reaction. Spectral characteristics and fluorescence intensity of estrogens.

Steroid	μg	Optim. conditions				Solvent	Spectral characteristics		Fluorescence intensity		
		H_2SO_4%	T°	min	H_2O ml		$\lambda_A$max/$\lambda_E$max nm	Variation $\lambda_A$max/$\lambda_E$max with H_2SO_4 concentrat.	530/550	530/560	Solvent ratio
Δ16-			100	15		TCE	536/550	40-75% 536-537/550	98		100
estra-								80-96% 538-542/552			
tetraen-	0.05	48			1	$CHCl_3$	538/550	40-70% constant	62		63
3-ol			120	3		TBE	544/558	40-60% constant		28	29
						TCE	536/550	57-96% 536-540/550-552	59		100
								only in highest conc.			
E_3	0.1	56	125	10	1.5	$CHCl_3$	540/550	40-66% 539-540/550	37		63
						TBE	544/558	40-63% constant		18	30
17-		50				TCE	536/550	36-70% constant	62		100
epi-	0.1	50	120	20	1.5	$CHCl_3$	540/550	40-57% constant	40		65
E_3		53				TBE	544/558	40-57% constant		18	29
16-		48				TCE	536/550		74		100
epi-	0.1	50	120	15	1.5	$CHCl_3$	540/550	40-57% constant	50		67
E_3		53				TBE	544/558			24	32
16,17-		48				TCE	536/550		104		100
epi-	0.1	50	120	5	1.5	$CHCl_3$	540/550	40-57% constant	70		67
E_3		53				TBE	544/558			33	32

Tab. 3/I.

Steroid	μg	Optim. conditions				Solvent	Spectral characteristics		Fluorescence intensity		
		H_2SO_4%	T°	min	H_2O ml		$\lambda_A$max/$\lambda_E$max nm	Variation $\lambda_A$max/$\lambda_E$max with H_2SO_4 concentrat.	$\frac{530}{550}$	$\frac{530}{560}$	Solvent ratio
16α-OH-		50	110	10		TCE	536/550	36-96% constant	64		100
E_1	0.1	50			1.5	$CHCl_3$	540/550	42-70% constant	46		72
		50				TBE	544/558	42-70% constant		18	28
16β-OH-		53			1.5	TCE	538/552	30-96% constant	57		100
E_1	0.1	53	120	15	2.0	$CHCl_3$	540/552	50-63% constant	31		55
3,16-acet.		56			1.5	TBE	545/560	50-63% constant		14	25
16-CO-		56	120	10		TCE	536/550	60-96% 536-540/552	57		100
E_2	0.1	56			1.5	$CHCl_3$	539/550	50-66% constant	36		63
		56				TBE	544/559	50-66% constant		15	26
16-CO-		56	120	10		TCE	536/550	70-96% constant	56		100
E_1	2.0	56			1.5	$CHCl_3$	540/550	45-66% constant	34		61
		56				TBE	545/560	50-66% constant		16	28

Tab. 3/II.

Steroid	μg	Optimum conditions				Solvent	Spectral characteristics		Fluorescence intensity		
		H_2SO_4% /v + v/	T°	min	H_2O ml		$\lambda_A max/\lambda_E max$ nm	Variations λmax with H_2SO_4 concentr.	$\frac{560}{594}$	$\frac{570}{600}$	Solvent ratio
2-CH_3O-E_1	1.0	45			1.5	TCE	426.566/594	Activ./emiss. peaks	149		100
		53	120	5	1.0	$CHCl_3$	428.566/596	are constant under	63		42
		50			1.0	TBE	430.576/602	varying conditions. Second typical activation peak		53	36
2-CH_3O-E_2-17β		45			1.5	TCE	426.566/594	A_2 = 426–428 nm	146		100
	1.0	53	120	5	1.0	$CHCl_3$	428.566/596	in TCE and $CHCl_3$	65		42
		50			1.0	TBE	430.576/602	and A_2 = 430 in TBE A_2/A_1 = 0.06–0,08		52	36
2-CH_3O-E_3		45			1.5	TCE	426.566/594	in the three solvents	65		100
	1.0	53	120	10	1.0	$CHCl_3$	428.566/596	in optimal conditions	35		57
		50			1.0	TBE	430.576/602			25	41

Tab. 3/III.

Steroid	μg	Optimum conditions				Solvent	Spectral characteristics		Fluorescence intensity		
		H_2SO_4% /v + v/	T°	min	H_2O ml		$\lambda_A max/\lambda_E max$ nm	Variations λmax with H_2SO_4 concentrat.	530/550	530/584	Solvent ratio
6-OH-E_3	1.0	68	120 125	20 10	1.0	TCE	440, 536/584	50-68% 440/536/584 70-96%: 538-540/552-554		63	100
						$CHCl_3$	440, 540/552	56-75%: 540/550 weak		16	25
						TBE	545/562	48-63%: 546/560		8	13
6α-OH-E_2-17β	1.0	72	120	10	2.0	TCE	440, 536/552	80-96%: 540/554 68-90%: peak F_3 440/463	98		100
						$CHCl_3$	440, 538/550	$F_3 = 0$	23		24
						TBE	544/560	48-85%: 544-546/558-560 90-96%: 548-550/562 $F_3 = 0$	16		16
7α-OH-E_2-17β	1.0	72	120	10	1.5	TCE	536/550 440, 536/552, 584	36% and 90% 50-75% transitory forms 68-90% peak F_3	40		100
						$CHCl_3$	540/550	Activ. peak at 440 nm very low	17		42
						TBE	544/560	absent	10		25

Tab. 3/IV.

Steroid	μg	Optimum conditions				Solvent	Spectral characteristics		Fluorescence intensity
		H_2SO_4% /v + v/	T°	min	H_2O ml		$\lambda_A$max/$\lambda_E$max nm	variations λmax with H_2SO_4 concentr.	
6-oxo-E_2	10	70	120	5	1.5	TCE	537/550	35-90%: constant, low, non distinct peaks	Low even in concentrations giving rise to *Kober* colours.
						$CHCl_3$	540/550		
						TBE	none		
6-oxo-E_3	10	53	120	10	1.5	TCE	536/550	35-90%: constant, low, non distinct peaks	Not useful for fluorimetry.
						$CHCl_3$	538/550		
						TBE	544/556		
6-OH-equilenin 3,6-dimethyl-ether	10	–	120	10	1.5	TCE	none	40-90%: no fluorescence	

Abbreviations:

Steroids: abbreviated trivial names

Solvents: TCE: 1,1,2,2-Tetrachloroethane; TBE: 1,1,2,2-Tetrabromoethane; $CHCl_3$: Chloroform — Each of the solvents containing p-Nitrophenol 2% (v/v) and ethanol 1% (v/v)

$\lambda_A$max/$\lambda_E$max (nm): wavelenghts of activation / emission peaks

Fluorescence intensity: ammeter readings measured at $\frac{\text{activ. } \lambda \text{ A}}{\text{emiss. } \lambda \text{ A}}$ (nm)

Measuring conditions: MPF 2A, Perkin-Elmer-Hitachi:
Light source: Xenon arc lamp OSRAM XBO 150 W/1
Detector: Photomultiplier R 136
Spectral bandpass: 2,5 nm for both excitation and emission monochromator
Sensitivity: S = 5 (= amplification 100x)
Same spectrofluorimeter response wetting with uranium glass rod for all determinations

Tab. 4. Relative fluorescence intensities / $F_{0,1\ \mu g\ E_3} = 100$/in optimum conditions of *Kibr* and spectral characteristics of 18 oestrogens in TCE.

Group	Type	Oestrogen Structure	Abbrev.	Relative intens.	Fluorescence Spectral changes under varying conditions of *KIBR*
I a	Epimeric oestriols	C16 OH C17 α β	E_3	100	Tab. 3/I, Fig. 1a Highly fluorogenic oestrogens. Analytic. range 10–100 ng. Fluorescence intensity highly dependent on optim. conditions. Excitation / emission spectra and their maxima at 536 / 550 nm are constant under varying conditions. Shifts of + 1 to + 4 nm with 85–96% H_2SO_4.
		α α	17-epi-E_3	105	
		β β	16-epi-E_3	125	
		β α	16,17-epi-E_3	176	
I b	Ring D α-ketols	. . . OH - O	16α-OH-E_1	109	
		-OAC - O	16β-OH-E_1 3,16-acetate	97	
		- O - OH	16-oxo-E_2	97	
I c	16,17-dione	- O - O	16-oxo-E_1	5	
	16-dehydro	16	Δ^{16}-estratetraenol	330	
II	2-MeO-oestrogens	2-CH_3O	2-CH_3O-E_1	22	Tab. 3/II, Fig. 16 Analytical range 100–1000 ng. Fluorescence intensity highly dependent on the reaction conditions. Constant activation/emission peaks shifted to longer wavelenghts 566/594 nm. Second typical activation peak A_2 at 426 nm.
			2-CH_3O-E_2	21	
			2-CH_3O-E_3	10	
IIIa	C6-OH	6ξ-OH	6ξ-OH-E_3	11	Tab. 3/III, Fig. 2,3,4 Analytical range 100–1000 ng. Fluorescence intensity highly dependent on *KIBR* conditions. Two pairs of activation/emission bands, highly dependent on *Kibr* condit. Typical emission peak F_3 at 440/463 nm, produced with 68–90% H_2SO_4, is absent in 6-OH-E_3.
		6α-OH	6α-OH-E_2	14	
IIIb	C7-OH	7α-OH	7α-OH-E_2	7	
IVa	6-oxo-oestrogens	6-oxo	6-oxo-E_2	0,5	Tab. 3/IV Weakly or non fluorescent oestrogens even in concentrations giving rise to *Kober*-colours not useful for fluorimetry. Atypical spectra with formation of plateau.
			6-oxo-E_3	0,5	
	Aromatic Rings AB	3,6-CH_3O-Oestra-1,3,5/10/,6,8-pentaen-17-on	6-OH-equilenin 3,6-dimethylether	0	

J. B. Brown's recent modification of the *Kober* reaction using higher heating temperature, shortened heating time and lower sulphuric acid concentration as well as a reduced extraction volume of tetrachloroethane has been described for the estimation of three classical oestrogens (*Brown* and coll., 1968).

In order to complete the findings of *J. B. Brown,* studies on the fluorescence of some newer oestrogens under varying conditions of the *Kober-Ittrich-Brown reaction, KIBR* have been undertaken by the authors.

In the first part (*Šťastný* and *Dubey,* 1970) fluorescence properties of some C6-substituted oestrogens have been demonstrated. In the recent investigation optimal conditions for 18 phenolic steroids have been established. The oestrogens have been classed into four groups according to their qualitative and quantitative fluorescence properties. (A preliminary account of this study was submited as advanced abstract to the VIII Acta Endocrinologica Congress, Copenhagen, July 1971.) Full details will be published elsewhere.

Material, methods and apparatus have been described elsewhere (*Šťastný* and *Dubey,* 1970).

Results

Optimal conditions of the *Kober-Ittrich-Brown*-Reaction, *KIBR,* for 18 phenolic steroids classed in four groups are listed in Tab. 3, I, II, III, IV.

Relative fluorescence intensities and qualitative spectral characteristics are summarized in Tab. 4.

Typical spectra are shown in Fig. 1a, 1b, 2, 3, 4.

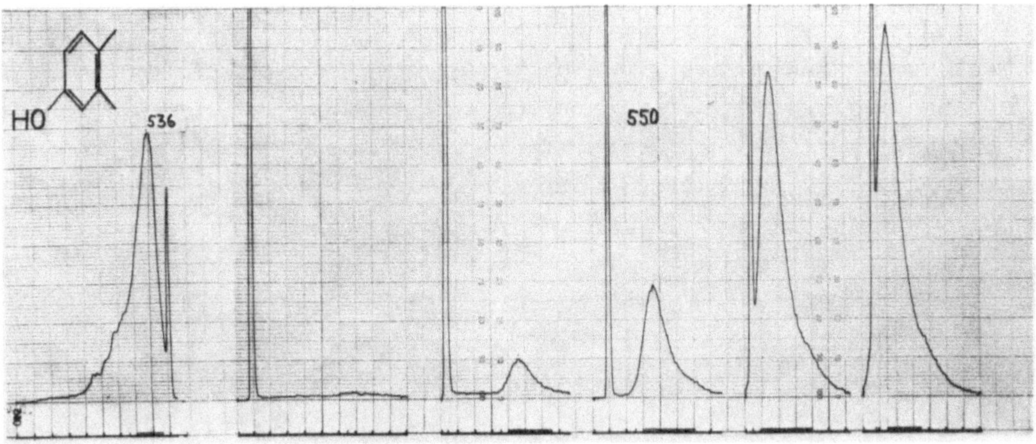

Fig. 1a. (upper part) Excitation and emission spectra of oestrogens listed in group I abc. /0,1 ug/0,6 ml TCE/
Excitation spectrum: one excitation peak A_1 at 536 nm.
Emission spectra: excitation at 440, 467, 500, 530 and 536 nm **develops** *constant* emission peaks at 550 nm of *different* intensities

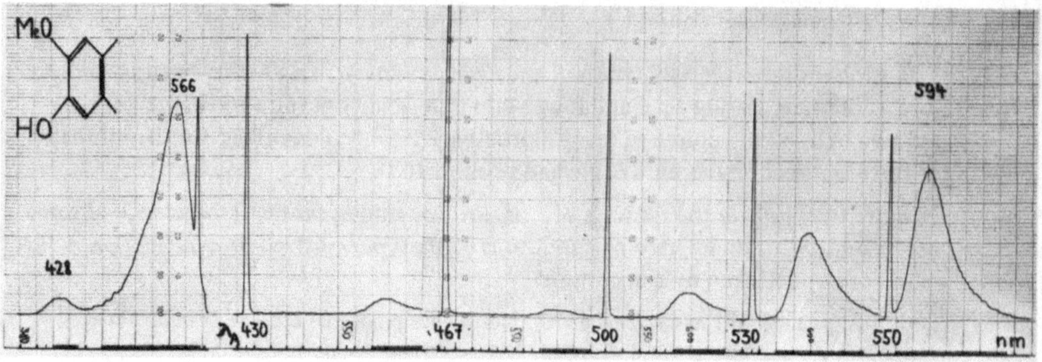

Fig. 1b. (lover part) Excitation and emission spectra of 2-Methoxyoestrogens /1,0 ug/0,6 ml TCE/
Excitation spectrum: two excitation peaks A_1 at 566 nm, A_2 at 428 nm.
Emission spectra: excitation at 430, 476, 500, 530 and 550 nm gives rise to *constant* emission peaks at 594 nm of *different* intensities

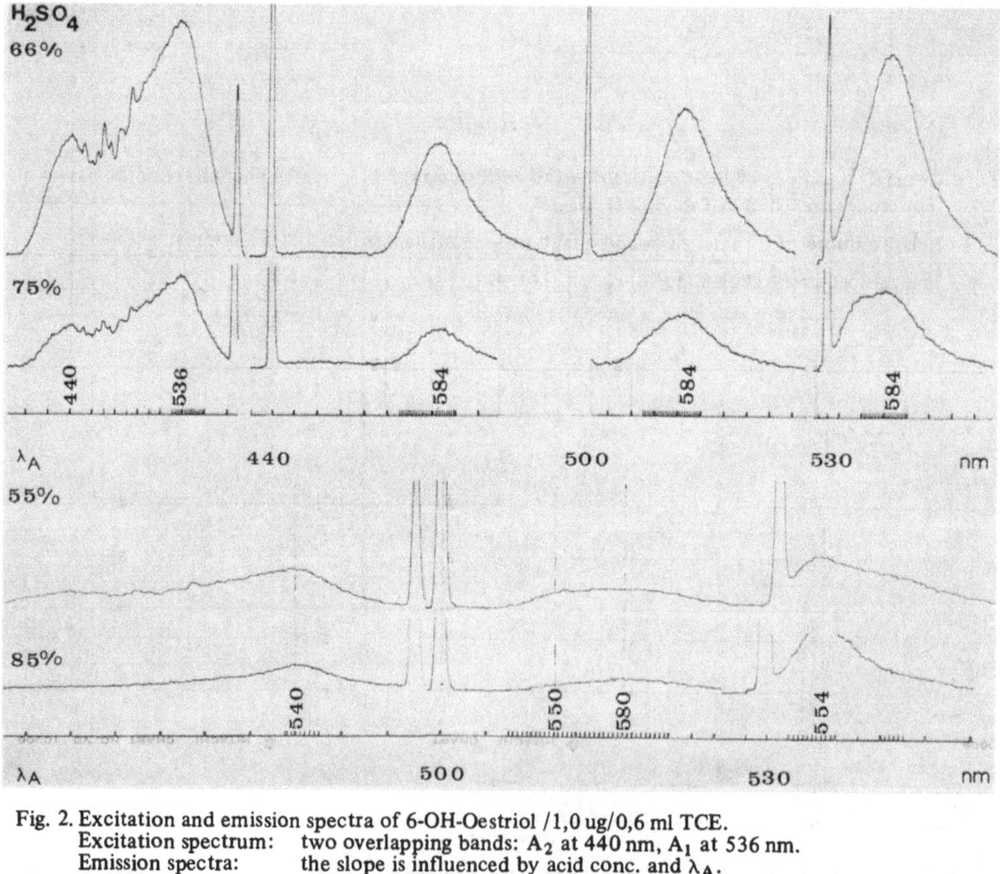

Fig. 2. Excitation and emission spectra of 6-OH-Oestriol /1,0 ug/0,6 ml TCE.
Excitation spectrum: two overlapping bands: A_2 at 440 nm, A_1 at 536 nm.
Emission spectra: the slope is influenced by acid conc. and λ_A.
66 % H_2SO_4: excitation at 400, 500 and 530 nm develops only one emission peak F_2 at 584 nm.
75 % H_2SO_4: deformation of the ascending shoulder of emission curves by the fluorogen F_1.
55 % and 85 % H_2SO_4: prevalence of the fluorogen F_1 develops peak F_1 at 554 nm

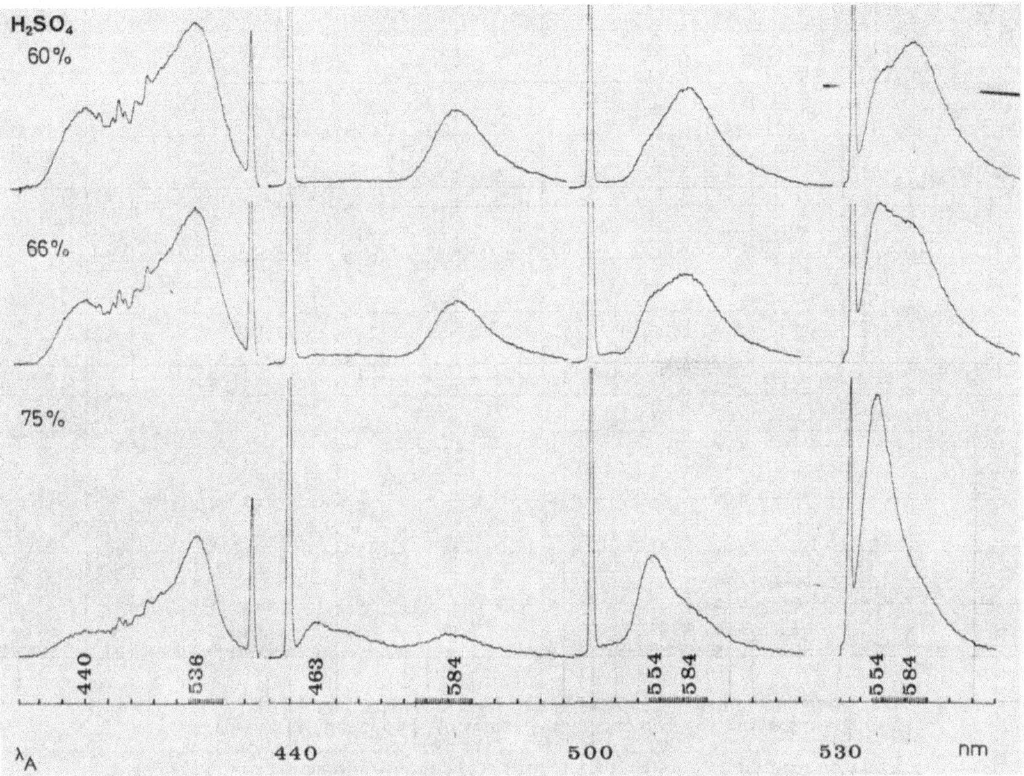

Fig. 3. Excitation and emission spectra of 6α-OH-E_2-17β /1,0 ug/0,6 ml TCE/

Excitation spectrum:	two overlapping bands: A_2 at 440 nm, A_1 at 536 nm.
Emission spectra	show the coexistence of two fluorogens.
60 % H_2SO_4:	excitation at 440 nm develops the emission peak at 584 nm, at 500 and 530 nm prevalence of F_2 at 584 nm, participation F_1.
66 % H_2SO_4:	excitation at 440 nm: pure peak F_2 at 584 nm excitation at 530 nm: transitory form with prevalence of F_1.
75 % H_2SO_4:	apparition of peak F_3 at 463 nm, pure peak F_1 at 554 nm

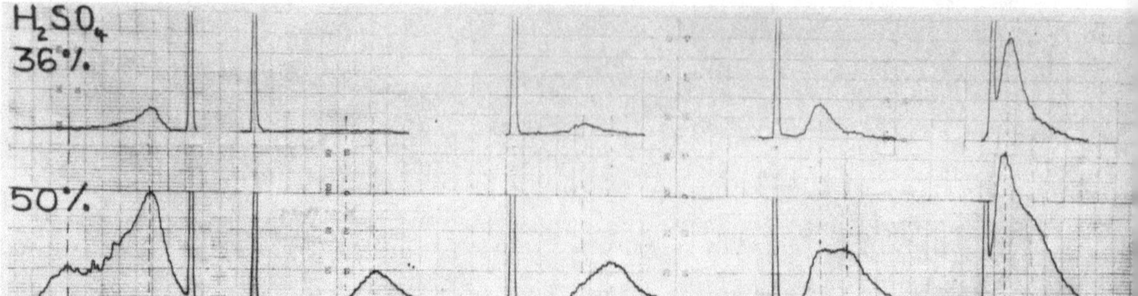

Fig. 4. Excitation and emission spectra of 7α-OH-E_2-17β /1,0 ug/0,6 ml TCE/

Excitation spectra: two overlapping bands: A_1 at 536 nm, A_2 at 440 nm.
A_2 in very low and ver high acid concentrations low.

Emission spectra: effect of sulphuric acid concentration and excit. wavelenght.

36 % and 80 % H_2SO_4: classical emission peaks F_1 at 554 nm.

50 % H_2SO_4: border line concentration developing transitory emission curves.

72 % H_2SO_4: optimum acid concentration develops *three* different emission peaks.
At 440 nm: peaks F_3 at 463 nm and F_2 at 584 nm.
Excitation at 500 nm and 530 nm develops peak F_1 at 554 nm

Discussion

The evaluation of qualitative and quantitative fluorescence properties of the 18 oestrogens allowed to distinguish four groups of compounds with similar qualitative properties. In order to demonstrate quantitative differences in terms of relative fluorescence, the fluorescence intensity of 100 ng oestriol – produced by heating at 120° 10 min with 56% H_2SO_4, diluted with 1,5 ml H_2O and extracted with 0,6 ml TCE containing 2% p-nitrophenol – has been used as reference. This fact as well as the optimalisation of reaction conditions for each steroid may change our figures in comparison with those published by other authors.

As far as the compounds listed in Tab. 3/I are concerned, the maxima recorded correspond to those found by authors performing the *Ittrich*'s extraction (*Strickler* 1961; *Scholler* 1966; *Eechaute* and *Demeester* 1965). Differences of 2 to 4 mm are due to lacking precision of some of the apparatuses used. On the other hand, we have not confirmed the results of *Scholler* who recorded maximum emission of 2-methoxy-oestrone as follows:

Author	Solvent	TCE	$CHCl_3$	TBE
Scholler et al.		583	585	591 (nm)
Šťastný, Dubey		594	596	602

The same authors found the C6- and C7-substituted oestrogens only barely fluorescent, while in our optimal conditions these compounds are of mediocre fluorogenity. Furthermore they have characteristic spectral properties demonstrating the probable existence of two independent fluorogenic systems. Their contribution to the resulting shape of the emission curve depends firstly on the ratio of both fluorogens produced under given conditions, secondly on their ratio extracted by the given solvent and thirdly on the activation wavelenght.

Different fluorescence properties of oestrogens under varying sulphuric acid concentrations have been found by *Bauld* and coll., 1960. The fluorescence has been measured in the *diluted acid phase,* without *Ittrich*'s extraction, in response to varying excitation wavelenghts. The 3 classical oestrogens and the epimeric oestriols develop fluorescence maxima at 480 mm, the ring Dα-ketols and 16-oxiestrone at 518–528 nm, 2-methoxyoestrone at 579 nm.

Although this modification seems to contribute to a differenciated specificity of the *Kober* reaction, its reliability in biological extracts has been shown as limited (*Ittrich,* 1958) and evidence for the superiority of the *Ittrich*'s extraction procedure over existing *Kober* modifications was given (*Ittrich,* 1960; *Strickler* et al., 1961; *Šťasný,* 1968; *Šťastný* et al., 1969).

The distinctive fluorescence properties of the four groups of oestrogens as delineated in the present study emphasize a differenciated specificity of the *Kibr* within the *Kober* group reaction for phenolic steroids and may be valuable as additional spectrofluorometric information in identification studies of oestrogens *isolated* from biological fluids.

On the other hand, in methods for *estimating* – as opposed to isolating – the newer oestrogens in biological fluids, phenolic steroids have each to be separated from interfering material as well as from one another. Combined procedures involving gel filtration and multiple chromatography on alumina, celite and thin layers have been designed for gas chromatographic methods which are known to require a high degree of extract purity (*Adlercreutz* et al., 1968; *Heikkila* et al., 1970). Some of them are applicable for clinical purposes. The purity of the final extracts as well as the concentrations of oestrogens listed in Tab. 2 justify the possible application of fluorometry for the final determination in conditions of the *Kober-Ittrich-Brown*-reaction as delineated in this paper, at least for determinations in late pregnancy urine, where the foetal well-being is a special focus of clinical interest.

References

Adlercreutz, H. and *T. Luukkainen* in: "Gas Phase Chromatography of Steroids." Eds. *K. B. Eik-Nes* and *E. C. Horning.* Springer-Verlag, New York (1968).

Adlercreutz, H. and *T. Luukkainen:* Annals clin. Res. 2 (1970) p. 365–380.

Breuer, H. in: "Research on Steroids", Vol. I. Poliglotta Vaticana Rome (1964).

Breuer, H.: Abhandl. Deut. Akad. Wiss., Med. 3 (1968) S. 51–67.

Brown, J. H., S. C. Mac Leod, C. Mac Naughtan, A. M. Smith, B. Smyth: J. Endocrinol. 42 (1968) p. 5.

Diczfalusy, E. and *Lauzitzen:* Östrogene beim Menschen. Springer, Berlin (1961).

Diczfalusy, E. and *Mancuso* in: Foetus and Placenta. Eds. *A. Klopper* and *E. Diczfalusy.* Blackwell, Oxford (1969).

Eechaute, W., G. Demeester and *I. Leussen:* Clin. Chim. Acta 12 (1965) p. 359.

Eechaute, W., G. Demeester and *I. Leussen:* Steroids 13 (1968) p. 101–120.

Heikkila, J. and *H. Adlercreutz:* J. Steroid Biochem. 1 (1970) p. 243–253.

Ittrich, G.: Z. phisiol. Chem. 312 (1958) p. 1.

Ittrich, G.: Acta Endocr. 35 (1960) p. 34–38.

Klopper, A. in: Foetus and Placenta. Eds. *A. Klopper* and *E. Diczfalusy.* Blackwell, Oxford (1969).

Lisboa, B. P.: Clin. chim. Acta 13 (1966) p. 179.

Nocke, V.: Biochem. J. 78 (1961) S. 593.

Nocke, V.: Abhandl. Deut. Akad. Wiss., Med. 3 (1968) S. 69–75.

Oakey, R. E.: Vitamines and Hormones 28 (1970) p. 1–36.

Scholler, R.: Acta Endocr. Suppl. 107 (1966).

Stoa, K. F.: Abhandl. Deut. Akad. Wiss., Med. 3 (1968) S. 101–109.

Šťastný, J. and *L. Dubey:* Z. Anal. Chem. 252 (1970) p. 309–322.

Šťastný, J. and *L. Dubey:* Acta Endocr. 67, Suppl. 155 (1971) p. 99.

Šťastný, J.: Abhandl. Deut. Akad. Wiss., Med. 3 (1968) S. 135–157.

Šťastný, J., J. Šponarová and *H. Stoklasová:* Acta Univ. Carol., Med. (1969).

Strickler, H. S., G. A. Wilson, R. C. Grauer: Anal. Biochem. 2 (1961) S. 486–496.

Preedy, J. R. K. in: Methods in Hormone Research I. *R. I. Dorfman* edit. Academic Press, New York (1962).

Bauld, W. S., M. L. Givner, L. L. Engel and *J. W. Goldzieher:* Can. J. Biochem. and Phisiol. 38 (1960) p. 213.

Abstract

18 different oestrogens have been studied under varying conditions of the *Kober-Ittrich-Brown*-reaction (KIBR) (*Brown,* 1968), by means of the Fluorescence Spectrophotometer MPF-2A Perkin-Elmer-Hitachi. Optimal conditions of the KIBR

have been established, in which oestrogens having been referred as barely fluorescent, develop analyticaly useful fluorescence. Characteristic spectral qualities have been found in oestrogens hydroxylated at C6 and C7. A possible coexistence of two independent fluorogens is demonstrated on typical examples of excitationand emission curves. The possible application to modern separation procedures is discussed on the basis of data reported for important oestrogen metabolites (*Adlercreutz* et al., 1970).

Acknowledgements

The authors wish to express their most sincere gratitude to Prof. de *Watteville* for the active support in apparative equipment and for favourable working conditions. For the generous gift of reference steroids we should like to thank Prof. *Klyne* and Dr. *Kirk*, British Medical Council London and Dr. *P. U. Zoller*, Perkin-Elmer AG Zürich.

Determination of Plasma Estriol Levels in Normal and Abnormal Pregnancies Near Term

Giulio Zucconi and *Mario Ciuffi*

Clinica Ostetrica e Ginecologica dell'Università, Firenze, Italia

On the basis of the recent studies on steroid metabolism we know that in pregnancy the biosynthesis of estriol takes place mainly in the feto-placental unit.

Estriol is transferred to the mother's circulation and is then eliminated in the urine, through the kidneys.

For many years the assay of urinary estriol, expressed by the creatinine-estriol ratio, has been used as an index of feto-placental function.

The advantages and limits of this method are well known.

Quite recently the interest has spread for the assay of estriol in the mother's blood using a method which needs 1 ml or even less of plasma.

Plasma-estriol determinations have at least three advantages over the analysis of urine in the evaluation of human pregnancy:

First: the need for the troublesome 24-hour-urine collection is eliminated.
Second: if necessary, 2 plasma samples may be drawn for analysis in a single day.
Third: in view of the short plasma estriol half-life, a rapid and marked decrease in estriol is reflected more rapidly in plasma than in urine, even one day before.

Ratanasopa et al. (1967), *Nachtigall* et al. (1968), *Schiffer* et al. (1971), have usually found a good correlation between the values of plasma estriol and the degree of fetal distress in toxemia.

For the essay of plasma estriol we use the method of *Nachtigall* et al. (1966), modified by *Goebelsman* and *Gorwill* (1970). It is based on the fluorimetric determination of estriol and the addition of $^{3}H\ E_3$ to each sample as intêrnal standard.

The method is relatively simple and needs only 1 ml of plasma. One technician can perform 5 duplicate assays in one working day.

We prepared the method only a few months ago. This is the reason for our small number of clinical cases. Till today only 32 observations with a total of 56 determinations in normal and toxemic pregnancies have been carried out.

No serious case of toxemia (eclampsia) has yet been observed.

From our data and mainly from the literature in this field, it is possible to show a good correlation between plasma and urinary estriol values in the same patient (*Gurpide* et al., 1971).

Diurnal variations in the plasma levels are frequently present, but the fall in maternal plasma estriol levels appears to be related to the recumbent position and probably reflects an altered blood flow through the liver and kidneys.

These changes are not constant and can vary about 25% at the most (*Selinger* and *Levitz*, 1969).

As regards day-today variations, the differences are 10% or less in almost 80% of the cases and was never more than 25% (*Macourt* et al., 1971).

The overal results are similar to those obtained when urinary estimations are performed.

Individual variations are very high and for this reason it is necessary to repeat the determinations, similarly to urinary estimation.

For clinical purposes it is more useful to have a curve rather than a single determination.

As can be seen in three of our own observations, there is a very rapid fall within a few hours after the fetal death in the uterus.

However on the basis of this very short communication and of the small number of our observations, we cannot deduce any conclusions. We can only call your attention to the usefulness of plasma estriol determination in normal and toxemic pregnancies.

This method is without any doubt more useful and more practical than urinary estriol determination.

References

Goebelsmann, W. and *R. H. Gorwill:* "The use of Silica gel impregnated glass fiber sheets in plasma estriol assays". Steroids 16 (1970) p. 635.

Gurpide, E., M. E. Giebenhaim, L. Tseng and *G. W. Kelly:* "Radioimmunoassay for estrogens in human pregnancy urine, plasma, and aminotic fluid". Am. J. Obstet. Gynec. 109 (1971) p. 897.

Macourt, D., C. S. Corker and *F. Naftolin:* "Plasma oestriol in pregnancy". J. Obstet. Gynaecol. Brit. Common. 78 (1971) p. 335.

Nachtigall, L., M. Basset, V. Hogsander, S. Slagle and *M. Levitz:* "A rapid method for assay of plasma estriol in pregnancy". J. Clin. Endocrinol. 26 (1966) p. 941.

Nachtigall, L., M. Bassett, V. Hogsander and *M. Levitz:* "Plasma estriol levels in normal and abnormal pregnancies: an index of fetal welfare". Am. J. Obst. Gynec. 101 (1968) p. 638.

Ratanasopa, V., A. E. Schindler, T. Y. Lee and *W. L. Herrmann:* "Measurement of estriol in plasma by gas-liquid chromatography". Am. J. Obst. Gynec. 99 (1967) p. 3, 295.

Schiffer, M. A., N. H. Ertel, L. M. Hellman and *M. Kobayashi:* "Combined method for evaluating fetal well-being by plasma estriol measurements and ultrasonography". Am. J. Obst. Gynec. 108 (1970) p. 1277.

Selinger, M. and *M. Levitz:* "Diurnal variation of total plasma estriol levels in late pregnancy". J. Clin. Endocrinol. Metab. 29 (1969) p. 995.

The Placenta

Hormonale und enzymologische Methoden zur Diagnose der Placentainsuffizienz bei EPH-Gestose

Paul J. Keller

Universitäts-Frauenklinik, Zürich

Ungeachtet zahlreicher neuer Erkenntnisse bleibt die Überwachung der gestotisch komplizierten Schwangerschaft schwierig; neue Methoden haben unsere Möglichkeiten immerhin erheblich verbessert. Da weder der Fetus noch die Plazenta unmittelbar zugänglich sind, ist die Kontrolle ihrer Funktion weitgehend auf indirekte biochemische Parameter beschränkt. Zur Diskussion stehen diesbezüglich zur Zeit die Östriolausscheidung im Urin, der Belastungstest mit Dehydroepiandrosteronsulfat (DHAS), die Pregnandiolausscheidung im Urin, das plazentare Laktogen (HPL) im Serum und die Aktivität der hitzestabilen alkalischen Phosphatase (HSAP) im Serum. Die ersten beiden Parameter sind als gemischte fetoplazentare Gradmesser zu betrachten, da die Biosynthese von Östriol in der Plazenta sehr weitgehend von der 16-Hydroxylierung der entsprechenden Vorläufer in der kindlichen Leber abhängt. Die drei letztgenannten Methoden spiegeln dagegen fast ausschließlich die plazentare Funktion.

In der vorliegenden Studie wurde versucht, die Aussagekraft der verschiedenen Parameter bei EPH-Gestose anhand des Zustandes von Fetus und Plazenta abzuschätzen.

Material und Methodik

Das Krankengut umfaßte 94 wegen EPH-Gestose stationär aufgenommene Patientinnen, bei denen Oedeme bestanden, der Ruheblutdruck im Liegen 140/90 überstieg und eine Proteinurie von mehr als 0.5 g/d vorlag. Der Gestoseindex erreichte somit in allen Fällen mindestens 4. Bei allen Patientinnen wurden wöchentlich ein- bis mehrmals Blutproben entnommen und 24-h Urin gesammelt. Die Östriolausscheidung wurde mit der halbautomatischen Methode nach *Brown* et al. (1968), der DHAS-Test nach *Lauritzen* (1969), die Pregnandiolausscheidung nach *Klopper* et al. (1955), die HPL-Aktivität im Serum nach *Keller* et al. (1970) und die HSAP im Serum mittels der Biochemica Kombination (Boehringer) nach fünfminütiger Erhitzung des Serums auf 65° bestimmt.

Östriol- und Pregnandiol- sowie HPL-Werte wurden als pathologisch klassiert, wenn sie unterhalb des 95% Normalbereiches lagen oder einen Abfall von mehr als 25% aufwiesen. Für den DHAS-Test wurde nach intravenöser Injektion von 50 mg ein Mindestanstieg der Östriolausgangswerte um 20% verlangt. Die HSAP-Werte wurden als pathologisch gewertet, wenn sie entweder über der 95% Normalstreuung lagen oder aber eine plötzliche, markante Trendänderung aufwiesen (*Bader* et al., 1971).

Um die biochemischen Resultate mit dem Zustand von Fetus und Plazenta korrelieren zu können, wurden katamnestisch zwei Gruppen gebildet. Eine schwere Beeinträchtigung wurde angenommen, wenn mindestens zwei der folgenden Kriterien erfüllt waren: Fortgesetzte pathologische Herzaktion in der cardiotokographischen Überwachung, fetale Azidose und grünes Fruchtwasser vor Wehenbeginn, extremer intrauteriner Wachstumsrückstand, intrauteriner Fruchttod sowie ausgeprägte Infarzierung der Plazenta. War keines dieser Symptome vorhanden, so wurde die Funktion der fetoplazentaren Einheit als normal klassiert, zweifelhafte Fälle und Zwischenstufen wurden ausgeschlossen.

Ergebnisse

Die Aussagekraft der verschiedenen Methoden bezüglich der gewählten Kriterien ist in Abb. 1 dargestellt. Bei gestörter fetoplazentarer Funktion war die HPL-Bestimmung am aussagekräftigsten, indem in allen Fällen pathologische Werte resultierten. Die Zuverlässigkeit der Östriolbestimmung, des DHAS-Tests und der HSAP-Aktivität war mit 69, 70 und 64% richtiger Ergebnisse zufriedenstellend, während die Pregnandiolausscheidung nur in 21% die Gefährdung anzuzeigen vermochte und demnach eine große Anzahl von falsch negativen Ergebnissen aufwies.

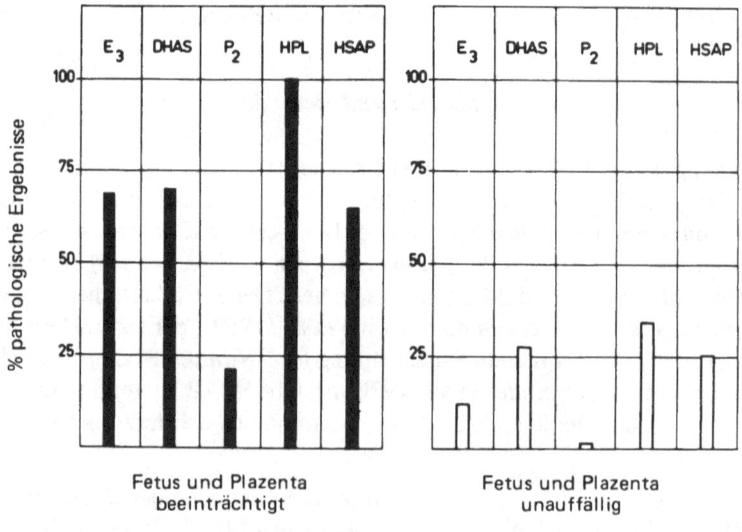

Abb. 1. Aussagekraft hormonaler und enzymologischer Methoden zur Diagnose der fetoplazentaren Insuffizienz bei EPH-Gestose

Bei ungestörtem Zustand von Fetus und Plazenta waren die Zahlen wesentlich anders verteilt. Östriol und Pregnandiol wiesen die geringsten Versagerquoten auf, nur 12 bzw. 2% der Ergebnisse waren als falsch positiv zu betrachten. Der DHAS-Test und die HSAP-Aktivität zeigten in 27 bzw. 25% der Fälle, das HPL sogar in 35% einen falsch positiven Ausfall.

Diskussion

Die Ergebnisse der Untersuchung zeigen, daß die platentare Insuffizienz und fetale Gefährdung heute auf biochemischem Wege recht gut erkannt werden können. Die am häufigsten verwendete Methode, die Bestimmung der Östriolausscheidung im Urin, zeigte eine beachtliche Versagerquote, indem fast ein Drittel der Fälle mit Zeichen eingeschränkter fetoplazentarer Funktion nicht reflektiert wurden, allerdings war andrerseits die Zahl der falsch positiven Ergebnisse sehr bescheiden. Der DHAS-Test wies unter den gleichen Bedingungen verhältnismäßig viele falsch positiven und falsch negativen Resultate auf, ebenso auch die HSAP-Aktivität im Serum. HPL erschien bei den pathologischen Fällen als idealer Parameter, die hohe Zahl von falsch positiven Ergebnissen zeigte hingegen, daß es sich offensichtlich um einen sehr empfindlichen Gradmesser handelt, der wohl auch auf leichte, mit einfachen makroskopischen Methoden nicht erkennbare und klinisch vorerst nicht bedeutungsvolle Einschränkung der Plazentarfunktion sehr bald anspricht. Die Pregnandiolausscheidung vermochte nur in Ausnahmefällen die kindliche oder plazentare Dysfunktion anzuzeigen, die Zahl der falsch positiven Ergebnisse war damit allerdings entsprechend gering.

Zusammenfassend ergibt sich, daß weitere Studien bezüglich des Aussagewertes der einzelnen Methoden äußerst wünschenswert sind, wobei neben den bisherigen, eher groben Kriterien wohl vor allem die plazentare Durchblutung und die histologischen und elektronenmikroskopischen Aspekte berücksichtigt werden sollten. Bis solche Resultate in genügender Zahl vorliegen, erscheint es uns empfehlenswert bei der Überwachung der durch EPH-Gestose gefährdeten Schwangerschaft zwei oder drei Parameter zu verwenden, beispielsweise die Östriolausscheidung und die HPL-Aktivität.

Literatur

Pader, P., U. Baertschi, P. J. Keller, J. Schmid: Schweiz. Z. Gynäk., Geburtsh. (im Druck).

Brown, J. B., S. C. McLeod, C. MacNaughtan, A. Smith, B. Smith: J. Endocr. 5 (1968) p. 42.

Lauritzen, C.: Horm. Metab. Res. 1 (1969) p. 46.

Keller, P. J., H. Greub, C. Gerber, W. E. Schreiner: Schweiz. Z. Gynäk. Geburtsh. 1 (1970) S. 149.

Klopper, A., E. A. Michie, J. B. Brown: J. Endocr. 12 (1955) p. 209.

Les vasculopathies placentaires et la pathologie foetale

I. I. Nubert, F. Munteanu

Clinique d.obstétrique et de Gynécologie, Laboratoire d'Anatomie Pathologique,
Institut de Médecine, Timisoara, Roumanie

Les anomalies et les lésions placentaires peuvent intervenir dans l'étiologie de la mortalité périnatale dans un pourcentage qui diffère selon divers auteurs, entre 25 et 60%. Les lésions placentaires sont déterminées ou aggravées en grandes parties par des vasculopathies primaires ou secondaires du placenta maternel ou foetal.

Les lésions placentaires consécutives à des perturbations de la circulation placentaire maternelle sont dues aux dérèglements fonctionels „spastiques", aux modifications anatomiques des artères utéro-placentaires, des lésions ischémiques de type infarctus, aux thromboses intervilleuses qui changent ainsi les conditions circulatoires à ce niveau. Ici s'y ajoute parfois la rupture des veines utéro-placentaires marginales.

En considérant l'importance de l'intégrité du système circulatoire et du trophoblaste villositaire dans le maintien de la vitalité du produit de conception, nous nous sommes proposés de suivre les changements placentaires dans les dysgravidies tardives, dans la maladie hypertonique, la pyélonéphrite chronique, le diabète, l'incompatibilité Rh.

Les placentas que nous avons étudiés proviennent de:

24 dysgravidies tardives, formes légères, sévères et graves,
5 pyelonéphrites chroniques,
6 gravides avec maladie hypertonique,
4 gravides diabétiques et
3 gravides Rh négatives.

On a prélevé de chaque placenta plusieurs fragments de diverses zones qui ont été analysées selon les techniques usuelles de fixation, inclusion et coloration trichrome et PAS.

Les lésions placentaires observées sur notre matériel peuvent être concrétisées par les aspects histologiques suivants:

thromboses intervilleuses,
nécroses ischémiques du tissu placentaire,
de vrais infarctus,
artériopathies dégénératives.

Les villosités placentaires réagissent à la modification du flux sanguin maternal par:

dilatation capillaire, villositaire,

dégénérescence du syncitiotrophoblaste,

dégénérescence du stroma villositaire (apparition de cellules, scléroses et dépôts de matériel PAS positif).

En même temps, dans la dysgravidie éclamptogène, lors d'hypertensions et glomérulonéphrites chroniques, on constate la persistance de quelques cellules Langhans, avec ralentissement de croissance des villosités, conduisant à une diminution du poids et du volume du placenta (hypoplacentose).

En ce qui concerne les modifications vasculaires du placenta foetal, elles consistent dans la thrombose des vaisseaux des troncs villositaires, la disparition des capillaires ou des artérioles des villosités terminales ou préterminales. On constate aussi une altération des conditions de l'hémodynamique et des villosités (chorangiomatose [6]).

La suppression complète de la circulation placentaire foetale, secondaire à la mort foetale „in utéro", constitute une situation plus complexe due au fait que le flux sanguin utéro-placentaire maternel, sans disparaître complètement diminue progressivement au cours de la rétention ovulaire.

La similitude histologique des placentas lors de diabète, isoimmunisation et hydrops, les caractères communs à la môle hydatiforme et les stades précoces de la rétention placentaire in utéro après la mort du foetus suggèrent l'intervention d'un facetur circulatoire dans la genèse des particularités lésionales.

Sans aucun doute toutes les lésions placentaires citées ont un rôle primordial dans la pathogénie des accidents foetaux. Il se produit une limitation de l'espace d'hématose placentaire qui peut apparaître brutalement (thrombus artériel placentaire, hématome rétroplacentaire) ou plus souvent lentement (thrombus intervilleux).

Les thrombus intervilleux favorisent la déposition de fibrine due à la stase circulatoire et isolent ainsi de grandes surfaces du trophoblaste villositaire de la circulation maternelle déterminant sa dégénérescence dans la sécrétion endocrine.

Tous ces éléments réduisent l'apport d'oxygène et de matériel nutritif au foetus en déterminant, d'une part l'apparition d'une hypoxie foetale (aigue ou chronique, compensée ou décompensée), et d'autre part des déficiences dans le transfer de diverses substances avec des répercussions sur le métabolisme foetal.

Dans les formes graves, aux lésions étendues, la mortalité in utéro, ante partum peut atteindre 35%. Les nouveaux-nés vivants présentent souvent un degré de dénutrition accentué à l'aspect hypotrophique [2].

La question qui se pose est la suivante: Laquelle des lésions placentaires mentionnées affecte particulièrement le foetus et pourquoi la souffrance foetale n'apparaît-elle pas dans les cas d'altérations histopathologiques de l'organe placentaire?

La conviction unanime que nous adoptons est que la réserve fonctionelle du placenta est très grande ce qui explique sa capacité d'assurer les substances nécessaires au foetus en développement même quand de larges portions ont été envahies par l'infarctisation.

D'autre part *Klostermann* et *Huidekoper* [4] ont montré que l'infarctisation étendue du placenta est associée avec la croissance de 40 fois du risque des morts périnatales „inexpliquées" en comparaison avec les placentas sans infarctus. Ces observations coincident avec celles de *Lillte* [5]. Souvent les placentas avec infarctus sont „tarés" antérieurement, présentent des atrophies ou des dépôts de fibrine qui peuvent atteindre leur réserve fonctionelle en rendant ainsi encore plus dangereux pour le foetus les infarctus éventuels qui apparaissent, menant à l'installation d'une insuffisance placentaire chronique (*Beltran-Driscoll* [1]).

Rien ne permet d'affirmer à priori que l'insuffisance pondérale du foetus, est due, pour une durée déterminée de la grossesse, à une altération de la fonction placentaire. Théoriquement il est possible qu'un manque de développement foetal soit dû à un trouble placentaire en outre un vice du métabolisme foetal mène à uné utilisation inadéquate des matériaux apportés en quantité et qualité normales par la membrane placentaire d'échange. D'ailleurs le placenta est un organe doté de multiples fonctions: nutritives, endocrines, enzymatiques et métaboliques qui ne varient pas toujours dans le même sens. Le terme d'insuffisance placentaire globale paraît, par suite être rejeté ou remplacé par un qualificatif qui montre la fonction placentaire qui est insuffisante: insuffisance nutritive, insuffisance métabolique, insuffisance endocrine, etc.

En conclusion, on peut affirmer que les vasculopathies primitives ou secondaires, de nature dystrophique, dégénérative ou toxique-allergique paraissent représenter le principal substrat étiopathogénique des états hypoxiques placentaires, donc des changements, qui une fois constitués pourraient réaliser un méchanisme d'auto-entretien se répercutant autant sur l'affection maternelle que sur les conséquences pathologiques de l'organisme foetal.

Nos observation confirment la nécessité d'étudier la déviation pathologique de l'angioarchitectonique de l'organe placentaire dans le but d'élucider quelques aspects pathogéniques de la morti-natalité.

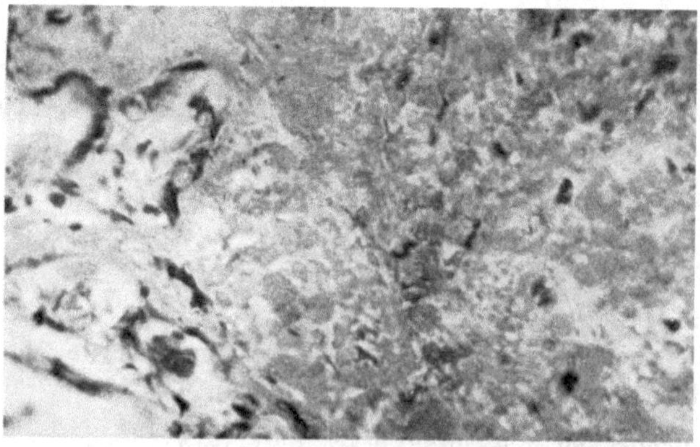

Fig. 1. Nécroses ischémiques de type infarct au niveau des villosités placentaires

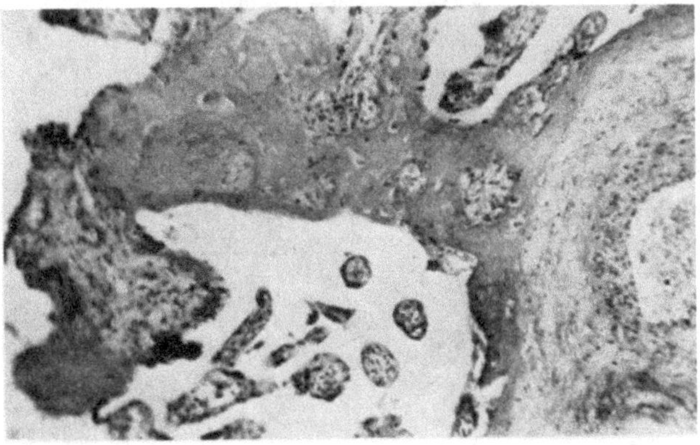

Fig. 2. Grossissement des arteriolles avec la hyalinisation des septes intercotylédonaires. Matériel fibrinoide englobant des villosités „fantôme". Prolifération des mvocvtes pariétales

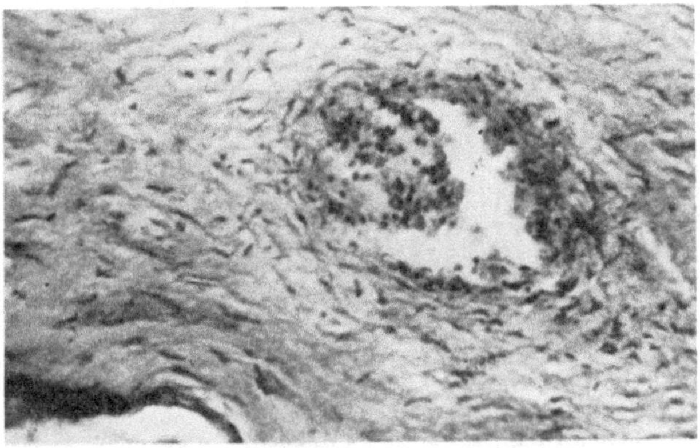

Fig. 3. Thrombus intraartériel obstruant partiellement le lumen du vaisseau

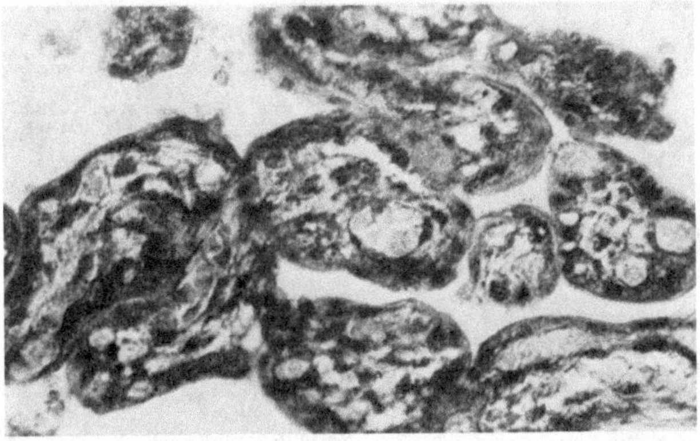

Fig. 4. Ectasie des capillaires villositaires. Cellules X

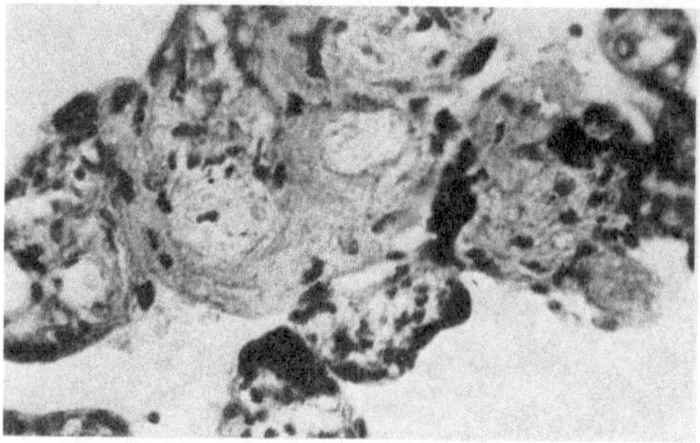

Fig. 5. Coloration trichrome: de grosses bandes de materiel fibrinoide perivillositaires. Bourgeons syncytiels

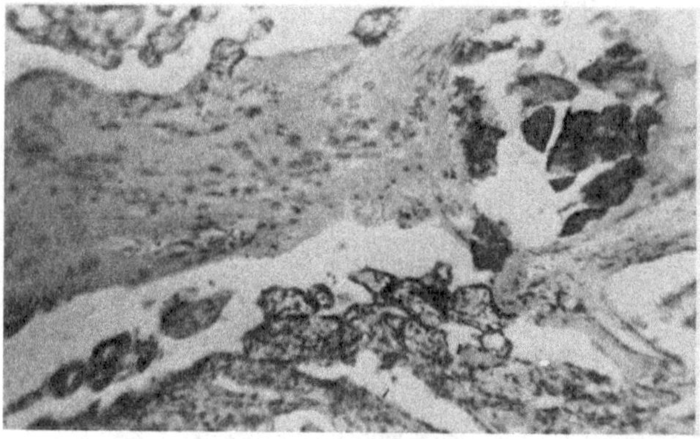

Fig. 6. Foyers de calcification au niveau de la plaque basale. Petites villosités, symphysées, constituant des conglomérats villositaires

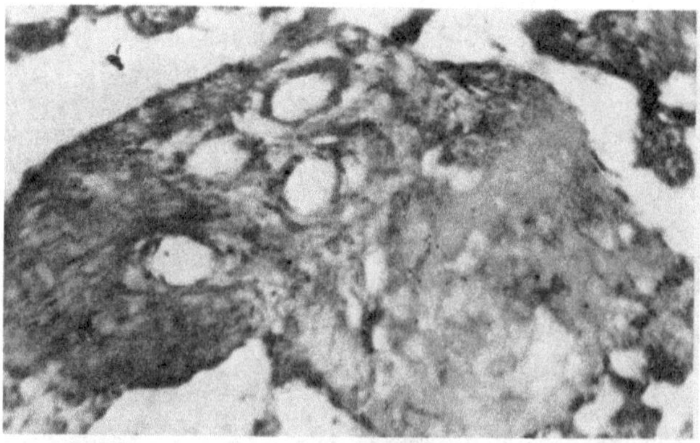

Fig. 7. Coloration PAS: dépôts marqués de matériel PAS-positif. Collagénisations

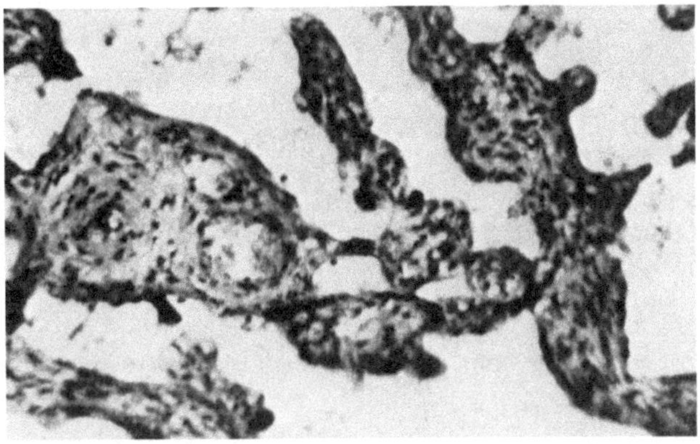

Fig. 8. Petites villosités, hypotrophiques avec microsymphyses. Artérite proliférative oblitérante

Résumé

On montre que le facteur placentaire intervient dans l'évolution foetale, entre autres, aussi par ses déficiences morpho-fonctionnelles. Ces dernières sont le plus souvent reliées à des troubles vasculaires ayant une pathologie propre notamment ceux qui surviennent au cours des dysgravidies tardives de la maladie hypertensive, des affections rénales ou du diabète.

Les auteurs présentent une série de preparations microscopiques obtenues à partir de l'organe placentaire dans de pareils cas. Sur ces préparations apparaissent des thromboses intervilleuses, des nécroses ischémiques, de vrais infarctus des artériopathies dégéneratives. On discute la manière dont ces lésions influent sur l'état du foetus.

Zusammenfassung

Verf. bemerken, daß sich der Faktor Placenta auf die Entwicklung der Frucht u. a. auch durch morphofunktionelle Mängel auswirkt. Diese sind meistens eine Folge vaskulärer Störungen mit eigener Symptomatologie, wie die im Laufe von Spätschwangerschaftsstörungen, im Verlaufe von Nierenerkrankungen oder eines Diabetes auftretenden Gefäßerkrankungen.

Verf. beschreiben eine Reihe mikroskopischer Präparate, die aus dem Plazentaorgan solcher Fälle stammen. An diesen kommen zwischen den einzelnen Zotten gelegene Thrombosen, ischämiebedingte Nekrosen, richtige Infarktbildungen und degenerative Arterienerkrankungen zum Vorschein. Verf. erörtern, in welcher Weise diese Schädigungen den Zustand der Frucht beeinflussen.

Le poids ou les poids du placenta. L'intérêt de normaliser les conditions précédant la pesée placentaire

E. Philippe

Institut d'Anatomie Pathologique, Hospices Civils, Strasbourg, France

Le poids du placenta constitute le critère le plus simple et le plus fidèle dans l'appréciation de la fonction placentaire et de ce fait du développement normal du foetus.

Il y a quelques années encore on pesait le placenta en totalité, membranes et cordon compris et on obtenait un poids moyen à terme d'environ 600 g. Puis, grâce à *Benirschke,* le placenta est pesé sans membranes ni cordon, à l'état frais ou, ce qui entraîne 5% du poids en sus, après fixation au formol pendant dix jours. Dans ces conditions le poids moyen du placenta à terme est d'environ 500 g. Ce type de pesée permet une meilleure corrélation des données pondérales et fonctionnelles en éliminant les annexes placentaires dont le poids est pratiquement constant au cours des dernières semaines de la grossesse, mais variable lors du travail par infiltration de liquide amniotique.

Le poids „normal" du placenta sans membranes ni cordon se situe cependant dans une fourchette trop large, puisque des poids proches de 300 g ou supérieurs à 700 g, sont considérés encore normaux à terme (Tab. 1). Ces variations pondérales dépendent en grande partie de la quantité de sang, foetal et maternel, retenu de manière différente d'un placenta à un autre (Tab. 2). Ainsi, la quantité de sang foetal placentaire est influencée par la section plus ou moins rapide du cordon à la naissance et par le drainage éventuel de la veine ombilicale avant la délivrance. La quantité de sang maternel retenu dans les espaces intervillositaires dépend en grande partie de la durée et de l'intensité des contractions lors du travail et lors de la période précédant l'expulsion du placenta.

En conséquence, le poids placentaire idéal est celui obtenu après élimination complète du sang maternel et foetal. On peut y aboutir par centrifugation (*Aherne*) au détriment cependant de toute étude histologique. On peut aussi y parvenir de manière satisfaisante, mais non complète, par section du placenta frais et vidange passive de son sang. Nous avons appliqué cette méthode en collaboration avec le Docteur *Guez,* à la Clinique Gynécologique et Obstétricale I (Directeur Prof. *R. Gandar*) du CHU de Strasbourg.

Tab. 1. Poids du placenta normal à terme.

		♂	♀
Placenta complet: *Hendricks*, 1964	610 g	620	600
Placenta sans membranes ni cordon: *Aherne, Dunnill*, 1966	488 g (391–723)	–	–
Institut de Pathologie de Strasbourg, 1967	495 g (320–750)	475	504
Boyd, Hamilton, 1970	508 g (310–880)	–	–
Placenta sans membranes, ni cordon, après section à l'état frais: Institut de Pathologie de Strasbourg, 1970	380 g (330–430)	380	380

Tab. 2. Les poids du placenta.

100 g	cordon et membranes
120 g	sang foetal (draîné par cordon) sang maternel (section placenta frais)
30 g	sang résiduel, maternel et foetal
320 g	eau
16 g	substances inertes
22 g	métabolites protéiques

Les modalités d'application sont les suivantes:

1. Vidange du sang veineux ombilical à l'extrémité placentaire pendant au moins 3 minutes, lors de la section du cordon à la naissance. Le sang recueilli peut être mesuré et servir, le cas échéant, à un examen sérologique.
2. Examen habituel du placenta frais et ablation des caillots récents, au moment de la délivrance.
3. Section du cordon et des membranes libres à 1 cm du placenta et éventuellement prise du poids placentaire sans membranes, ni cordon.
4. Section du placenta frais en tranches parallèles de 2 cm allant de la plaque choriale à la plaque basale. Cette opération est effectuée de préférence dans la demi-heure qui suit l'expulsion du placenta, mais peut être retardée de 24 heures en conservant le placenta à + 4°.

5. Pesée de l'ensemble des tranches placentaires quelques minutes après la section, afin de permettre l'écoulement du sang maternel et foetal (vaisseaux allanto-choriaux surtout en cas de ligature immédiate du cordon à la naissance).
   Le poids placentaire normal à terme est de l'ordre de 380 g ± 50 g.

6. Fixation éventuelle de l'ensemble des tranches dans du formol à 10% en vue de l'examen par le pathologiste. On aura soin d'éviter la déformation des tranches en les plaçant dans une cuvette assez large ou dans des sacs en plastique.

Cette technique entraîne quelques inconvénients: perte de temps (assez réduite par l'expérience), servitude matérielle (affûtage fréquent du couteau), nécessité de reconnaître les lésions sur le placenta frais. Contrairement à l'opinion de *Benirschke,* l'interprétation des anomalies macroscopiques du placenta frais est relativement aisée. En pratique le placenta normal est de structure homogène, sans anomalies, en dehors parfois de quelques foyers de nécrose ischémique villositaire, de calcifications, de thromboses sous-choriales peu étendues, de quelques thromboses intervilleuses, lésions facilement reconnaissables par la sage femme ou les médecins après un entraînement sur une centaine de cas. Le placenta pathologique ou porteur d'autres anomalies nécessite, au contraire, l'examen par le pathologiste.

La section du placenta frais élimine les variations pondérales consécutives aux perturbations hémodynamiques de la circulation placentaire au cours du travail et de la période précédant l'expulsion du placenta. Elle permet aussi de normaliser les données macroscopiques et histologiques du placenta et d'établir des corrélations réellement significatives entre l'état du placenta et le développement intra-utérin du foetus. Le poids du placenta varie ainsi dans des limites raisonnables (± 50 g) et la courbe de répartition des poids des placentas normaux n'empiète pas largement sur la courbe des poids des placentas pathologiques.

De plus, l'examen histologique des placentas est nettement amélioré: bonne fixation, examen rapide, appréciation valable des conditions hémodynamiques du placenta avant l'accouchement (degré de dilatation et d'affaissement des espaces maternels intervilleux et des vaisseaux foetaux) et par conséquence réduction des artéfacts atteignant les villosités terminales. En effet, la congestion aiguë des vaisseaux villositaires entraîne un déplissement du syncytiotrophoblaste, l'affaissement des vaisseaux villositaires, la contraction du syncytiotrophoblaste et l'apparition de nombreux amas nucléaires trophoblastiques.

Enfin, la section du placenta frais permet d'étudier valablement, par des méthodes histométriques, les rapports entre les différentes structures du placenta (Tab. 3) et l'hypotrophie réelle du trophoblaste en cas d'insuffisance placentaire.

Ainsi, en éliminant une grande partie du sang maternal et foetal par section de l'organe frais avant sa pesée et sa fixation, on normalise les données pondérales et histologiques du placenta. Ces données devront toujours être rapportées en fonction de l'âge de la grossesse et le cas échéant, du sexe de l'enfant.

Tab. 3. Les structures du placenta (modifié d'après *Aherne* ct *Dunnill*, 1966).

21%	plaque choriale et basale vaisseaux villositaires 0,1 cm septum intercotylédonnaire		
36%	espace intervilleux		
	capillaires	10%	
43%	conjonctif	20%	villosités
	trophoblaste	13%	

A Correlation between Serum and Placental Enzymes in EPH-Gestosis

Mohamed B. Sammour, B.Sc. (Oxford), F.R.C.S., M.I.A.C.
Mohie A. Ramadan, Ph.D. and *Fawzia M. Khalil,* M.Sc.

From the Department of Obstetrics and Biochemistry, Faculty of Medicine,
Ain Shams University, Cairo, Egypt

Introduction

In EPH-gestosis placental infarcts and scattered areas of degenerated trophoblast are consistently found. When a toxemic syndrome becomes clinically evident, this means that cellular enzymes are liberated from the damaged placenta, exactly as they are released from the infarcted heart muscle.

Cory in 1934 was the first to demonstrate that serum alkaline phosphatase was elevated in late pregnancy. This fact was also confirmed by the work of others as *Carryla* and *Fabre* in 1935, *Bayer* in 1963 and *Neale* in 1965.

The alkaline phosphatase from the placenta is heat stable at 56°C, whereas phosphatases from other sources are heat labile. *Neale* in 1965 found a sharp rise in the heat stable alkaline phosphatase readings in patients with mild preeclampsia more than in normal pregnancy. *Tennant* in 1970 after studying serum and placental alkaline phosphatase in normal pregnancy and in preeclampsia concluded that the circulating enzyme in the serum during late pregnancy was of placental origin. The numerous pathological conditions which are accompanied by elevation of serum lactate dehydrogenase (S.L.D.) are all associated with tissue injury and breakdown. A placental source for the lactate dehyrogenase was proposed by *Little* (1959) who found definite elevation of the S.L.D. in placental infarcts.

Much has been published about the choline esterase of the blood. Chronic liver damage as cirrhosis entails a greater decrease in the level of enzymes especially the choline esterase.

The purpose of our present investigation is to study the level of certain enzymes in the serum and to compare their concentrations in the placental extract in a group of EPH-gestosis patients with the idea to find a correlation between the placental and serum levels, then we can use the latter as an index of placental sufficiency.

Materials and Methods

This study was carried on 47 cases divided into three groups:
1. Fifteen cases of normal pregnancy used as a control sample.
2. Twelve cases of mild EPH-gestosis.
3. Twenty cases of severe EPH-gestosis.

We followed the classification of mild and severe EPH-gestosis as standardized in the Paris Meeting of the Organisation Gestosis and we estimated the Gestosis-Index according to such classification.

The detailed description of our cases is mentioned in Tab. 1.

Tab. 1. Description of 32 cases of EPH-Gestosis (Preclampsia) and 15 Normal Pregnancies submitted for Enzyme Estimations of the Serum and Placenta.

Diagnoses	No. of cases	Average age (years)	Parity			Blood pressure		Gestosis Index.
			primip. %	Grand-mult. %	Average No. of deliveries	Systolic (mm Hg)	Diastolic (mm Hg.)	
Normal Pregnancy	15	28.1	20.8	20.8	2.5	120.0	78.5	–
Mild EPH-Gestoses	12	29.1	25.0	23.8	1.2	143.1	91.1	3.8
Severe EPH-Gestoses	20	29.3	41.6	29.2	3.2	177.1	109.3	8.5

All our patients were hospital cases and we unified the time of collecting all samples taking the third stage of labour as the proper time to obtain both maternal blood samples and to excise a wedge of the placenta constituting the whole thickness from the centre to the periphery. All our cases were delivered vaginally with no difficult interferrence and anaesthesia if needed was either local infiltration or pudendal block anaesthesia.

The following enzymes were estimated both in the serum of the blood sample and in the extract of the frozen placenta:

1. The alkaline phosphatases, by the method of *Kind* and *King* (1954).
2. The lactate dehydrogenase by *Wroblewki* and *Ruggiero* method (1958).
3. The choline esterase by the method followed by *Huerga, Yesinnick* and *Dapper* (1952).
4. The transaminase, both the serum glutamic oxalacetic transaminase (S.G.O.T.) and the serum glutamic pyruvic transaminase (S.G.P.T.) following the *Reitman* and *Frankel* method (1957).

Results

I. *Alkaline Phosphatases:*

1. The total alkaline phosphatase in the 15 normal pregnancy cases ranged between 6 and 16 King Armstrong Units (K.A.U.) in the serum with an average mean 10.26 ± 0.951 K.A./100 ml, while in the placenta, it ranged between 6–15 with an average of 10.46 ± 0.756 K.A./100 mg tissue.
2. In the group of mild EPH-gestosis, the serum level ranged between 15–20 with an average of 17.5 ± 0.484 K.A./100 ml while the placental level varied between 17–23 with a mean value of 20.16 ± 0.627 K.A./100 mg tissue.
3. In the group of severe EPH-gestosis, the serum values were varying between 17–23 with a mean of 22 ± 1.574 K.A./100 ml and the placental readings were from 19–62 with a mean of 37.45 ± 2.360 K.A./100 mg tissue.

These results are detailed in Tab. 2.

Tab. 2.

	Alkaline Phosphatase					
	K.A./100 ml Serum			K.A./100 mg. tissue		
	Normal Pregnancy	Preeclampsia Mild	Preeclampsia Severe	Normal Pregnancy	Preeclampsia Mild	Preeclampsia Severe
No of cases	15	12	20	15	12	20
Range	6-16	15-20	15-39	6-15	17-23	19-62
Mean ± S.E.	10.26 ± .951	17.50 ± .484	22.00 ± 1.57	10.46 ± .756	20.16 ± .627	37.45 ± 2.36
Significance test (P)	Normal–Mild: 0.001	Mild–Severe: 0.01	Normal–Severe: 0.001	Normal–Mild: 0.001	Mild–Severe: 0.001	Normal–Severe: 0.001
Correlation Coefficient (R) Serum X Placenta	Normal: 0.1	Mild: Not significant	Severe: 0.001			

0.001 = Significance
0.01 = Slightly significance
0.1 = Not significance or at level of 10%

II. *Lactate Dehydrogenase:*

1. In normal pregnancy, the serum levels were 112–114 with a mean of 131.66 ± 3.23 I.U./litre while the placental readings were 112–145 with a mean value of 128.90 ± 2.36 I.U./gm.
2. In mild EPH-gestosis the serum levels varied between 138–263 with an average mean of 184.16 ± 11.73 I.U./litre while the placental levels varied between 142–245 with a mean of 182.50 ± 10.13 I.U./gm.

3. In severe EPH-gestosis, the serum values were 372–500 with a mean of 423.75 ± 6.75 I.U./litre and the placental readings were 380–490 with a mean of 434.50 ± 6.69 I.U./gm.

The above results are summarized in Tab. 3.

Tab. 3.

	Lactate Dehydrogenase					
	I.U./ Litre Serum			I.U./ gram Placenta		
	Normal Pregnancy	Preeclampsia Mild	Preeclampsia Severe	Normal Pregnancy	Preeclampsia Mild	Preeclampsia Severe
No. of cases	15	12	20	15	12	20
Range	112-154	138-263	372-500	112-145	142-245	380-490
Mean ± S.E.	131.66 ±3.23	184.16 ±11.73	423.75 ± 6.75	128.90 ± 2.36	182.50 ±10.13	434.50 ±6.69
Significance test (P)	Normal × Mild: 0.002	Mild × Severe: 0.001	Normal × Severe: 0.001	Normal × Mild: 0.001	Mild × Severe: 0.001	Normal × Severe: 0.001
Correlation Coefficient (R) Serum X Placenta	Normal: 0.01	Mild: 0.001	Severe: 0.1			

0.001 = Significance
0.002 = Slight significance
0.01 = Small significance
0.1 = Not significant or at 10% level

III. *Choline Esterase:*

1. In cases of normal pregnancy, the serum levels were 216–310 with a mean of 279.13 ± 6.43 U./100 ml while, the placental enzyme levels were 76–131 with a mean of 112.33 ± 6.96 U./100 mg placenta.
2. In mild EPH-gestosis, the levels in the serum were 240–293 with a mean of 274 ± 4.69 U./100 ml and the levels in the placental extract were 77–157 with a mean value of 108.41 ± 6.90 U./100 mg placenta.
3. In severe EPH-gestosis, the serum value varied between 200–300 with a mean of 244.45 ± 5.39 U./100 ml while the placental figures were 52–175 with a mean of 103.20 ± 6.96 U./100 mg placenta.

Tab. 4 summarizes these results.

Tab. 4.

	Choline Esterase					
	Units / 100 ml Serum			Units / 100 mg Placenta		
	Normal Pregnancy	Preeclampsia Mild	Preeclampsia Severe	Normal Pregnancy	Preeclampsia Mild	Preeclampsia Severe
No. of cases	15	12	20	15	12	20
Range	216-310	240-293	200-300	76-161	77-157	52-175
Mean ± S.E.	279.13 ±6.43	274.00 ±4.69	244.45 ±5.39	112.33 ±6.96	108.41 ±6.90	103.20 ±6.96
Significance test (P)	N.S. (Normal vs Mild); N.S. (Normal vs Severe)	N.S. (Mild vs Severe)		N.S. (Normal vs Mild); N.S. (Normal vs Severe)	N.S. (Mild vs Severe)	
Correlation Coefficient (R) Serum X Placenta	N.S. (Normal)	N.S. (Mild)	N.S. (Severe)			

IV. *Transaminases:*

A. *Glutamic Oxalacetric Transaminases (G.O.T.)*

1. In normal pregnancy, the serum levels were 9–18 with a mean of 13.13 ± 0.72 I.U./litre, while in the placenta the levels were 11–19 with a mean of 13.86 ± 0.568 I.U./gm placenta.

2. In mild EPH-gestosis, the serum values were 12–20 with a mean of 16.41 ± 0.570 I.U./litre while the placental readings were 16–21 with a mean value of 16.83 ± 0.927 I.U./gm placenta.

3. In severe EPH-gestosis, the serum estimations were 11–55 with a mean value of 25.55 ± 2.88 I.U./litre and the placental readings were 21–41 with an average mean of 29.85 ± 1.68 I.U./gm placenta.

B. *Glutamic Oxalacetic Transaminase (G.P.T.)*

1. In the group of normal pregnancy, the serum levels were 2–9 with a mean of 5.20 ± 0.564 I.U./litre and the placental readings were 3–9 with a mean of 6.66 ± 0.58 I.U./gm placenta.

2. In mild EPH-gestosis, the serum values were 4–10 with a mean of 7.00 ± 0.673 I.U./litre and the placental estimations were 5–11 with a mean of 8.08 ± 0.557 I.U./gm placenta.

3. In severe EPH-gestosis, the serum contained 3–15 U. with a mean value of 8.75 ± 0.714 I.U./litre, while the placental contents were 3–13 U. with an average mean of 7.60 ± 0.45 I.U./gm placenta.

Tab. 5 and 6 summarizes the results of the transaminases.

Tab. 5.

	Glutamic Pyruvic transaminase					
	I. U./Litre Serum			I.U./gram Placenta		
	Normal Pregnancy	Preeclampsia Mild	Preeclampsia Severe	Normal Pregnancy	Preeclampsia Mild	Preeclampsia Severe
Nº of cases	15	12	20	15	12	20
Range	2-9	4-10	3-15	3-9	5-11	3-12
Mean ±S.E.	5.20 ±.564	7.00 ±.673	8.75 ±.714	6.66 ±.585	8.08 ±.557	7.60 ±.454
Significance test (P)	Normal–Mild: 0.1; Normal–Severe: 0.001	Mild–Severe: 0.1		Normal–Mild: 0.1 N.S.; Normal–Severe: N.S.	Mild–Severe: N.S.	
Correlation Coefficient (R) Serum X Placenta	Not significant	Not significant	0.05			

0.1 = N.S.
0.001 = Significance
0.05 = Slightly significance

Discussion

The statistical analysis of our estimations of the total alkaline phosphatases both in the placenta and in the serum of patients suffering from EPH-gestosis points to the fact that the increase in this enzyme was significant in the different grades of toxaemia. On obtaining the correlation between the total alkaline phosphatases in the serum and in the placenta, it was high in severe EPH-gestosis while in the mild type no such correlation was obtained. Our results are similar to those obtained by *Birkett* (1966) who explained the increase in the serum alkaline phosphatases in pregnancy toxaemia by the increase of the enzyme activity in the placenta. In our series the elevation in the total alkaline phosphatases in EPH-gestosis showed a direct relation to the severity of the case and there was a correlation between the serum and the placental enzymes.

Tab. 6.

	Glutamic axalacetic transaminase					
	I. U./ Litre Serum			I.U./ gram Placenta		
	Normal Pregnancy	Preeclampsia Mild	Preeclampsia Severe	Normal Pregnancy	Preeclampsia Mild	Preeclampsia Severe
No. of cases	15	12	20	15	12	20
Range	9-18	12-20	11-55	11-19	10-21	21-41
Mean ± S.E.	13.13 ±.725	16.41 ±.570	25.55 ±2.88	13.86 ± .568	16.83 ±.926	29.85 ± 1.68
Significance test (P)	Normal vs. Mild: 0.002; Normal vs. Severe: 0.001	Mild vs. Severe: 0.001		Normal vs. Mild: 0.01; Normal vs. Severe: 0.01	Mild vs. Severe: N.S.	
Correlation Coefficient (R) Serum X Placenta	Normal: Not significant	Mild: 0.001	Severe: Not significant			

0.001 = Significant
0.002 = Slightly significant
N.S. = Not significant
0.01 = Small significance

As far as the lactate dehydrogenase enzyme is concerned, its level was significantly high in both the mild and severe EPH-gestosis and the figures between the serum and the placenta were highly correlated. Previously, *Hagerman* and *Wellington* (1959) ascribed the increase in the maternal L.D.H. to enzyme release from degenerating placental cells.

The results of the choline esterase estimations did not show any significant variations between normal and toxaemic pregnancies. The analysis of our data in case of G.O.T. showed significant increase in the serum of severe EPH-gestosis patients. The correlation of the results between the serum and the placental levels was only observed in mild EPH-gestosis. The only significant finding in case of S.G.P.T. was in the severe EPH-gestosis with no correlations between the serum and the placental enzyme levels.

As a conclusion, one can see that with excessive placental damage as in severe EPH-gestosis, there was a high level of the total alkaline phosphatases, of the lactate dehydrogenase and of the transaminases especially the glutamic oxalacetic transaminase. The indication that the high level of such enzymes in the serum of toxaemic patients would mean a serious placental insufficiency is further supported by the fact that in 3 cases of concealed accidental hemorrhage associating severe EPH-gestosis we obtained the highest serum and placental levels of alkaline phosphatases, and lactate dehydrogenases. In the 3 cases the foetuses were stillbirths. One can suggest that repeated estimations of such enzymes in the serum in cases of EPH-complex would help in deciding the time of termination of the pregnancy for fear of placental insufficiency. The continuous rising serum levels of alkaline phosphatases, lactate dehydrogenase and the GOT form a proper index for the placental function (Fig. 1).

Summary and Conclusions

The alkaline phosphatases, the lactate dehydrogenase, the choline esterase and both types of transaminase (SGPT and SGOT) were estimated in the serum and placenta of 32 cases of EPH-gestosis and 15 normal pregnancies.

There was a significant rise in the serum and placental alkaline phosphatases in both mild and severe EPH-gestosis as compared to the normal pregnancy. There was also a significant correlation between the serum and placental levels.

The lactate dehydrogenase was significantly high in the serum and placenta of mild and severe EPH-gestosis with a significant correlation coefficient of serum and placenta.

The choline esterase did not show any significant difference either in the serum or in the placenta. The glutamic pyruvic transaminase manifested a slight significant rise in the serum in EPH-gestosis cases as compared to the normal pregnancy. The glutamic oxalacetic transaminase showed a significant rise in the serum of both the severe and mild EPH-gestosis, with a significant correlation between the serum and placental levels of both types of EPH-complex.

It is suggested that estimations of the above enzymes would help in the diagnosis of placental damage and its effect on the outcome of the newborn.

References

Bayer, S. H.: Science 1484 (1963).

Birkett, D. J., J. Done and *F. C. Neale:* Brit. Med. J. 1 (1966) p. 1210.

Corryla, J. and *F. Fabre:* Conpt. Rend. Soc. Biol. 120 (1935) p. 748.

Dela Huerga, J., S. Yesinnick and *H. Dapper:* Am. J. Clin. Path. 22 (1952) p. 1126.

Hagerman, D. D. and *F. M. Wellington:* Amer. J. Obstet. Gynec. 77 (1959) p. 348.

Kind, P. R. N. and *E. J. King:* J. Clin. Path. 7 (1954) p. 322.

Little, W. A.: Obstet. and Gynec. 13 (1959) p. 152.

Neale, F. C., J. S. Clubb and *S. Pasen:* J. Clin. Path. 18 (1965) p. 359.

Reitman, S. and *S. Frankel:* Amer. J. Clin. Path. 28 (1957) p. 56.

Tennant, R.: Obstet. and Gynec. 36 (1970) p. 4, 535.

Wròblenski, C. and *A. Ruggiero:* Am. J. Clin. Path. 30 (1958) p. 234.

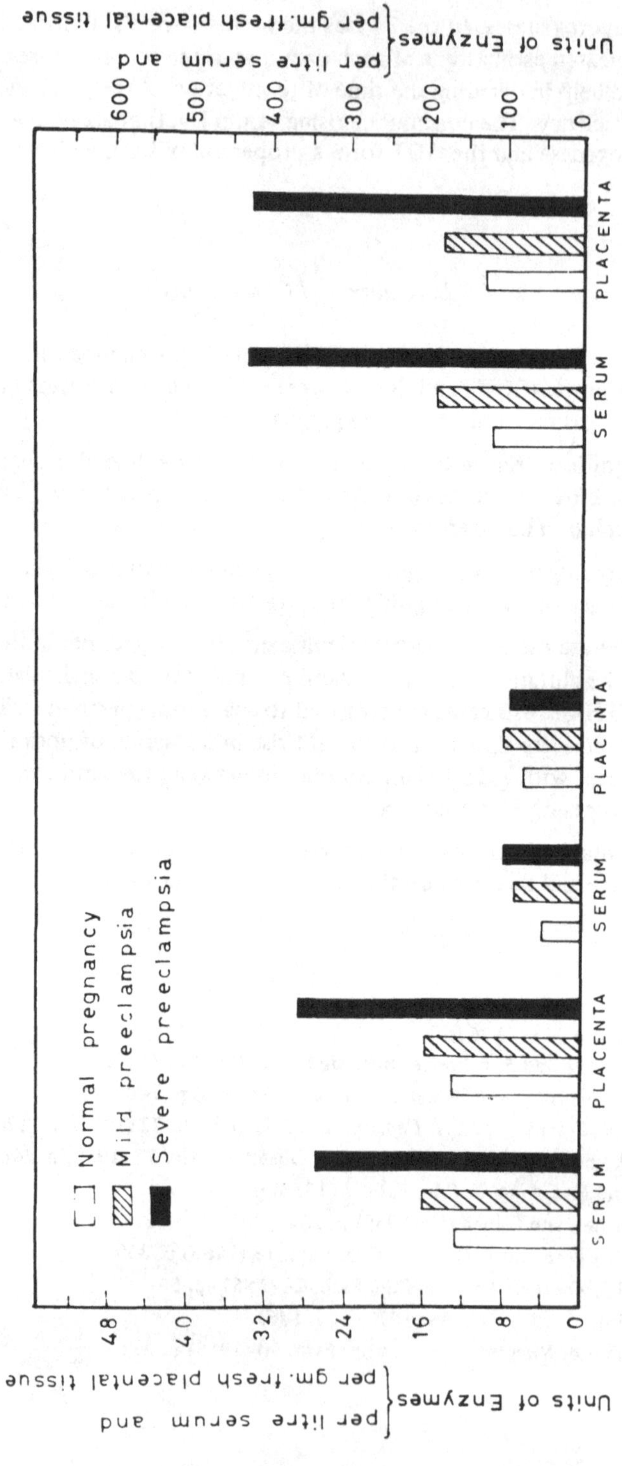
Units of Enzymes per litre serum and per gm. fresh placental tissue
0 100 200 300 400 500 600
0 8 16 24 32 40 48
Normal pregnancy
Mild preeclampsia
Severe preeclampsia
SERUM PLACENTA
G.O.T
SERUM PLACENTA
G.P.T
SERUM PLACENTA
L.D.H

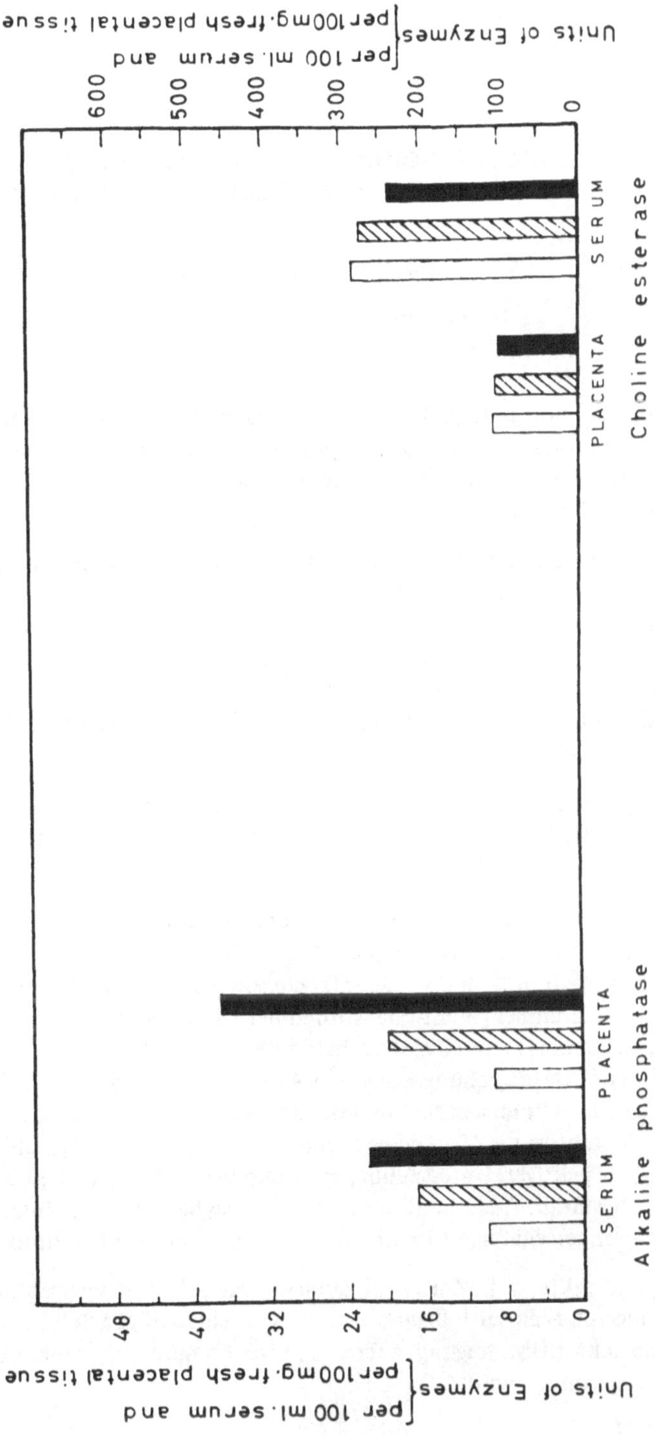
Units of Enzymes per 100 ml. serum and per 100 mg. fresh placental tissue
0
100
200
300
400
500
600
PLACENTA
SERUM
Choline esterase
SERUM
PLACENTA
Alkaline phosphatase
0
8
16
24
32
40
48
Units of Enzymes per 100 ml. serum and per 100 mg. fresh placental tissue

Fig. 1

Placentabefunde bei EPH-Gestose, eine phasenkontrastmikroskopische Untersuchung

Ch. Werner, G. Schwartz

Universitäts-Frauenklinik, Düsseldorf, BRD

Eine Vielzahl von morphologischen Veränderungen an der Placenta werden der Praeeklampsie zugeschrieben. Im Folgenden geben wir eine Zusammenstellung über die am häufigsten von uns erhobenen Befunde bei Praeeklampsie und setzen sie in Beziehung zu einigen klinischen Daten.

1. An der Universitätsfrauenklinik in Düsseldorf wurde bisher eine Hypertonie über 140/90 mm/Hg, eine Proteinurie über 1‰ und Ödeme mit einer Gewichtszunahme von mehr als 500 g/Woche, abhängig vom Schweregrad der Symptome, als Praeeklampsie leichten oder schweren Grades bezeichnet. Von der essentiellen Praeeklampsie wurde die symptomatische Form abgegrenzt beim Vorliegen eines praeexistenten Grundleidens, d. h. wenn eine Nierenerkrankung oder eine Hypertonie vor der Schwangerschaft bestanden.

Alle Geburtsplacenten werden routinemäßig makroskopisch und phasenkontrastmikroskopisch untersucht. Bei den ersten 1000 unausgewählten Placenten war die Schwangerschaft 180 mal durch eine Praeeklampsie kompliziert.

Bei der makroskopischen Beurteilung der frischen Geburtsplacenta wurde besonders die Größe und Zahl der Infarkte berücksichtigt. Alle Zeichen der maternen Durchblutungsstörung, d. h. rote und weiße Infarkte sowie intervillöse Thrombosen haben wir als Infarkte zusammengefaßt. Sie wurden bei 180 Placenten aus Schwangerschaften mit einer Praeeklampsie nur 12 mal nachgewiesen, das sind 6,6%, in den übrigen 820 Placenten des Untersuchungskollektivs 47 mal, das sind 5,7%. Somit liegt die Infarkthäufigkeit im untersuchten Material unabhängig davon, ob eine Praeeklampsie vorlag oder nicht, etwa bei 6%. Dieses Ergebnis wurde durch *Becker* unlängst an dem Material des prospektiven Untersuchungsprogrammes der Deutschen Forschungsgemeinschaft bestätigt. Auch in dieser Untersuchung bestand kein Zusammenhang zwischen Schwangerschaftsgestose und dem Vorkommen von Placentainfarkten.

Abb. 1. Mikroinfarkte, d. h. Zottenspitzennekrosen u. U. mit Verklebung von mehreren Zotten und intervillöser Fibrinablagerung sind ein häufiger Befund, der bei Gestosen und echter Übertragung, aber auch nach komplikationslosem Schwangerschaftsverlauf gefunden wird.

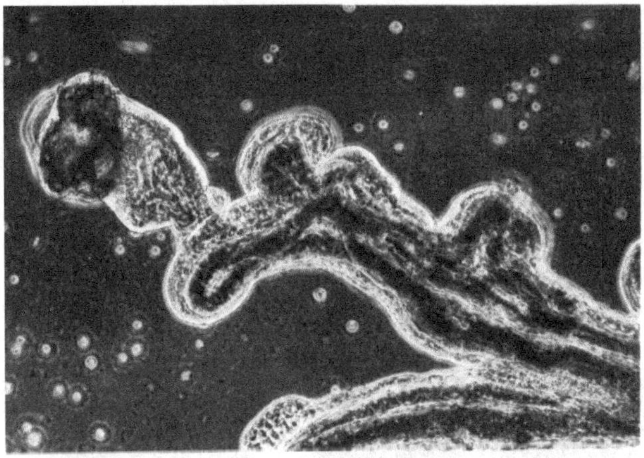

Abb. 1. Phasenkontrastmikroskopische Aufnahme eines Mikroinfarktes (Vergr. 63 : 1)

Im Vordergrund unserer Untersuchung steht die Reifediagnostik der Placenta angelehnt an die nach *Alvarez* und *Becker* zusammengestellten Reifekriterien und den daraus erkennbaren Placentareifungsstörungen. Abb. 2.

Phasenkontrastmikroskopische Reifezeichen

I. Präpartale Verkleinerung der Zottendurchmesser
II. Umwandlung der Kapillaren in Sinusoide unter Verdrängung des lockeren Zottenstromas
III. Kernverschiebung des Syncytiotrophoblasten und Ausbildung von Stoffwechselmembranen
IV. Abnahme der Sprouts (Trophoblastknospen)

Formen der Plazentareifungsstörungen

I. Vorzeitige Plazentareifung bei unreifem Kind (M. präcox pl.)
Ursache: z. B. kleine Plazenta, Infarktplazenta
→ plazentogene Frühgeburt

II. Unreife Plazenta bei reifem Kind
a) essentielle Reifungsretardierung (M. retardata pl.)
Ursache: ?
→ plazentogene Übertragung in ihrer Belastbarkeit eingeschränkte Pl.
b) symptomatische Reifungsretardierung
Ursache: z. B. Rh-Inkompatibilität, Diabetes mellitus, Präeklampsie, Lues
→ in ihrer Belastbarkeit eingeschränkte Pl.

Abb. 2. Phasenkontrastmikroskopische Reifezeichen und Formen der Placentareifungsstörungen

Die Placenta reagiert auf verschiedenste bekannte und unbekannte Noxen mit einer gewissen Monotonie, die gekennzeichnet ist durch eine Reifungsretardierung, welche das morphologische Substrat einer Placentainsuffizienz darstellt. Die Funktionseinschränkung einer reifungsretardierten Placenta bei Praeeklampsie wird bei der Gegenüberstellung zu einer reifen Terminplacenta deutlich (Abb. 3 u. 4). Die Praeeklampsie stellt einen Faktor dar, welche die nach einem ökonomischen Prinzip ablaufenden Reifungsvorgänge behindern. Die Diffusionsstrecke zwischen mütterlichem und kindlichem Blut ist erheblich verlängert, dies führt zu einer Behinderung des schnellen und für den Fetus notwendigen Gasaustausches und kann Ursache einer Placentainsuffizienz sein.

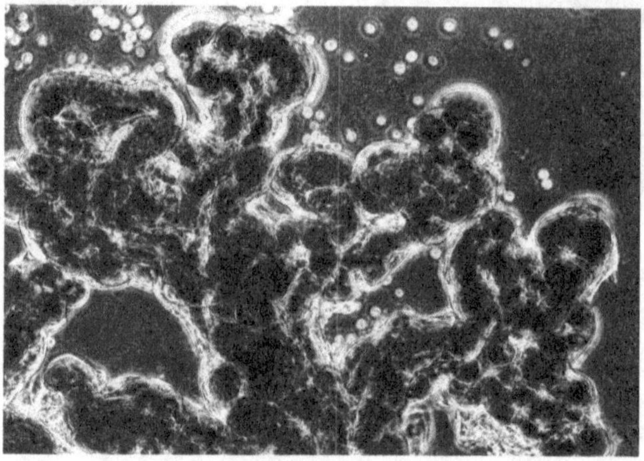

Abb. 3. Phasenkontrastmikroskopische Aufnahme einer reifen Terminplacenta (Vergr. 63 : 1)

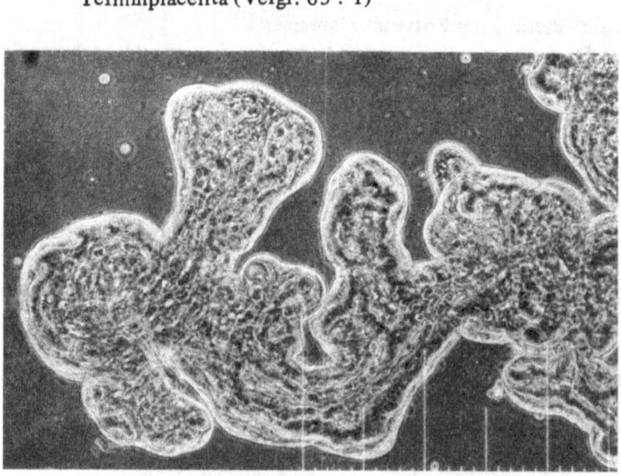

Abb. 4. Phasenkontrastmikroskopische Aufnahme einer reifungsretardierten Placenta bei Präeklampsie (Vergr. 63 : 1)

Abb. 5. Das folgende Diagramm gibt einen Überblick über die Verteilung der Reifediagnosen im Gesamtmaterial (weiße Säulen) und der Fälle, bei denen eine Praeeklampsie bestand (schwarze Säulen), dargestellt in Relativzahlen. Besonders hervorzuheben ist der hohe Anteil an reifen Placenten bei Vorliegen einer Praeeklampsie, diese Placenten ließen morphologisch keine Beeinträchtigung ihres Reifungsverhaltens durch die Schwangerschaftstoxicose erkennen. Ein zweites wichtiges Ergebnis dieser Untersuchungen ist, daß Formen der leichten und schweren Reifungsretardierung bei der Praeeklampsie nahezu doppelt so häufig vertreten sind wie im Restkollektiv.

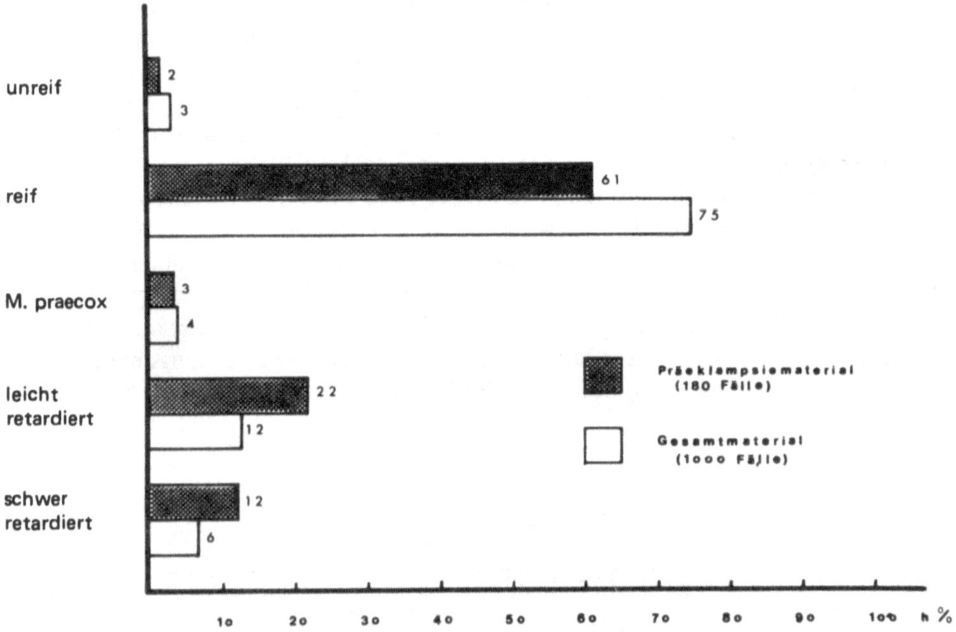

Abb. 5. Verteilung der Placenta – Reifediagnosen im Gesamtmaterial (weiße Säule) und im Präeklampsiekollektiv (schwarze Säule)

2. Der Einfluß der essentiellen und der symptomatischen Praeeklampsie auf die dargestellten Reifediagnosen war kaum unterschiedlich, so daß wir beide Formen zusammenfassen konnten.

Um die Placentabefunde einigen klinischen Daten gegenüber zu stellen, haben wir die Reifediagnosen ihrem Funktionswert entsprechend in drei Gruppen gegliedert (Tab. 1, Abb. 6).

Gruppe 1 umfaßt die unreifen und die reifen Placenten, sie sind zeitgerecht entwickelt und nicht pathologisch. In Gruppe 2 haben wir die M. praecox und die leicht retardierten Placenten zusammengefaßt, ihnen kommt nach der klinischen Erfahrung eine mäßig pathologische Bedeutung zu. In der 3. Gruppe befinden sich die schwer retardierten Placenten, deren Funktion am stärksten eingeschränkt ist. Wir haben versucht, einzelne klinische Daten in 3 sinnvolle Wertigkeitsgrade einzuteilen und diese den

Placentareifediagnosen gegenüberzustellen. Die beste Übereinstimmung besteht zwischen Placentamorphologie und Geburts-CTG sowie dem akt. pH-Wert, die schlechteste zwischen Morphologie und Apgar-Score. Eine volle Übereinstimmung ist nicht zu erwarten, da die angeführten Untersuchungsmethoden keine reinen Placentafunktionsteste sind, sondern auch andere Faktoren als die Placentafunktion in die Daten miteingehen, wie z. B. eine mütterliche Acidose oder Nabelschnurkomplikation.

Die Untersuchungen ergeben, daß der Praeeklampsie in der zugrundegelegten Definition eine sehr unterschiedliche pathologische Bedeutung hinsichtlich ihrer Auswirkung auf die Placentamorphologie und die angeführten klinischen Daten zukommt. – Die Infarkthäufigkeit ist die gleiche wie in dem Vergleichskollektiv. 61% der Placenten aus einer Schwangerschaft mit Praeeklampsie zeigen morphologisch keine pathologischen Veränderungen. Nur die Placentareifungsstörungen sind deutlich gegenüber dem Restkollektiv vermehrt, so daß angenommen werden muß, daß die Reifungsstörung ein wichtiges Indiz einer placentaren Schädigung ist. Es bleibt offen, wieweit Beginn und Dauer der Praeeklampsie eine Wirkung auf die Placentamorphologie und damit auf die Placentafunktion haben. – Weiter zeigt sich, daß die morphologische Placentadiagnostik eine gute Übereinstimmung mit klinischen Daten der Placentafunktion und des Kindszustandes ergibt, insbesondere zum ET, so daß diese Untersuchungsmethoden der Placentamorphologie zugeordnet werden können, um sie morphologisch zu untermauern.

Tab. 1. (Abb. 6)

Zusammenfassung der Placentareifediagnosen	Wertigkeit	DHEA-S Test	Plac. morph	Geburts-CTG	Plac. morph	akt pH Wert	Plac. morph	AS 1 Min	AS 5 Min	Plac. morph
unreif reif	nicht pathologisch	29%	50%	56%	69%	68%	53%	84%	98%	64%
M. praecox leicht retardiert	mittelgradig pathologisch	45%	32%	20%	23%	17%	32%	10%	1%	26%
schwer retardiert	schwer pathologisch	26%	18%	24%	8%	15%	15%	6%	1%	10%
		n = 38		n = 114		n = 53		n = 172		

Lysosomes and Lysosomal Enzymes in Normal and Gestosis Placentas

B. Zsolnai, J. Somogyi

2nd Obstetric Clinic and Experimental Research Department,
University Medical School, Budapest, Hungary

In spite of several reports on placental metabolism, the mechanism of different transport processes in the human placenta has not been clarified. In this relation our attention has been drawn to the possible role of lysosomes in the mediation of placental transport processes. As a first step it seemed to be necessary to characterise the lysosomes and lysosomal enzymes of the human placental tissue.

We should like to talk about the results of our electronmicroscopic and biochemical studies in which 4–12 and 39–40 weeks old placentas were used. Immediately after the interruptions of healthy pregnancies or after completed deliveries, appropriate pieces of placental tissues were fixed for electronmicroscopic examinations or they were homogenized after several washings in isotonic sucrose using a *Potter* type tephlon glass homogenizer. The free and total activities of different lysosomal enzymes were estimated in homogenates using triton-x-100 for liberation of bound hydrolases. In other experiments the homogenates were centrifuged at 20 000 x g for 60 minutes and the enzyme activities were assayed in the soluble and particular fractions, respectively.

Based on light microscopic examinations the following hypothesis was developed. As the syncitiotrophoblasts forms a continous layer on the surface of the free villi, this layer might function as an obligate filter for substances transported across the placenta. Contrary to syncitium cells the Langhans cells do not form a continous layer. If lysosomes play an importent role in the placental transport, it might be expected that their number and cytoplasmic localisation are different in the two types of cells. Indeed, this hypothesis could be verified by electronmicroscopic examinations.

In Fig. 1 a part of a syncitiotrophoblast from a 8 weeks old human placenta can be seen. These cells contain a relative great number of osmiophil granule which are mainly localised near the intervillous space. These granules are probably secondary lysosomes. A lot of dense bodies can be also observed in the slide. In contrast to this, the number of lysosomes in the Langhans cells is less, and the localisation is more diffuse, than in the syncitium cells. On one half of Fig. 2 a part of a syncitium cell and on the lower half, a part of a Langhans cell can be seen. This Langhans cell contain only a few dense bodies and no secondary lysosomes.

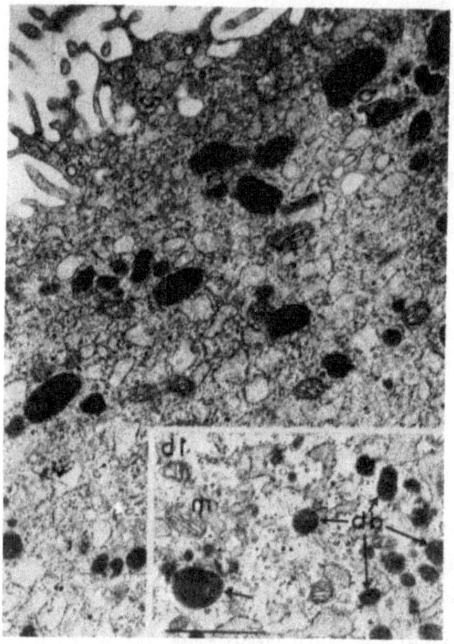

Fig. 1

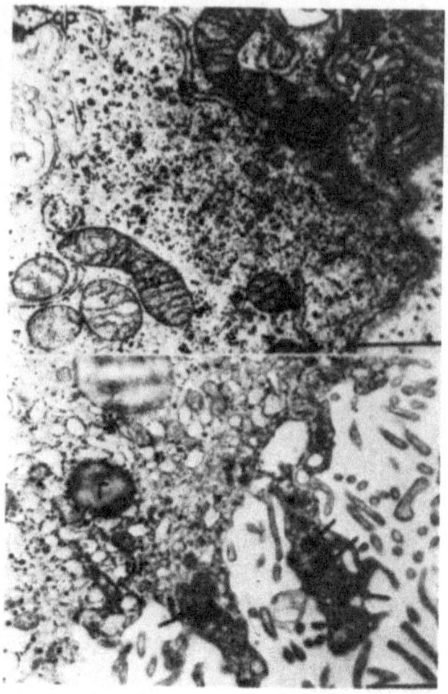

Fig. 2

It is generally accepted that during pregnancy the placental transport processes show a considerable qualitative and quantitative change. If our hypothesis were correct, this changes should be reflected in the biochemical and morphological properties of the placental lysosomes.

In Fig. 3 the total activity of a few acid hydrolases of placental homogenates is presented. As can be seen, the activity of different lysosomal enzymes change during pregnancy. The total activity of one group of hydrolases decreases, and that of others, increases in the course of pregnancy. The total activity of acid phosphatase, cathepsin D and cathepsin B is considerably lower, the activity of acid ribonuclease and beta-glucuronidase is much higher in the old than in the young tissue. Fig. 4 demonstrates the ratio of the different total activities. For the calculation the acid phosphatase activity was chosen as 100 per cent both in the young and old placentas. In relation to acid phosphatase the proportions of cathepsin B and cathepsin D were identical in the young and old placentas, on the other hand this ratio was different in case of acid ribonuclease and beta-glucuronidase.

The intracellular distribution of the lysosomal hydrolases was also dependent of the age of the placentas. The ratio of the bound to free activities decreased significantly in the case of all lysosomal enzymes tested. This is presented in Fig. 5 in cases of acid phosphatase, beta-glucuronidase and acid ribonuclease. Fig. 6 shows that the cathepsin activities of particular fractions decrease and the activities in the soluble fractions increase during the pregnancy.

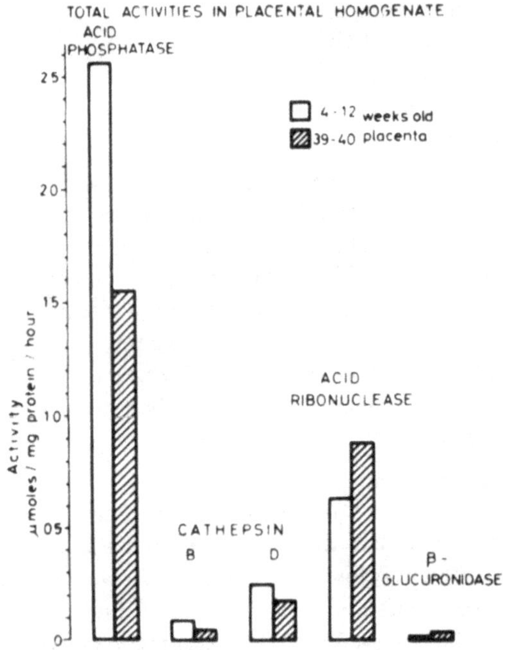

Fig. 3. Total activities in placental homogenate

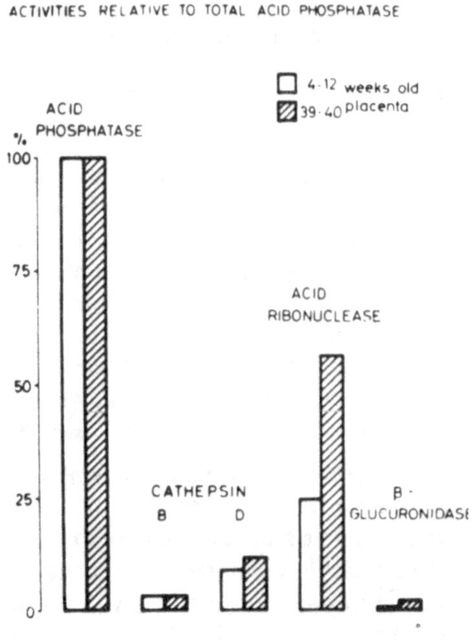

Fig. 4. Activities relative to total acid phosphatase

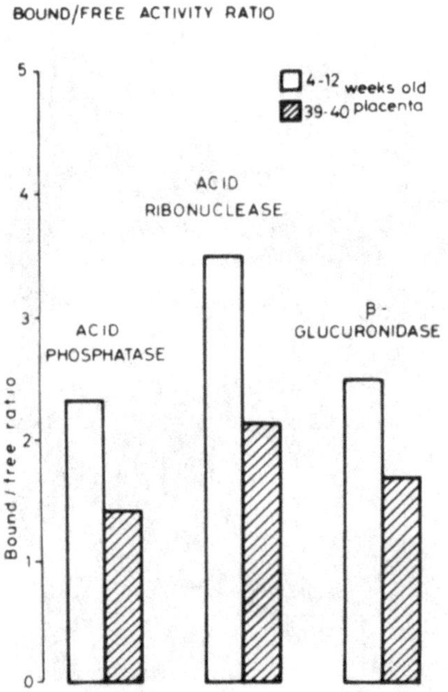

Fig. 5. Bound/free activity ratio

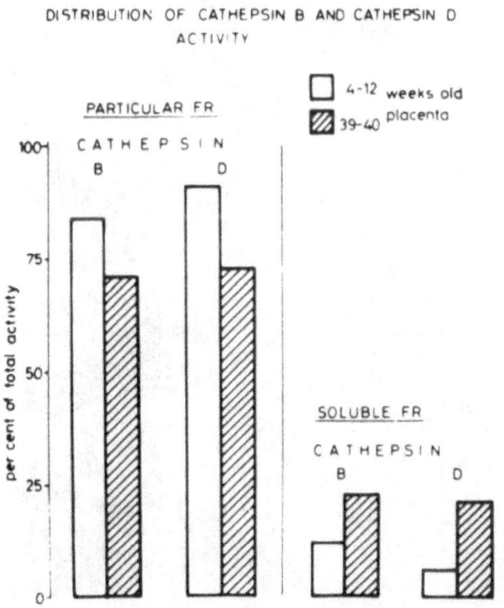

Fig. 6. Distribution of cathepsin B and cathepsin D

Judged from these changed bound per free activity ratios, it seems reasonable to suppose, that the integrity of lysosomes can be changed also during the pregnancy, and the loss of enzymes from the lysosomes must be responsible for the increase in the free enzyme activity detected. However the next slide indicates, that in addition to this process the number of lysosomes also decreases.

In Fig. 7 only a few lysosome can be dedected near the *Golgi* region of a 40 weeks old syncitium cell. The lower part of the slide demonstrates that the lysosomes have lost their characteristic homogenous structure. The osmiophil substances are absent partly in these lysosomes. On the other hand, in the placental macrophag cells, in the so cold *Hofbauer* cells, no alteration could be observed either in the number or in the integrity of lysosomes. The results presented here indicate that during normal pregnancy substantial changes occur both in the number and integrity of placental lysosomes. It is likely that these alterations may be related to the changed intracellular digestion and transport processes of placental tissue during pregnancy.

Based upon the presented biochemical and electronenmicroscopic observation of placenta tissue derived from normal pregnancies, it could be supposed, that these ratios may be more pronounced in gestosis-placentas, that in normal ones. Indeed, in these cases the bound/free activity ratios of different lysosomal hydrolases showed a very decreased value. Parallel with the biochemical alterations the changes in the number and intergrity of lysosomes could also be observed in the electronmicroscopic picture. This is demonstrated in Fig. 8, which originated from a 39 weeks old gestosis-placenta.

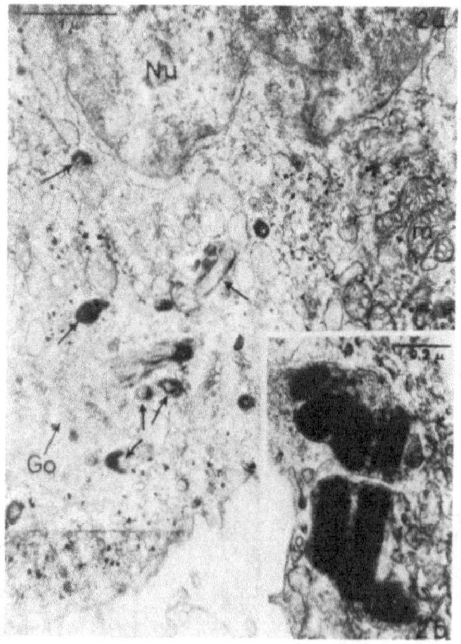

Fig. 7

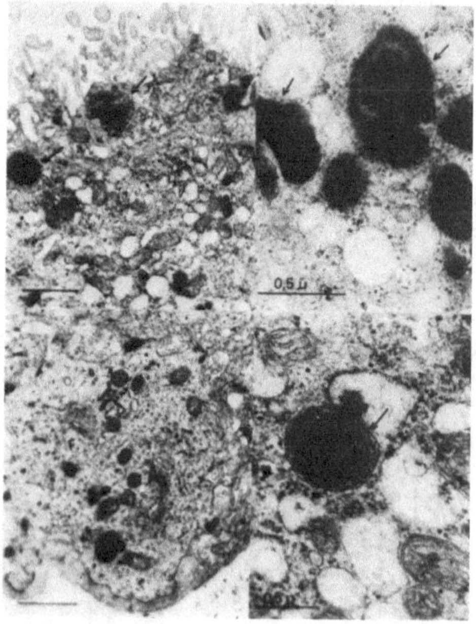

Fig. 8

On this slide only a few secondary lysosomes can be seen. The density of these lysosomes is very inhomogenous. It seems that the electrodense substances are partly dissolved from the particles, especially around the lysosomal membranes. It is also characteristic that the lysosomal membranes have partialy lost their continuities. These changes have been observed in normal mature placentas too, but these changes in integrity and number of lysosomes were significantly more pronounced in cases of EPH-gestosis.

Summing up, it seems that lysosomes and lysosomal enzymes play an important role in the transport processes of human placentas. We could demonstrate that their biochemical and morphological properties change during normal pregnancy. These changes are more pronounced in cases of EPH-gestosis. These alterations are probably also related to changes of lysosomal functions.

However, the exact nature and significance of this altered lysosomal function requires further detailed investigations.

References

B. Zsolnai, J. Somogyi, Z. Szarvas, L. Székely: Die eiweißspaltenden Enzyme in der Schwangerschaft. III. Die Aktivität und subcelluläre Lokalisation von Leucinaminopeptidase, Kathepsin-B und Kathepsin-D in der unreifen und reifen Placenta. Arch. Gynäk. 205 (1967) S. 1–11.

B. Zsolnai, J. Somogyi, Z. Szarvas, E. Papp, L. Székely, J. Hámori: Lysosome und lysosomale Enzyme in der jungen und in der reifen menschlichen Plazenta. Acta chir. Acad. Sci. hung. 10 (1969) S. 191–205.

B. Zsolnai, J. Somogyi: Changes in activity and localization of lysosomal enzymes in human placentas during normal pregnancy. Fourth annual meeting of the European Society for Çlinical Investigation. Abstracts of Papers (1970) p. 74.

Vaginal Cytology in EPH-Gestosis

Vaginal Cytology in Preclampsia before and after Progesterone Therapy

Mohamed B. Sammour, B.Sc. (Oxford), F.R.C.S., M.I.A.C.

Assistant Professor, Department of Gynaecology and Obstetrics,
Ain Shams University, Cairo, Egypt

Introduction

Exfoliative vaginal cytology is a good reflection to the balance of the female hormones. Its procedure is simple and could be easily performed in the antenatal clinic without any inconvenience to the patient.

Papanicolaou in 1925 was the first to describe the navicular cells in the vaginal smears of pregnant women. The navicular cell is intermediate between the superficial and the basal cell, has a dense cytoplasm and an elongated nucleus with dark thickened borders. *Sammour* (1964 and 1967) in his study of the vaginal smear during pregnancy has described 4 stages:

1. The smear of early pregnancy, the morphology of the smear is similar to the picture of the late secretory phase of the menstrual cycle with abundent navicular cells.

2. The placental phase which covers the duration from 16–38 weeks; all smears showed a similar picture described as "the typical pregnancy smear".
   More than 80% of the cells were of the navicular type arranged in compact grouping. The Karyopyknotic index never exceeded 15%. Cytolysis is a feature in 70% of the smears collected during the second half of pregnancy (Fig. 1).

3. The antepartum phase covering the last two weeks of pregnancy; the navicular cells were no longer predominent, being replaced by the intermediate cell, the cells were discrete, and cytolysis had markedly disappeared from the smear (Fig. 2).

4. The "at term" smear is characteristic of pregnancy which has reached term. The cells are intermediate, discrete clean background and absent cytolysis (Fig. 3).

The purpose of this study is to describe the vaginal smear in preclamptic toxaemia of pregnancy, to correlate it with the placental insufficiency and to demonstrate the changes in the smear pattern after progesterone administration to a group of preclamptic patients.

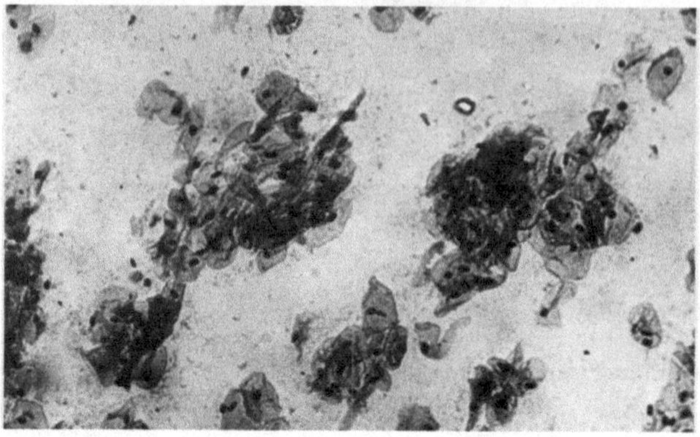

Fig. 1. Typical pregnancy smear, compact groups of navicular cells. x 150

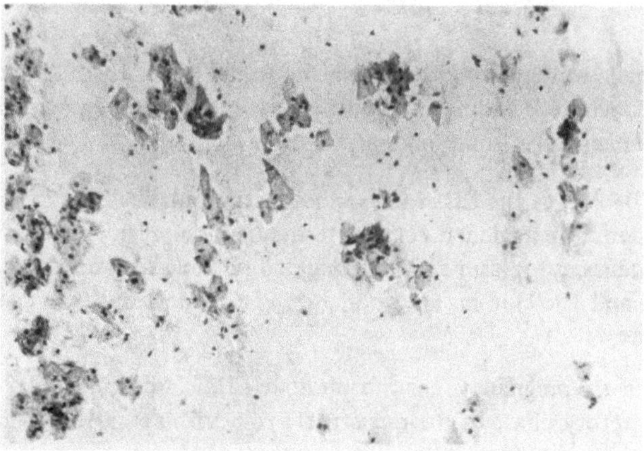

Fig. 2. A pregnancy smear at 39 weeks. x 150

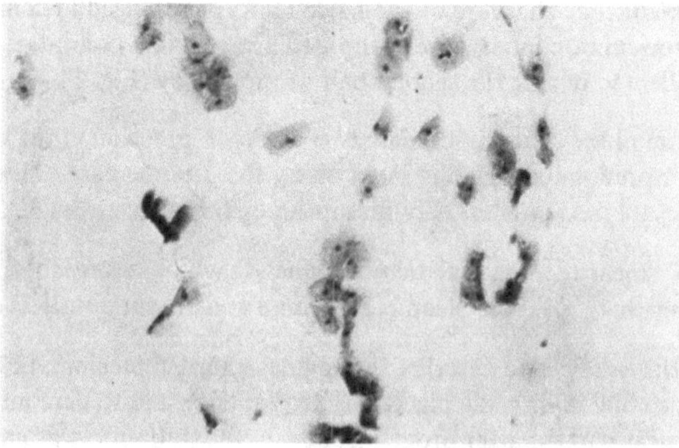

Fig. 3. The "At Term" smear. x 250

Material and Methods

The vaginal smear was collected by scraping of the lateral vaginal wall. The smear was fixed in a mixture of 3% acetic acid in 95% ethyl alcohol, then stained by the *Papanicolaou* stain using *Harris* haematoxyline as counter-stain. The vaginal smear was collected every 2–3 weeks until the onset of labour. We examined 850 smears, collected from 372 patients suffering from preclampsia. The duration of pregnancy varied between 30 and 36 weeks.
The smears were examined mainly for:

1. The dominent type of cells.
2. The cellular arrangement.
3. The karyopyknotic index.
4. Cytolysis.

A group of 40 pregnant women, their pregnancy complicated with preclampsia, were treated with natural progesterone at a dose of 200 mgs daily for a period varying from two to three weeks. The duration of the pregnancy varied from 30–36 weeks. Vaginal smears were obtained weekly by scraping the lateral vaginal and a total of 250 smears were collected.

Results

The cytological picture deviated from the typical smear of pregnancy in 85.7% of the mild preclamptic patient and in 97.5% of the severe preclamptic group.

The following are our findings:

1. *The type of cell:*
   The navicular cell was replaced by the superficial and intermediate cells and the navicular index ranged between 35–50% in all slides examined. The appearance of some superficial squamous with eosinophilic cytoplasm was frequently encountered.
2. *Cellular arrangements:*
   The cells were discrete in 75% of the specimens examined while 25% of the smears showed thick groups of cells (Fig. 4).
3. *The karyopyknotic index:*
   It remained unchanged in most of the smears.
4. *Cytolysis:*
   The phenomena of cytolysis was absent in 60% of the smears. The cells had a well defined outline and well developed cytoplasm with clear background. In the remaining 40%, cytolysis was present with the smear background full of leucocytes and histiocytes (Fig. 5). Tab. 2 summarises the cytological results in the 850 smears collected. From the table the difference in the smear description is slightly variable between the mild and the severe preclampsia. Most of the 850 smears collected conform to the picture of the "at term" smear which is composed of discrete

intermediate and navicular cells, clear background of the smear, limited or no cytolysis and a slight rise in the karyopyknotic index. Basal cell infiltration of the smear was encountered in eleven of the 372 cases of preclampsia examined. This basal cell infiltration is considered as a serious sign in the smear as far as the foetal salvage is concerned (Fig. 6).

5. *Cytological changes after progesterone therapy:*

   a) Increase in the number of the navicular cells, exceeding 50% of the total cell count, was demonstrated in 32 cases out of the 40 preclamptic patients examined i.e. 80%.

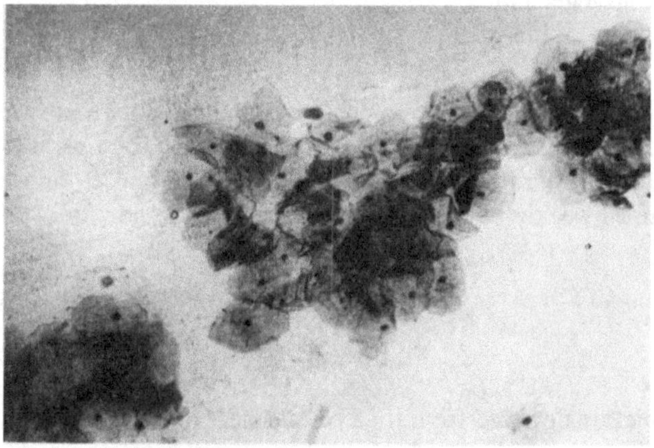

Fig. 4. A smear at 32 weeks from pregnancy complicated with severe preclampsia. x 350

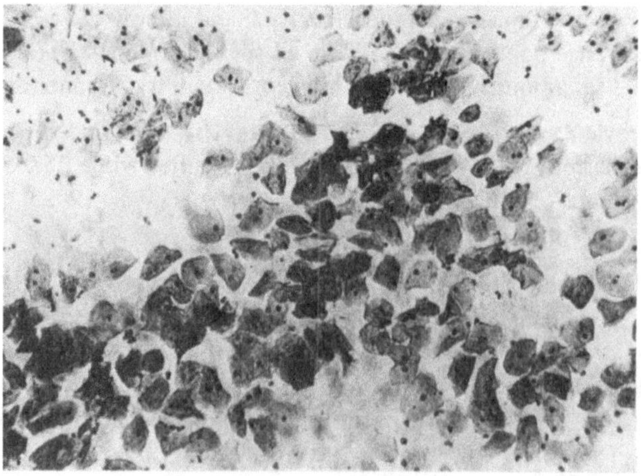

Fig. 5. A smear at 28 weeks from pregnancy complicated by severe preclampsia, note the clean background inspite of the high navicular index. x 150

b) The discrete arrangement of the cells was changed into the normal pregnancy pattern of thick groups in 85% of the smears examined after progesterone medication.

c) There was a mild drop in the karyopknotic index from 12 to 5% after progesterone therapy.

d) Cytolysis was established in almost all the smears that were examined after progesterone therapy (Fig. 7).

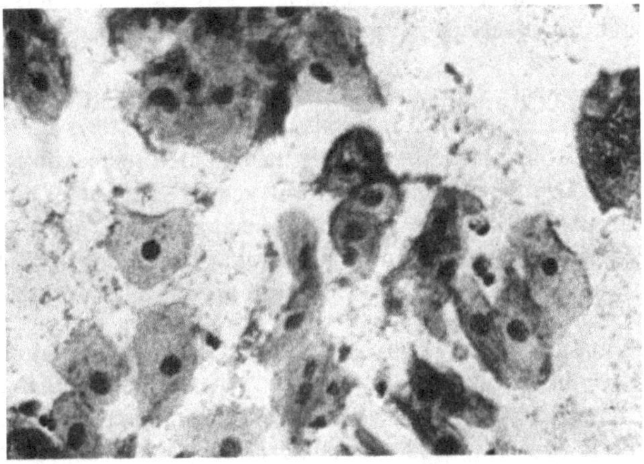

Fig. 6. A smear at 38 weeks from a pregnancy complicated with severe preclampsia, pregnancy ended in stilbirth, note the basal cell infiltration. x 350

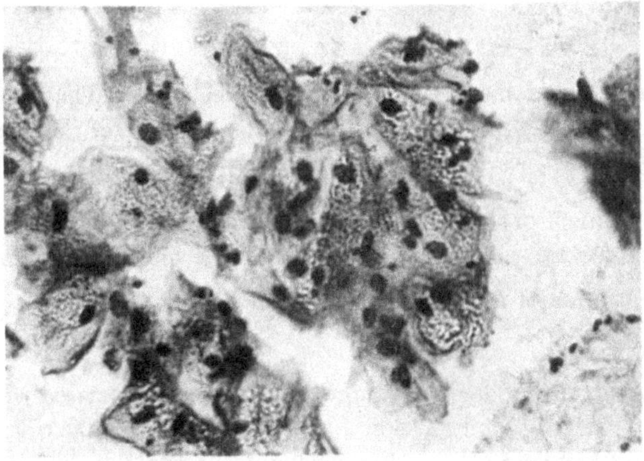

Fig. 7. A smear at 34 weeks after progesterone therapy in preclampsia, note the thick groups of navicular cells. x 350

Discussion

There is good reason to suppose that vaginal cytology can now be added to the diagnostic procedures in preclampsia and it is becoming an established test as far as the foetal prognosis is concerned. The picture of the normal mid pregnancy smear is well defined and any variation from the normal would certainly mean some defect in the hormonal production from the placenta (*Pundel,* 1959, *Von Haam* and *Schwallenberg,* 1959). Such a simple test might well save many babies from intrauterine or perinatal death. The perinatal mortality is corresponding to the changes in the vaginal smear.

Vaginal cytology can provide a new and a comparatively simple method of selecting those cases for induction of labour to avoid placental insufficiency.

These changes in the vaginal cells in preclampsia are qualitative and not quantitative and more than one smear collected at intervals of two or three days are necessary for describing the smear pattern and for evaluating the case before deciding on termination of the pregnancy for fear of severe placental insufficiency. The use of progesterone therapy in the treatment of preclampsia is not a recent attempt (*Ragab* and *Sammour,* 1971). It was suggested that the high cornification index in the vaginal smear of preclamptics would mean a low progesterone production from the placenta.

Progestational domination was considered responsible for the typical mid-pregnancy smear pattern. This would explain the conversion of the vaginal smear in preclampsia to the typical mid-pregnancy smear after progesterone administration. The changes in the vaginal smear were also associated with clinical improvement in the form of diuresis, drop in the blood pressure and marked improvement in the blood biochemistry.

Summary

The vaginal smear was examined in 372 patients of preclampsia. The cytological picture deviated from the typical smear of pregnancy in 85.7% of the cases examined. The karyopyknotic index was of no significance.

The discrete arrangement of the cells, the disappearance of cytolysis and the abundent superficial squamous were the essential characters of the smear in preclampsia.

The basal cell infiltration of the vaginal smear is associated with a high perinatal mortality.

Progesterone administration in 40 preclamptic patients was associated with a conversion of the vaginal smear to the typical mid-pregnancy smear in 80% of cases examined and treated by natural progesterone. This changes in the smear pattern accompanied profound clinical response in the form of hypotension, diuresis and improvement of the renal function.

References

Papanicolaou, G. N.: The diagnosis of early human pregnancy by the vaginal smear method. Proc. Soc. Exper. Biol. & Med. 22 (1925) p. 436.

Pundel, J. P.: Vaginal Cytology as prognostic method in pregnancy disorders. Acta Cytol. 3 (1959) p. 231.

Ragab, I., M. B. Sammour, H. El-Kabarity and *R. Hegazy:* Progesterone, A treatment for preclamptic toxemia. Ain Shams Medical Journal 22, 1 (1971) p. 9–24.

Sammour, M. B.: Vaginal Cytology during normal pregnancy its role in determination of the approximate date of confinement, Obst. Gynec. 24 (1964) p. 682.

Sammour, M. B.: Vaginal Cytology as a Guide to Prognosis in threatened Abortion, Northwest Medicine, p. 360–364 April (1967).

Von Haam, E. and *R. Schwallenberg:* Symposium on hormonal cytology during pregnancy and the postpartum period. Acta cytol. 3 (1959) p. 218.

Die Möglichkeiten der Zytodiagnostik bei der Beschädigung des Kindes bei EPH-Gestose

J. Zidovsky, B. Vedra

Research Institute for the Care of Mother and Child, Prag, CSSR

Bis heute haben sich nur wenige Autoren mit der Problematik der EPH-Gestose aus dem Standpunkt der Zytodiagnostik beschäftigt, obwohl es um eine wichtige Schwangerschaftspathologie geht, die mit einer erhöhten antenatalen und perinatalen Mortalität verbunden ist.

Bei der zytologischen Analyse unseres EPH-Gestose Materials gehen wir von der bekannten Tatsache aus, daß die regressiven Vorgänge in der Placenta bei der Spätgestose offensichtlich wesentlich früher beginnen als im Laufe einer normalen Schwangerschaft. Der Grad der placentaren Regression und der damit verbundenen Dysfunktion ist offenbar von dem Zustand der EPH-Gestose abhängig.

Der Hauptspender der energetischen Quellen für das Leben des Foeten – die Placenta – ist zu gleicher Zeit ein Regulator der hormonellen Verhältnisse in der Schwangerschaft. Diese metabolische und hormonelle Funktionen der Plazenta sind eng verbunden mit den Bedingungen, in denen sich die Frucht befindet im Sinne der foeto-plazentaren Einheit. Infolgedessen bringt jedwede Änderung oder Störung der metabolischen Funktion der Placenta zu gleicher Zeit eine Störung im hormonellen Gleichgewicht der Schwangerschaft mit sich. Diese hormonelle Abweichungen werden dann natürlicherweise auch in dem Zielorgan – in der Scheide – widerspiegelt, wo man sie mit Hilfe der vaginalen Zytologie ablesen kann.

Auf diesem Prinzip beruht die zytologische Diagnostik der biologischen Bereitschaft der Frau zur Geburt (das heißt Bestimmung des Geburtstermins) und pathologischer Abweichungen im Sinne einer Schwangerschaftsverlängerung (Übertragung), oder Schwangerschaftsabkürzung (Frühgeburt). Mit Hilfe des gleichen Prinzips gewinnen wir auch zytologischen Informationen über den Zustand der Placenta und damit auch des Foeten bei den EPH-Gestosen im Sinne der foeto-placentaren Abhängigkeit.

Die regressiven Änderungen der Placenta im Laufe einer EPH-Gestose werden durch eine hormonelle und metabolische Störung charakterisiert, die ihren Ausdruck im Zytogramm findet:

Der Abstrich verändert sich von den günstigen Zytotypen I, beziehungsweise II in die ungünstigen Terminzytotypen III oder IV.

Methodik und Resultate

59 Frauen mit der Diagnose einer Spätgestose wurden der zytologischen Analyse unterworfen. *In 25 Fällen* handelte es sich um *schwere Formen der EPH-Gestose.* Die *restlichen 34 Frauen* hatten einen leichten, monosymptomatischen Verlauf der Gestose (d. h. Ödeme oder Hypertension), der leicht therapeutisch beeinflußbar war. Diese monosymptomatische Gruppe bewerten wir darum als eine Kontrollgruppe mit der Zytologischen Reaktion, die ähnlich ist derjenigen bei normalem Verlauf der Schwangerschaftsende.

Abb. 1. Hier werden die zytologischen Befunde bei schweren Formen der EPH-Gestose mit dem Zeitfaktor, das heißt mit der Länge der Schwangerschaft, und mit dem Zustand des Foeten korreliert. Die gesunden Früchte sind durch weiße Ringe, beschädigte und hypotrophische Früchte durch schwarz-weiße, und abgestorbene Früchte durch schwarze Ringe bezeichnet. Aus der Abbildung kommt eine klare Abhängigkeit zwischen dem Zustand des Foeten, dem Zytogramm und der Länge der Schwangerschaft hervor. Alle beschädigte (d. h. 6 Hypotrophiker und 2 schwere Alterationen der Herztöne) und tote Früchte (5 Fälle), im ganzen dreizehn Foeten, finden wir *schon vor der 38. Woche* der Schwangerschaft und in der Zone der „Terminzytotypen" III und IV, obwohl die Geburt zu dieser Zeit noch nicht erwartet wurde. Bei einer physiologischen Schwangerschaft finden sich diese „Terminzytotypen" vor der 38. Woche normalerweise nicht. Praktisch alle unsere gesunden Kinder (10 von 12) befinden sich zwar in der Zone des III. beziehungsweise IV. Zytotyps, jedoch schon *nach dem Zeitlimit* der *38. Woche.* Das heißt also zu einer Zeit, wo, bezogen auf die Reife des Foeten und den Beginn der physiologischen Seneszenz der Placenta, die Zytotypen III und IV normalerweise erwartet werden. Von den zwei Fällen gesunder Kinder, die in der Zone des III. und IV. Zytotyps waren und vor der 38. Woche geboren wurden, kann ein Fall als Mißerfolg der Zytodiagnostik beurteilt werden. In dem zweiten Falle wurde die Schwangerschaft künstlich durch Geburtsinduktion mit Hilfe von Oxytocininfusion beendet.

Abb. 2. Analog wie auf der ersten Abbildung, werden hier Zytogramme auch mit der Dauer der Schwangerschaft und mit dem Zustand des Kindes korreliert. Es handelt sich um die Gruppe der 34 Frauen mit leichter Form der monosymptomatischen Gestose. Alle Kinder wurden gesund geboren. 29 Frauen hatten zwar den Zytotyp III und IV, dies jedoch nach der 38. Schwangerschaftswoche, das heißt schon in der Zone „Schwangerschaft am Ende". Eine Frau hat ein gesundes Kind kurz vor der 38. Woche geboren. Vier weitere Frauen haben gesunde Kinder geboren in der Zone „günstiger" Zytotype I und II: Hier wird die plazentare Insuffizienz und deswegen auch eine Beschädigung der Frucht nicht vorausgesetzt, ohne Rücksicht auf die Länge der Schwangerschaft. Zwei von den erwähnten Frauen haben vor, und zwei nach der 38. Woche geboren.

Zusammenfassend kann man zur Abb. 2 sagen, daß bei allen Fällen den zytologischen Kriterien gemäß, Geburten gesunder Kinder erwartet werden konnten. Bei 30 Frauen hat man zwar „ungünstige" Terminzytotype III und IV gefunden, jedoch schon im

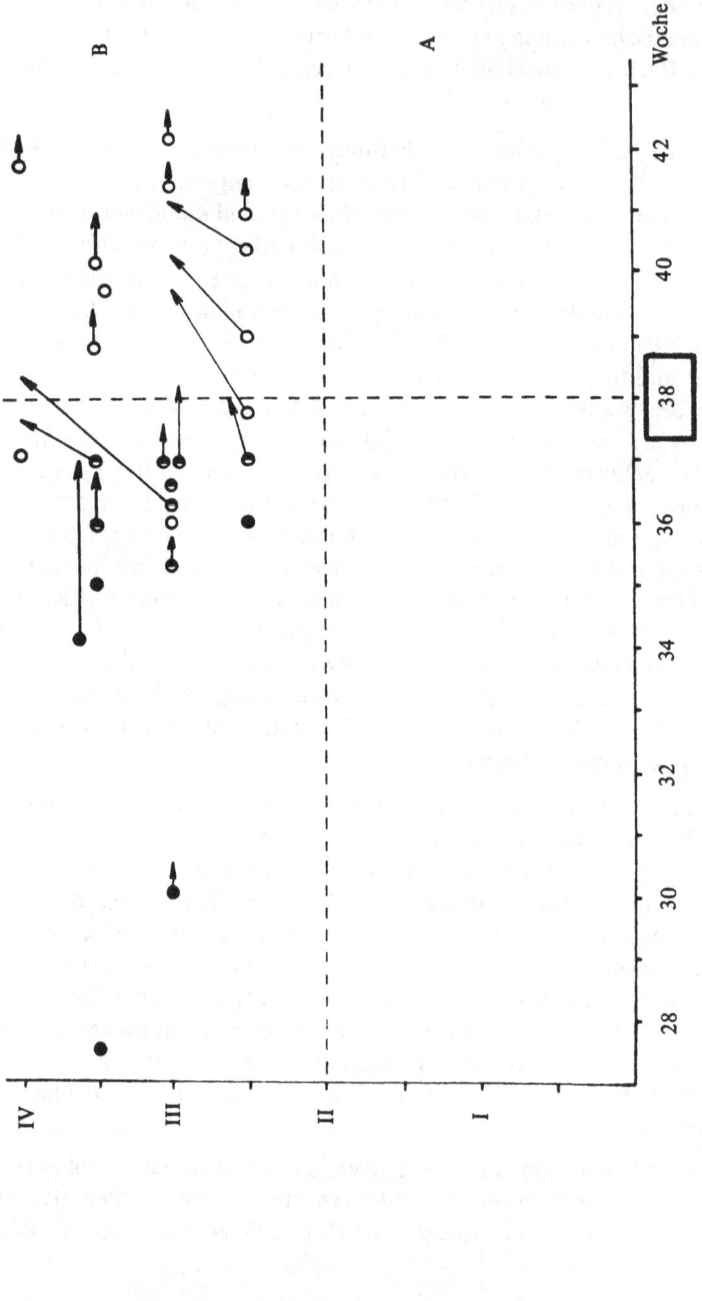

Abb. 1. Zytotypus I. „Fortgeschrittene Schwangerschaft". Bei EPH-Gestose (vor der 38. Woche) ist dieser Zytotypus prognostisch ein „günstiger" Zytotypus

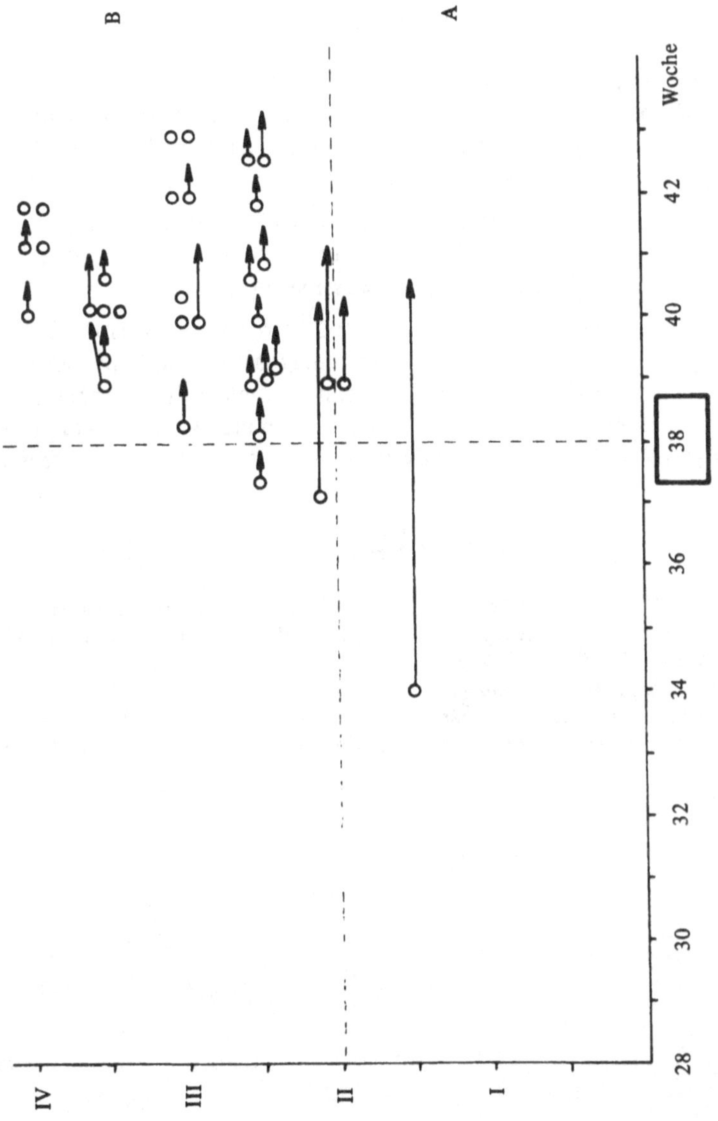

Abb. 2. Zytotypus II. „kurz vor dem Termin“. Bei EPH-Gestose (vor der 38. Schwangerschafts-woche) ist wieder ein „günstiger“ Zytotypus.

richtigen Zeitabschnitt, das heißt *nach der 38. Woche.* Bei weiteren 4 Fällen hat man günstige Zytotypen I und II gefunden, die eine Äußerung der funktionsfähigen Placenta sind und wo man eine Beschädigung der Frucht nicht erwartet ohne Rücksicht auf das Alter der Schwangerschaft.

Zusammenfassung

1. Der Befund eines ungünstigen Zytogramms (d. h. Zytotyp III und IV, resp. II bis III) bei den EPH-Gestosen *vor der 38. Woche* der Schwangerschaft *ist pathognomonisch* und beweist eine Störung in der foeto-plazentaren Einheit. Die Wahrscheinlichkeit einer Beschädigung der Frucht ist hoch signifikant.

2. Der Befund eines *günstigen* Zytogramms (Zytotyp I und II) *vor und nach der 38. Woche* der Schwangerschaft bedingt nicht eine Induktion der Geburt. Die Möglichkeit einer Beschädigung der Frucht kann ausgeschieden werden.

3. Nach der 38. Schwangerschaftswoche bei EPH-Gestosen gelten für die ungünstigen Zytogramme (Zytotyp III und IV) dieselbe zytodiagnostische Kriterien als bei physiologischen Schwangerschaften, das heißt Notwendigkeit einer dynamischen Kontrolle der Zeitlimiten einzelner Zytotype. Das Überschreiten dieser Limite – das heißt *6 Tage* für das Zytotyp *III* und 3 Tage für das Zytotyp *IV* – ist schon *pathognomonisch.*

Literatur

Židovský, J., B. Vedra, J. Mareš, S. Horská: Cytodiagnostics of damage to the foetus in potential foetal distress from intrauterine asphyxia. Excerpta Medica Monograph: Intrauterine Danger to the foetus, Prague (1966) p. 291–295.

Židovský, J., B. Vedra, J. Mareš, S. Horská: The foeto-placental unit assessed by colpocytology during normal and pathological pregnancy. Excerpta Medica Monograph Proceeding of the International Symposium on Foeto – Placental Unit, Milano, 1968, Amsterdam (1969) p. 371–375.

Research in Therapy

Kann man durch Complamin-Retard die Placentafunktion beeinflussen?

N. A. M. Bergstein

Frauenklinik, Ziekenhuis, Zevenaar, Holland

Ein klarer Einblick in die Ursachen der Spätgestosen besteht noch nicht; deshalb ist es auch nicht möglich, eine spezifische Therapie zu betreiben. Es wird des weiteren noch über die Vorteile der konservativen gegenüber der aktiven Behandlung diskutiert. Durch Verordnung von Bettruhe, salzloser Diät, Diuretika und blutdrucksenkender Pharmaka nimmt die Möglichkeit des Auftretens einer eclampsia convulsiva zwar ab, aber keine dieser Behandlungsmethoden darf als spezifisch für diese Erkrankung betrachtet werden.

Falls die niedrigen Oestriol- und Pregnandiolwerte im Harn, welche manchmal bei Toxikosepatientinnen vorgefunden werden, einen Hinweis für das Bestehen eines foetalen Notzustandes und einer nicht gut funktionierenden Placenta darstellen, so würde sich nach wirksamer Behandlung – vorausgesetzt, daß die Placentadurchblutung verbessert werden könnte – eine Steigerung der Oestriol- und Pregnandiolausscheidung im Harn zeigen. Auch die hitzestabile Fraktion der alkalischen Phosphatase, die bekanntlich in der Placenta gebildet wird, würde bei einer besseren Durchblutung (besseren Funktion) der Placenta in diesen Fällen steigen.

Es ist bekannt, daß Complamin-Retard einen günstigen Einfluß auf erkrankte Gefäße ausübt. Dabei verbessert Complamin-Retard die metabole Funktion im „kranken" Gewebe. Wenn man nun annimmt, daß die Anomalien, die man bei Patientinnen mit einer Spätgestose vorfindet, direkt oder indirekt im Zusammenhang mit einer Durchblutungsstörung und einer metabolen Störung in der Placenta, den Nieren und der Leber stehen, so könnte man sich vorstellen, daß – wenn diesen Patientinnen ein Medikament verabreicht wird, das die pathologischen Gefäßveränderungen verbessert oder normalisiert – die Wirkung dieses Pharmakon sich in einer Steigerung der Hormonproduktion der Placenta manifestieren würde.

Material und Methodik

Unseren Patientinnen mit Spätgestose wurde Bettruhe und eine salzlose Diät verordnet. Bei dieser Patientinnengruppe wurde Oestriol- und Pregnandiolausscheidung im Harn bestimmt. Weiterhin wurde die hitzestabile alkalische Phosphatase, das Kreatinin, die

Harnsäure, der Serum-Cholesteringehalt und das Serum-Eiweißspektrum, sowie die B.S.P.-Ausscheidung durch die Leber kontrolliert.

Daraufhin wurde diesen Patientinnen während 8 Tagen oder kontinuierlich bis zur Geburt 2000 mg Complamin-Retard/die verabreicht.

Aus dieser Vorstudie gewannen wir den Eindruck, daß bei Verabreichung von Complamin-Retard an Patientinnen mit Spätgestose der Effekt desto signifikanter war, je höher der Serum-Kreatininspiegel war. Nach diesem Gesichtspunkt eingeteilt, ergibt sich für unser Patientengut folgende Tabelle (Tab. 1):

Bei unseren weiteren Untersuchungen haben wir unsere Patientinnen in drei Gruppen aufgeteilt.

Gruppe I : Kontrollgruppe,

Gruppe II : Patientinnen mit erniedrigter Oestriolausscheidung. (Erniedrigung tritt allmählich auf.)

Gruppe III: Patientinnen mit niedrigen Ausgangswerten für Oestriolausscheidung.

Als Kontrollgruppe nahmen wir Patienten, die wegen Varizen Complamin-Retard in derselben Dosierung erhielten wie Gruppe II und III. Bei diesen Patientinnen bestand kein Verdacht auf eine Spätgestose. Bei ihnen zeigten sich folgende Resultate: (Tabelle 2, S. 326)

Bei der Gruppe II mit abfallenden Oestriolwerten handelt es sich um Patientinnen mit Spätgestose, die schon mit Bettruhe und salzloser Diät behandelt worden waren. Während der Beobachtungszeit wurde festgestellt, daß die Oestriolausscheidung sich verringerte, deshalb wurde Complamin-Retard verabreicht.

Die dritte Gruppe umfaßt jene Patientinnen, welche wegen Spätgestose eingewiesen wurden. Ihnen wurde ebenfalls Bettruhe und salzlose Diät verordnet. Bei dieser Gruppe wurden wiederholt niedrige bis zu niedrige Oestriolausscheidungswerte festgestellt. Nach Verabreichung vom Complamin-Retard zeigte sich ein Effekt, der anhand folgender vier Beispiele dargestellt sei:

Zusammenfassung der Beobachtungen

In der Kontrollgruppe fanden wir keinen Effekt von Complamin-Retard. In der Gruppe II (mit allmählicher Senkung der Oestriolwerte) zeigte sich (Fig. 12), daß in allen Stadien der Gravidität nach Verabreichung von Complamin-Retard eine Verbesserung der Oestriolwerte auftritt. Auch in Gruppe III (mit initial niedrigen Werten) zeigte sich in allen Stadien der Gravidität eine Steigerung der Oestriolausscheidung nach Verabreichung von Complamin-Retard (Fig. 13).

Tab. 1.

Patient no.	Uric acid	Creatinine	Before treatment			During treatment			After treatment			Birth weight (g)	Placental weight (g)	Patient no.
			Estriol	Pregnandiol	Alkaline phosphatase	Estriol	Pregnandiol	Alkaline phosphatase	Estriol	Pregnandiol	Alkaline phosphatase			
P 66-21	4.1	5.5	18.4	50.2	–	20.6	51.1, 46.5	–	–	–	–	–	–	P 66-21
Z 65-38	5.9	6.0	11.5, 12.9	30.2, 41.1	1.2	13.9	–	2.2	15.7	43.4	2.8	3750	500	Z 65-38
Z 66-78	3.6	7.0	17.4	37.3	1.6, 3.6	21.6, 20.1	31.4, 44.5	3.4	–	–	4.0	–	–	Z 66-78
P 67-45	5.0	7.0	8.4, 8.2	20.3, 40.8	4.0	9.1, 19.7	28.9	5.6, 10.2	20.6	26.8	10.8	3400	700	P 67-45
Z 67-338	3.0	7.0	13.1	58.4	6.6	13.5, 16.6	38.4, 79.2	9.2	21.5	63.5	11.0	3110	550	Z 67-338
Z 66-492	4.7	7.5	24.6, 22.0	35.7, 57.6	5.2, 6.0	30.6	25.2	8.4	27.5	20.8	–	3700	700	Z 66-492
Z 67-312	6.9	8.0	2.8, 8.3, 8.9	–	1.0, 2.2	12.5	17.3	3.2	13.3	–	–	3110	550	Z 67-312
Z 67-253	7.2	8.0	6.7, 8.7	123.0, 83.9	6.8	7.4, 13.4	62.9, 70.9	7.0	12.1	64.5	12.0	3790	640	Z 67-253
Z 67-336	6.4	8.0	5.1	42.8	10.4	16.5, 24.9	27.2, 8.7	16.2, 23.0	–	–	–	2790	550	Z 67-336
Z 65-14	3.5	8.0	14.0, 16.5	44.1	5.2	20.8	54.4	6.4	14.8	26.2	–	3990	675	Z 65-14
Z 67-278	6.9	8.0	12.4	18.7	3.0	18.3	23.4	–	–	–	–	3020	575	Z 67-278
Z 65-145	4.5	10.5	5.4	13.2	0.4	11.2	25.8	1.2	–	–	–	–	–	Z 65-145
Z 67-292	8.9	10.0	3.0, 3.3, 3.0	46.1, 19.9	4.8, 8.0, 8.8	13.9	–	25.4	–	–	18.2	2950	580	Z 67-292
Z 67-409	6.7	10.0	7.7, 7.9	18.1	10.0	14.6, 17.4, 22.9	26.8, 27.5, 25.6	11.6	30.0	58.2	22.4	3250	475	Z 67-409
Z 67-345	8.4	12.0	14.1	36.6	11.2	13.4, 29.8	15.9, 55.4	10.8, 11.6, 12.0	36.0	24.3	–	3020	500	Z 67-345

Tab. 2. Control group.

patient no.	uric acid	creat.	dose	indication	Complamin before after	weight child	weight placenta
P 66-21	4.1	5.5	2000 mg continue	varices	18.4-↓18.1-20.6-21.6-20.6	3840	600
Z 67-231	4.0	5.7	2000 mg continue	varices	23.0-↓22.5	3130	550
Z 65-38	5.9	6.0	2000 mg continue	varices	11.5-↓12.1-15.7	3750	500
P 68-119	5.2	7.0	2000 mg continue	varices	14.2-15.2-↓17.0-16.5-20.7	3070	575

Tab. 3. Toxicose with falling values for Estriol.

patient no.	uric acid	creat.	dose	Complamin before after	weight child	weight placenta
Z 67-277	4.3	7.0	2000 mg continue	18.5 → 8.0 ↓→ 15.5	2140	500
Z 68-138	4.4	7.0	2000 mg continue	19.5 → 11.5 ↓→ 25.0	3100	470
P 67-45	5.0	7.0	2000 mg 8 days	11.6 → 8.2 ↓→ 20.6	3400	700
Z 66-492	4.7	7.5	2000 mg 8 days	24.6 → 22.0 ↓→ 30.6	3700	700
P 65-53	5.2	7.6	2000 mg continue	20.0 → 10.5 ↓→ 30.0	3830	670
Z 66-498	5.2	7.8	2000 mg continue	31.0 → 22.0 ↓→ 30.0	3100	460
P 68-36	5.7	7.8	2000 mg continue	16.0 → 9.5 ↓→ 39.0	3110	390
Z 67-292	9.4	9.5	2000 mg 8 days	7.0 → 5.5 ↓→ 13.9	2950	580

Weitere Untersuchung

Nach dieser „Pilot-Studie“ wurden die Ergebnisse in einem Doppelblindversuch überprüft. Die Kriterien für die Patientenauswahl waren:

a) Zweimaliger erniedrigter Oestriol-Harn-Wert.
b) Kreatinin- und Harnsäurespiegel im pathologischen Bereich (Kreatinin 7,5% mg), Harnsäure 5,6–7,5% mg in der 36.–40. Woche.

Jede Patientin erhielt dieselbe Diät mit standardisiertem niedrigem Na-Gehalt (400 mg). In der Complamingruppe befanden sich 8 Patientinnen, die Placebogruppe betrug 9 Patientinnen.

Tab. 4. Toxicose with low values for Estriol.

patient no.	uric acid	creat.	dose	Complamin before → after	weight child	weight placenta
Z 67-338	3.2	7.0	2000 mg 8 days	13.1 → 21.1	3110	550
Z 66-78	3.6	7.0	2000 mg continue	17.4 → 21.6	4180	580
Z 67-274	4.9	7.2	2000 mg continue	19.0 → 31.0	4370	780
P 66-110	4.5	7.3	2000 mg continue	19.0 → 46.0	3860	600
Z 67-220	3.7	7.5	2000 mg continue	16.5 → 31.5	3900	610
Z 65-14	3.5	8.0	2000 mg 8 days	14.0 → 20.8	3990	675
Z 67-336	6.4	8.0	2000 mg 8 days	5.1 → 24.9	2790	550
Z 67-312	6.9	8.0	2000 mg 8 days	8.3 → 13.3	3110	550
Z 67-278	6.9	8.0	2000 mg 8 days	12.4 → 18.3	3020	575
Z 67-253	7.2	8.0	2000 mg 8 days	6.7 → 13.4	3790	640
Z 67-409	6.7	10.0	2000 mg 8 days	7.7 → 30.0	3250	475
Z 67-310	7.9	10.0	2000 mg 8 days	5.8 → 24.6	3980	590
Z 67-409	8.4	12.0	2000 mg 8 days	14.1 → 36.0	3020	500

Zu Beginn der Untersuchung waren die Patientinnengruppen größer, da aber viele den oben genannten Kriterien nicht entsprachen (z. B. kein zweiter Oestriolwert, bevor Anfang der Therapie), konnten wir sie (12) nicht mehr in die Untersuchung aufnehmen.

In der Complamingruppe ist häufiger eine höhere Oestriolausscheidung zu verzeichnen (Statistische Signifikanz gesichert: p = 0,06). Daraus die Schlußfolgerung, daß zwingende Argumente annehmen lassen, daß die Steigerung der Oestriolausscheidung bei der Complamingruppe größer ist als in der Kontrollgruppe (Fig. 14).

Die Kinder der Complamingruppe haben durchwegs ein höheres Geburtsgewicht (Durchschnitt 3402 g, gegen 2885 g in der Kontrollgruppe).

Theoretische Schlußfolgerung

Bei dieser Studie sehen wir eine Verbesserung der Oestriol- und Pregnandiolausscheidung, eine Senkung des Cholesterins und eine Erhöhung der hitzestabilen alkalischen Phosphatase nach Verabreichung von Complamin. Dies könnte darauf hinweisen, daß der Complamin-Effekt eine deutliche Verbesserung des Symptomenkomplexes der Spätgestose bewerkstelligt. Alle Schwangerschaften wurden mit der Geburt eines gesunden Kindes mit normalem Geburtsgewicht beendet (hoher Apgar-Score).

Zusammenfassend meinen wir, daß Complamin-Retard ein wesentlicher Fortschritt bei der Behandlung von Patientinnen mit Spätgestose darstellt.

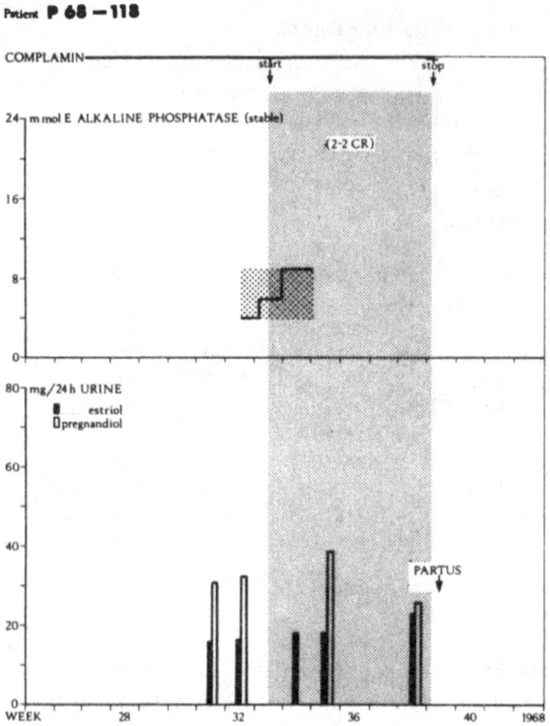

Fig. 1. Patient P 68–118

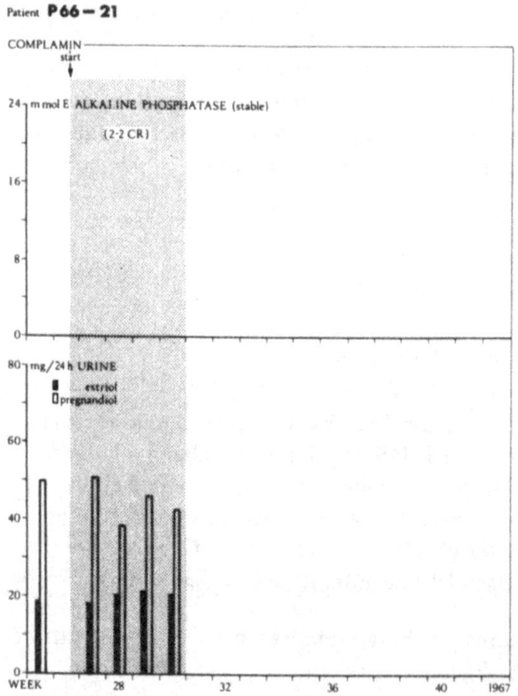

Fig. 2. Patient P 66–21

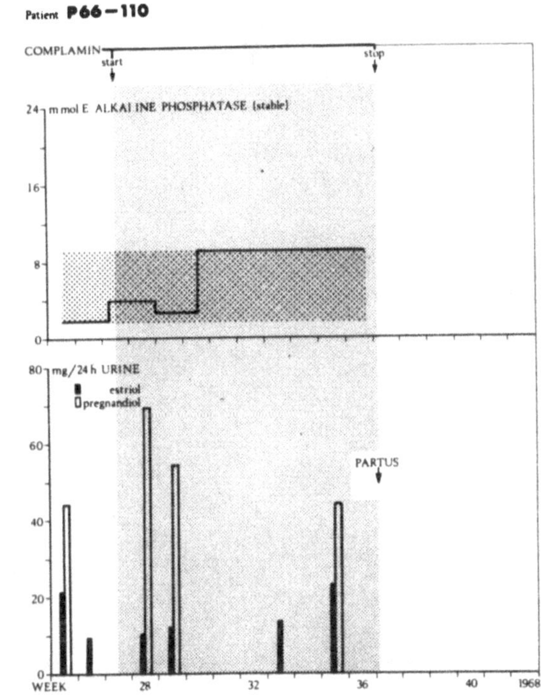

Fig. 3. Patient P 66–110

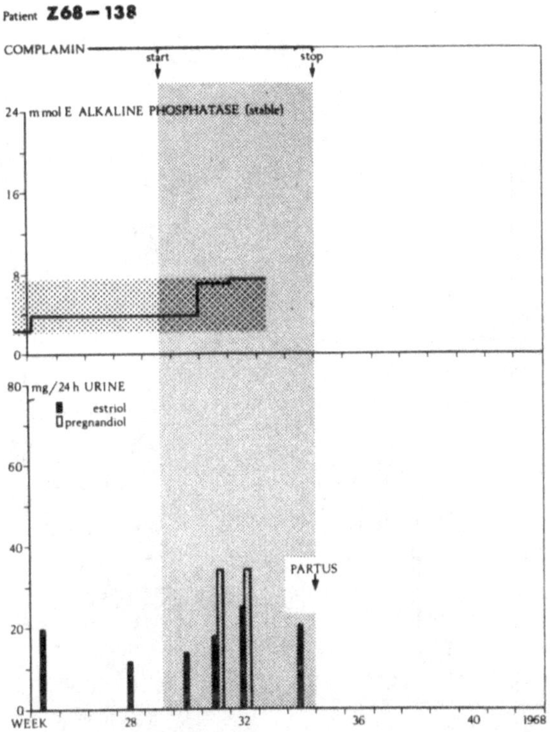

Fig. 4. Patient Z 68–138

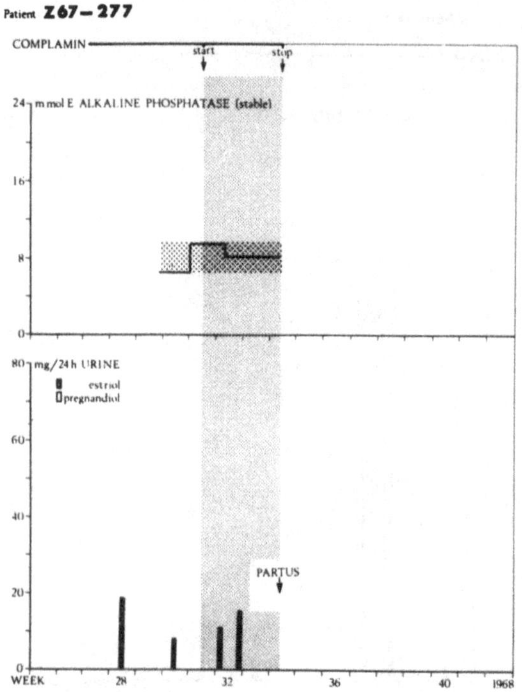

Fig. 5. Patient Z 67–277

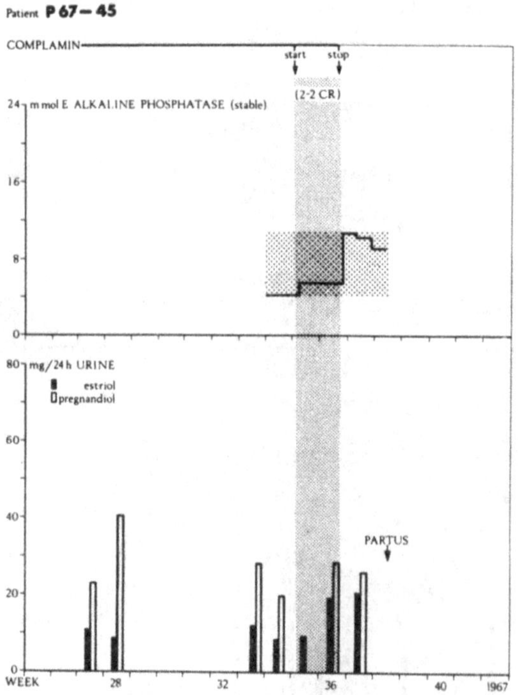

Fig. 6. Patient P 67–45

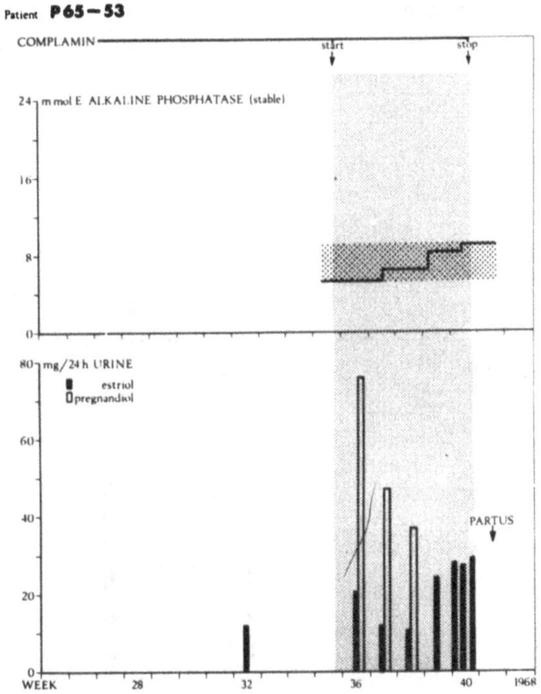

Fig. 7. Patient P 65–53

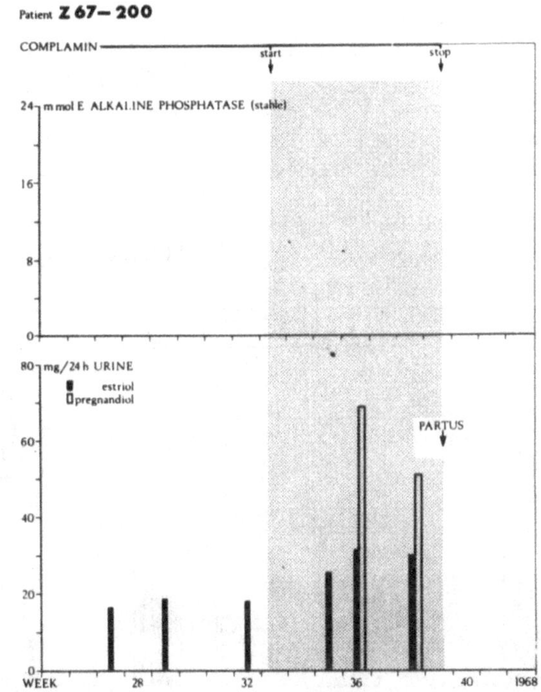

Fig. 8. Patient Z 67–200

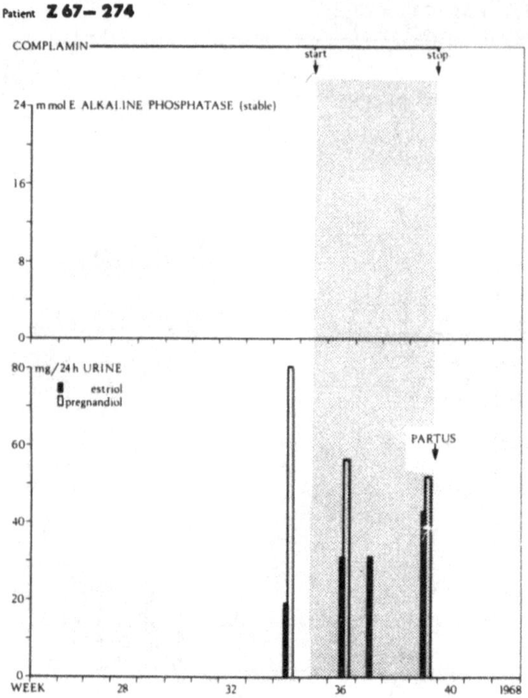

Fig. 9. Patient Z 67–274

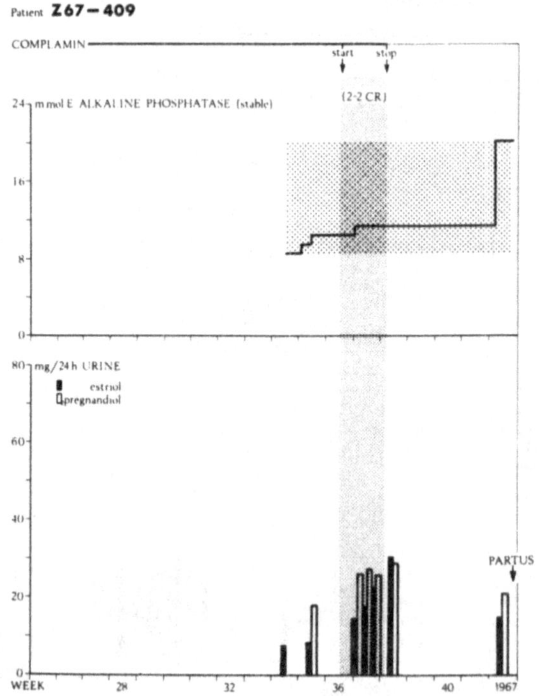

Fig. 10. Patient Z 67–409

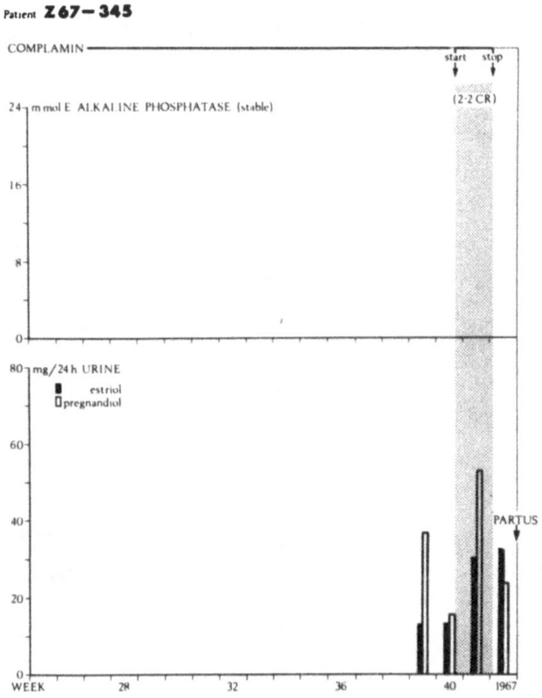

Fig. 11. Patient Z 67–345

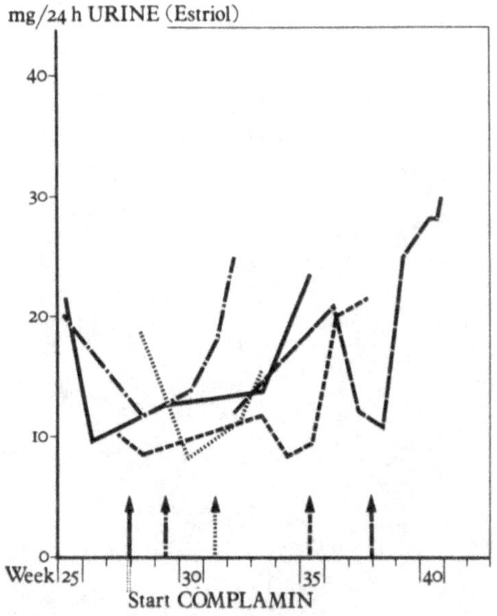

Fig. 12

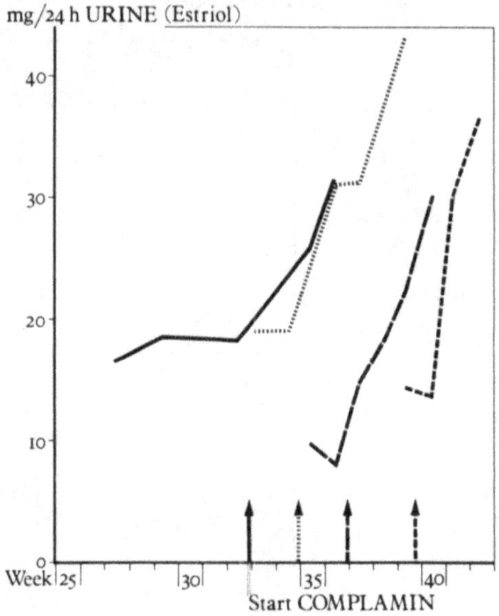
mg/24 h URINE (Estriol)
40
30
20
10
0
Week 25
30
35
40
Start COMPLAMIN

Fig. 13

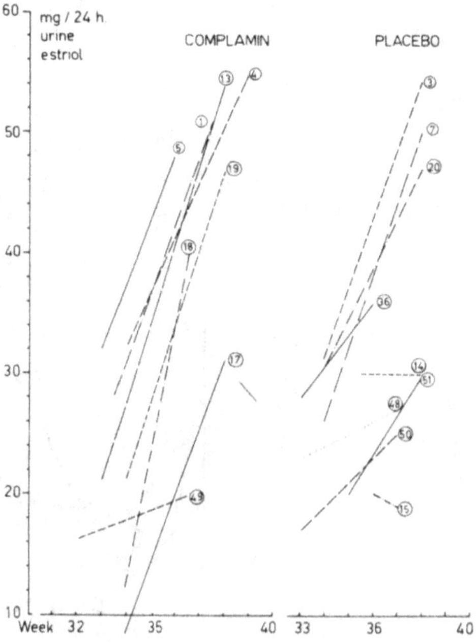
60
mg / 24 h
urine
estriol
COMPLAMIN
PLACEBO
13
4
1
5
19
18
17
43
3
7
20
36
14
51
48
50
15
50
40
30
20
10
Week 32
35
40
33
36
40

Fig. 14

The Effect of Spironolactone on Sodiumdiuresis in Normal and Hypertensive Pregnancy

P. J. Boodt, A. C. Drogendijk

VU Ziekenhuis, afd. Verlosk/Gynaec., Amsterdam, Holland

In pregnancy much emphasis has been laid on the sodium and water metabolism since the beginning of this century. The hypothesis that every pregnant woman retains sodium in her tissue was untenable since it was shown by isotopetechniques that the amount of sodium required in pregnancy is quite proportional to the demands made by the conceptus (*F. E. Hytten* and *I. Leitch*, 1964).

Only in toxaemia of pregnancy the amount of sodium retained has been proven to exceed the physiological demands (*Plentl* and *Gray*, 1959; *Mahran*, 1961).

One of the hormones that has a very powerful and well known effect on water and sodium metabolism is aldosterone. However the exact role of aldosterone in normal and toxaemic pregnancy is still unknown. In normal pregnancy the secretion rate of aldosterone is high whereas in toxaemia, a condition associated with retention of abnormal great amounts of sodium the secretion rates generally found are low (*Watanabe* at al., 1963; *Watanabe* et al., 1965).

These and other observations did cast some doubt whether aldosterone does play a role at all in maintaining sodium metabolism in pregnancy (*Drucker* et al., 1963; *Stark*, 1970).

In order to try to elucidate some of the features of aldosterone in pregnancy we made an investigation about its role. If the increased aldosterone secretion should be responsible for maintaining sodium balance in pregnancy, a blockade of its peripheral action on the renal tubule should result in an increased sodium diuresis.

An inhibition of the sodium-retaining quality of aldosterone is relatively simple with the use of the specific aldosterone-antagonist: spironolactone (trade-name: Aldactone-A) (*Liddle*, 1958; *Barnes* and *Buckingham*, 1958).

Methods

14 women in the last trimester of their pregnancies were studied. All were hospitalized and strictly confined to bed and put on a daily constant low sodium-intake. Ample care was taken to ensure that a "steady-state" was reached before starting the investigations. A requirement was a constant renal excretion of sodium for at least five days.

Total 24 hour urines were collected and checked for completeness of collection by creatinine-estimations. Sodium-content was measured by flame-photometer. After the initial period spironolactone, as Aldactone-A was given orally during three days; 200 mg per day – divided in 4 equal doses with an interval of six hours.

The excretion of sodium in the period of five days following the first dose of spironolactone was compared with the excretion in the five days prior to and after the medication.

Subjects participating, were divided into three groups.

Group I consisted of non-toxaemic pregnancies:
Patients A and E had normal pregnancies. The other five pregnancies were characterized by fetal growth retardation.

Pat.	Age years	Grav.	Para	Week of medication	Aldactone-A mg/day	Daily sodium intake mmole
A	27	III	II	34	200	23
B	28	II	0	35	200	30
C	26	V	I	33	200	23
D	18	I	0	36	200	29
E	26	II	I	30	200	20
F	34	I	0	36	200	31
G	20	I	0	34	200	18

Fig. 1. Non-toxaemic pregnancy

Group II consisted of four patients with pre-existing hypertension. The only abnormal symptom here was a blood-pressure of 140 systolic over 90 diastolic or over, measured on more than one occasion.

Pat.	Age years	Grav	Para	Week of medication	Aldactone-A mg/day	Daily sodium intake mmole
H	29	II	I	35	200	25
I	27	I	0	31	200	19
J	35	III	II	31	200	20
K	25	I	0	36	200	21

Fig. 2. Pregnancy with pre-existing hypertension

Group III, three patients, all showing hypertension, albuminuria, i.e. a protein-excretion of at least 100 mg in 24 hour urine – and elevated serum creatinine and uric-acid levels. In this group only one patient (patient N) was treated with an hypotensive drug – namely α-methyl-dopa in a dosage of 350 mg/day.

Pat.	Age years	Grav	Para	Week of medication	Aldactone-A mg/day	Daily sodium intake mmole
L	25	III	II	36	200	20
M	30	II	I	33	200	20
N	22	I	0	34	200	19

Fig. 3. Toxaemic pregnancy

Results

Fig. 4 gives you an impression of the typical sodium-balance during spironolactone-medication, we saw in all patients of group I.

From Fig. 5 it is clear that in group I a significantly greater sodium diuresis occurs during Aldactone-A-medication compared to the period prior to it. This difference is highly significant (Students t-test $p < 0.005$ = highly significant).

Comparision of the five days excretion prior to and following the spironolactone administraticn shows a rebound-phenomenon. Statistically significant (Student's t-test $p < 0.01$).

Fig. 6 gives an example of the sodium-balance in group II. Again a significant increase of sodiumdiuresis occurs during spironolactone.

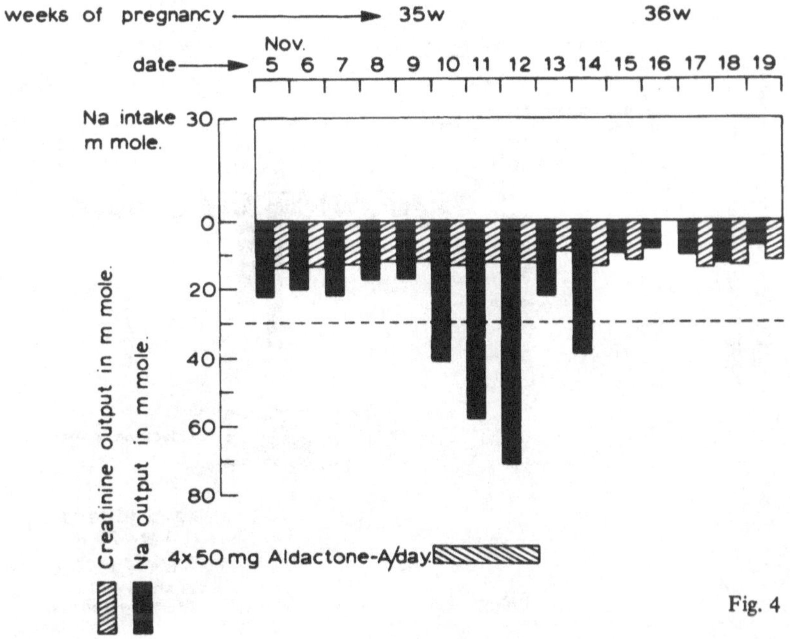

Fig. 4

From Fig. 7 it is evident that a statistically significant (Student's t-test $p < 0.005$) elevated sodium-excretion occurs during spironolactone-medication as compared to the period prior to it. In this aspect there is no difference between normal pregnancy and pregnancy with preexisting hypertension in our investigation. No clear rebound-phenomenon can be seen.

Fig. 8 is an example of the reaction on spironolactone in group III. From Fig. 9 the impression is obtained that the difference between the period prior to and during spironolactone-medication, in these patients is rather small. A statistical analysis is impossible because of the too small number of observations.

Pat.	Sodium diuresis total amount mmole/5 days in relation to Aldactone-A-administration		
	before	during	after
A	85	104	38
B	98	231	45,5
C	49	193	34
D	56	162	60
E	101	232	39
F	55	176	57
G	43	120	16

Fig. 5. Non-toxaemic pregnancy

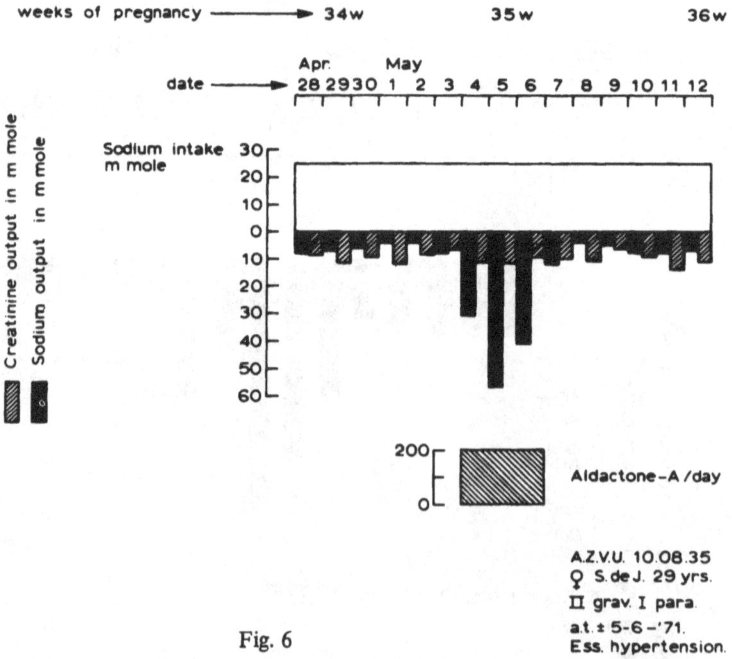

Fig. 6

Pat.	Sodium diuresis total amount mmole/5 days in relation to Aldactone-A-administration		
	before	during	after
H	29	145	40
I	43	116	23
J	49	165	50
K	60	144	41

Fig. 7. Pregnancy with pre-existing hypertension

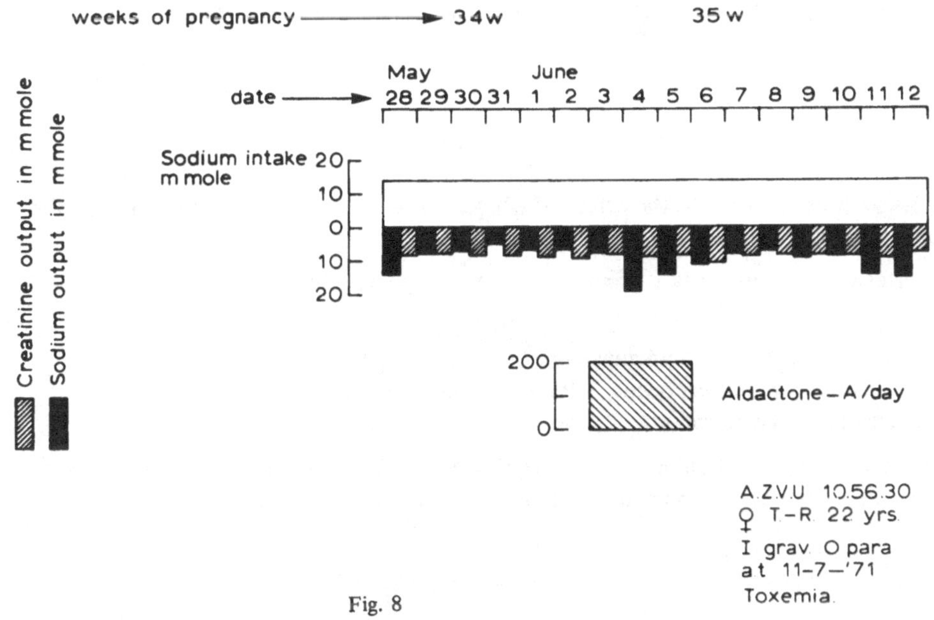

Fig. 8

Pat.	Sodium diuresis total amount mmole/5 days in relation to Aldactone-A-administration		
	before	during	after
L	13	18	21
M	40	55	22
N	35	60	54

Fig. 9. Toxaemic pregnancy

Discussion

Our results are in accordance with those of *Barnes* and *Buckingham* (1958) and prove that in non-toxaemic pregnancy a significant sodium diuresis occurs during spironolactone-medication. It too proves that aldosterone does act on sodium metabolism in normal and hypertensive pregnancy.

The conclusion of *Stark* (1970) that aldosterone must be biologically inactive during pregnancy is not justified.

The absence of a significant response in sodium-diuresis during spironolactone in toxaemic pregnancy is again in accordance with *Barnes* and *Buckingham* (1958). The explanation of this small reaction could be that aldosterone secretion rate in toxaemic pregnancy is not as high as in normal pregnancy. In other words, in toxaemia of pregnancy the sodium retention is only partially accounted for by the action of aldosterone.

Summary

A research was made into the effect of a blockade with spironolactone of the peripheral action of aldosterone on the renal tubule in pregnancy.

Fourteen women in the last trimester of their pregnancies were studied under steady-state conditions.

In normal pregnancy and pregnancy with pre-existing hypertension a significant increased sodium diuresis occurs with spironolactone. In toxaemic pregnancy only a very small increase in sodium diuresis is seen.

The results prove that aldosterone must play a role in maintaining sodium-balance in normal pregnancy and pregnancy with pre-existing hypertension.

References

Barnes, A. C. and *J. C. B. Buckingham:* Electrolyte balance studies with the antihormones. Am. J. Obst. Gynec. 76 (1958) p. 955.

Druckner, W. D., A. Hendrikx, J. H. Laragh, N. P. Christy and *R. L. vande Wiele:* Effect of administered aldosterone upon electrolyte excretion during and after pregnancy in two women with adrenal cortical insufficiency. J. Clin. Endocr. 23 (1963) p. 1247.

Hytten, F. E. and *I. Leitch:* The physiology of human pregnancy. Blackwell, Scient. Public., Oxford (1964).

Liddle, G. W.: Aldosterone Antagonists. Arch. Int. Med. 102 (1958) p. 998.

Mahran, M.: Sodium-metabolism in gynecology and obstetrics. J. Obstet. Gynaec. Brit. Cwlth. 68 (1961) p. 597.

Plentl, A. A. and *M. J. Gray:* Total body water, sodium space and total exchangeable sodium in normal and toxemic pregnant women. Am. J. Obst. Gynec. 78 (1959) p. 472.

Watanabe, M., C. I. Meeker, M. J. Gray, E. A. H. Sims and *S. Solomon:* Secretion rate of aldosterone in normal pregnancy. J. Clin. Invest. 42 (1963) p. 1619.

Watanabe, M., C. I. Meeker, M. J. Gray, E. A. H. Sims and *S. Solomon:* Aldosterone secretion rates in abnormal pregnancy. J. Clin. Endocr. 25 (1965) p. 1665.

Progesterone Therapy in EPH-Gestosis

Mohamed B. Sammour, B.Sc. (Oxf.), F.R.C.S.E., M.I.A.C.,
H. El-Kabarity, M.CH. and *A. S. Khalifa,* M.D.

From the Departments of Obstetrics and Paediatries
Faculty of Medicine, Ain Shams University, Cairo, Egypt

Introduction

One of the physiological functions of progesterone is to normalise the blood pressure in pregnancy.

Harrison [9] found that in cases of renal hypertension the blood pressure declined spontaneously during the last few days of pregnancy, and rose again gradually after delivery until it reached the original level. *Corbit* [2] showed that pregnancy produced about a 20 per cent reduction of the systolic pressure both in normal and in renal hypertensive rabbits. The blood pressure returned to the pre-pregnancy level gradually after labour. *Foa* [4] found that the systolic blood pressure of renal hypertensive rats was sharply reduced during pregnancy. After delivery the systolic blood pressure rose again to the pre-pregnancy levels. They suggested that the drop of blood pressure might be due to an endocrine mechanism. *Grollman* [7] demonstrated a tendency for the blood pressure to decline during pregnancy in renal hypertensive dogs, rabbits and rats, but that pseudo-pregnancy was not accompanied by a change in the blood pressure. *Page* [17] found that when pregnancy was superimposed upon desoxycorticosterone hypertension the blood pressure and fluid balance were not affected, in contra-distinction to renal hypertension where a fall of blood pressure occured. *Gross* [8] showed that circulating renin, angiotensin and alsosterone levels were increased in renal hypertension, but were reduced in desoxycorticosterone hypertension. The purpose of the present investigation is to study the effect of progesterone administration on pregnancy complicated by EPH-gestosis.

Material and Method

Type of patients:

1. A group of 40 pregnant women with the pregnancy ranging from 34 to 40 weeks, suffering from EPH-gestosis, were given natural progesterone as the only line of treatment for their toxaemia. This group included:

A. Nineteen cases of mild EPH-gestosis whose blood pressure varied between 135–160 mm/Hg systolic and 90–100 mm/Hg diastolic. The oedema was limited to the lower limbs and their proteinuria was mild.

B. Sixteen cases of severe EPH-gestosis as indicated by a systolic blood pressure above 160 mm/Hg and a diastolic blood pressure of 100 mm/Hg or more, pitting oedema of the lower limbs and abdominal wall and heavy albuminuria.

C. Five cases of fulminating toxaemia of a short duration of symptoms and high blood pressure reaching over 180 mm/Hg systolic and 110 mm/Hg diastolic, intensive oedema, and heavy albuminuria.

2. A group of 10 normal pregnant women at the 34th–38th week of pregnancy, were taken as control cases for studying the effect of natural progesterone administered in doses similar to those used in toxaemic cases.

Tab. 1 shows the full description of the cases under study.

Tab. 1. The description of 40 cases of EPH-Gestosis and 10 normal pregnancies treated by progesterone.

Type of patient	No. of cases	Average age „years"	Primi-para %	Grand multipara %	Average No. of deliveries	Mono-sym-ptomatic	Poly-sym-ptomatic	Mean value gestosis index.
Mild EPH-Gestosis	19	23.9	41.6	11.2	1.6	14.7%	85.3%	2.4
Severe EPH-Gestosis	21	25.3	32.1	16.5	3.1	0%	100%	8.1
Normal pregnancy	10	30.6	30.0	27.2	3.5	–	–	–

Progesterone: we used the natural progesterone which was given deep intramuscularly in the gluteal region.

In order the obtain a constant high level of progesterone, the drug was given in 4 divided doses of 50 mg each, at six-hour intervals.

The administration of the drug continued according to the clinical response of every individual case, the maximum length was six weeks. The earliest response was obtained after 36 hours from the start of treatment.

Women pregnant at the 38th week or more were given the drug until the onset of labour. Cases pregnant at the 36th week were given the drug for two weeks, then, the pregnancy was terminated.

Follow up investigations:

All patients were admitted to hospital and were kept in bed for 24 hours, during which regular recording of the blood pressure was carried out every 6 hours in order to register the basal blood pressure.

After the elapse of the first 24 hours, progesterone therapy was started. In the fulminating group progesterone was administered immediately on admission in order to avoid further complications.

The following tests and investigations were carried out:

1. *Weight:* The estimation was repeated every 24 hours at 7.30 a.m. before breakfast. The extent of the oedema was tested daily.
2. *Blood pressure:* It was recorded every 6 hours in all cases, and every 2 hours in the fulminating group.
3. *Urine:* The 24-hour urine was measured and tested for specific gravity, sugar, pus cells and total protein content.
4. *Blood urea:* It was estimated before starting the treatment and when the patient responded to it.
5. *Urea clearance:* During this work the urea clearance was calculated as a percentage of the normal. It was estimated before starting the treatment, when the patient showed any response, and on the 10th day of therapy.
6. *Serum uric acid: Mc Farlane* [15] considered the level of uric acid in serum to be the most sensitive test for renal function, particularly in the diagnosis of kidney insufficiency associated with toxaemia of pregnancy. The serum uric acid level was estimated at the start of treatment when the patient showed any response and on the 10th day of therapy.
7. *Serum sodium and potassium:* These were estimated by flame photometry, before starting the treatment, when the patient responded to it and on the 7th day of therapy.

Results

A. *Effect of Natural Progesterone Therapy on EPH-gestosis.*

I. *Clinical Response:*

32 out of the 40 cases (80%) treated by natural progesterone showed evident clinical response.

1. *Blood pressure:*

The earliest drop in the systolic blood pressure was noticed 24 hours after the onset of treatment, while the maximum drop was reached on the 4th day of treatment. The systolic blood pressure dropped from a mean of 170 mm/Hg to 130 mm/Hg.

Three out of the five cases of the fulminating toxaemia responded to treatment, while in the remaining two cases the response was minimal.

The drop in the systolic blood pressure was rapid during the first 3 or 4 days of treatment, after which the pressure was maintained at 130 mm/Hg, and never dropped below that level inspite of the continued progesterone therapy.

Fig. 1 shows a scattergram of the systolic blood pressure of the 32 cases of EPH-gestosis under natural progesterone therapy. It demonstrates the rapid drop of the systolic blood pressure during the first few days of treatment and its maintenance around 130 mm/Hg.

There was a drop of the diastolic blood pressure in 34 out of 40 cases that received the progesterone therapy (85%). The earliest change appeared 72 hours after medication, later than the drop in the systolic pressure. It was then maintained at about 85 mm/Hg with the continued administration of progesterone.

The lowest diastolic pressure was obtained on the 7th day of treatment, i.e. the maximum response was achieved 3 days later than that of the systolic blood pressure.

Fig. 2 shows a scattergram of the changes in the diastolic blood pressure in 34 cases of EPH-gestosis under the effect of natural progesterone.

2. *Volume of urine:*

All the 40 cases responded to progesterone therapy by diuresis.

The volume of urine in the first 24 hours of treatment was at least double the amount of the day before, with an average of 1500 cc, even in those cases where the daily volume of urine had never exceded 400 ccs before treatment. The manifest oedema of the lower limbs was reduced. It completely disappeared within a period of 7 days.

These patients were not restricted to bed, which would have otherwise accounted, at least in part, to the subsidence of the oedema.

Fig. 3 demonstrates the changes in the volume of urine as compared with the changes of blood pressure and body weight under the effect of natural progesterone.

3. *Weight of the patient:*

The average drop in weight per week was 1.25 Kg. Those who continued therapy for 3 weeks manifested a total drop of 4–6 Kgm.

4. *Albuminuria:*

In spite of the marked increase of urinary output, decrease of blood pressure, body weight and oedema, the albuminuria persisted.

II. *Biochemical changes:*

1. *Changes in the serum sodium:*

In 28 out of 40 cases (70%) of EPH-gestosis which responded to natural progesterone therapy, the serum sodium dropped starting from the 3rd day of treatment. In some cases it dropped from a level of 180 mEq/litre to 150 mEq/litre, which is very near the normal figure. In other cases it dropped to 130 mEq/litre. This reduction was gradual and maintained throughout the course of treatment and was associated with diuresis and subsidence of oedema.

Four remarkable cases responded to therapy by increase of the daily output of urine and reduction of the oedema, but, their high serum sodium continued unresponsive for two weeks of progesterone administration.

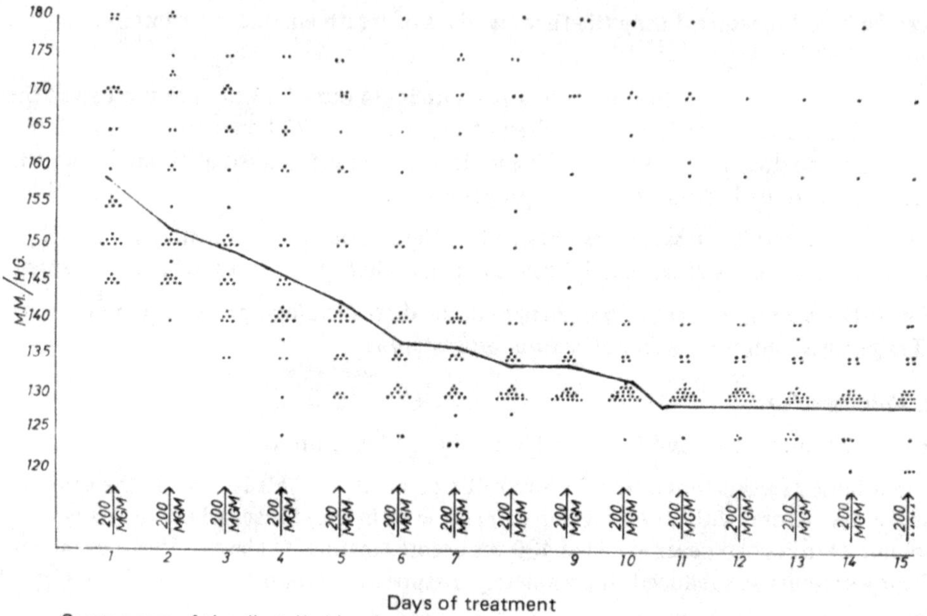

Scattergram of the diastolic blood pressure changes on natural progesterone therapy for toxaemic patients

Fig. 1

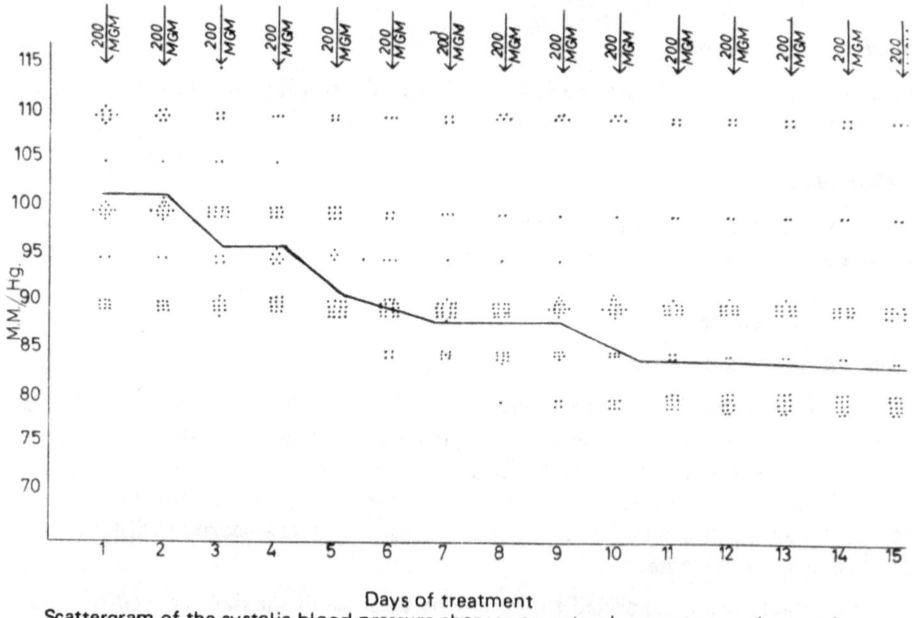

Scattergram of the systolic blood pressure changes on natural progesterone therapy for toxaemic patients

Fig. 2

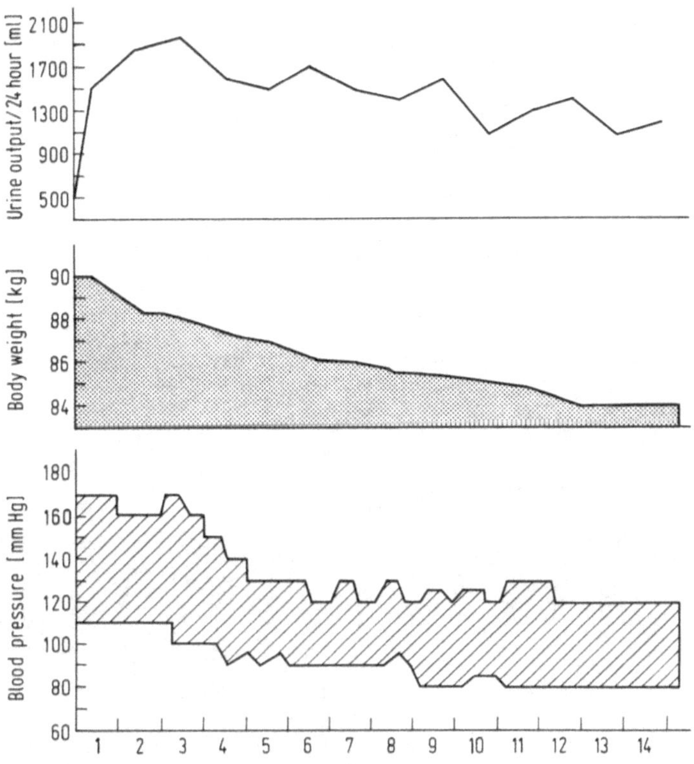

Days of treatment
Blood pressure, body weight and urinary output changes in severe preeclampsia on natural progesteron therapy

Fig. 3

Even worse were 2 cases of EPH-gestosis whose blood pressure was not markedly reduced and whose serum sodium was raised from 140 mEq/L. to 145 mEq/L. in one case and from 152 mEq/L. to 155 mEq/L. in the other case.

Fig. 4 demonstrates the variations in the serum sodium of EPH-gestosis patients under treatment with natural progesterone.

2. *Changes in the serum potassium:*

Only in 12 cases (30%) of EPH-gestosis treated with progesterone did the serum potassium drop. The reduction never exceded 0.2 mEq/L. In two cases the reduction was marked. In 19 cases (47.5%), there was no demonstrable change in the serum potassium for 2 weeks under treatment and inspite of the drop of blood pressure, the increase of volume of urine, the subsidence of oedema and the drop of the serum sodium. In 3 cases, the serum potassium had slightly increased under progesterone therapy.

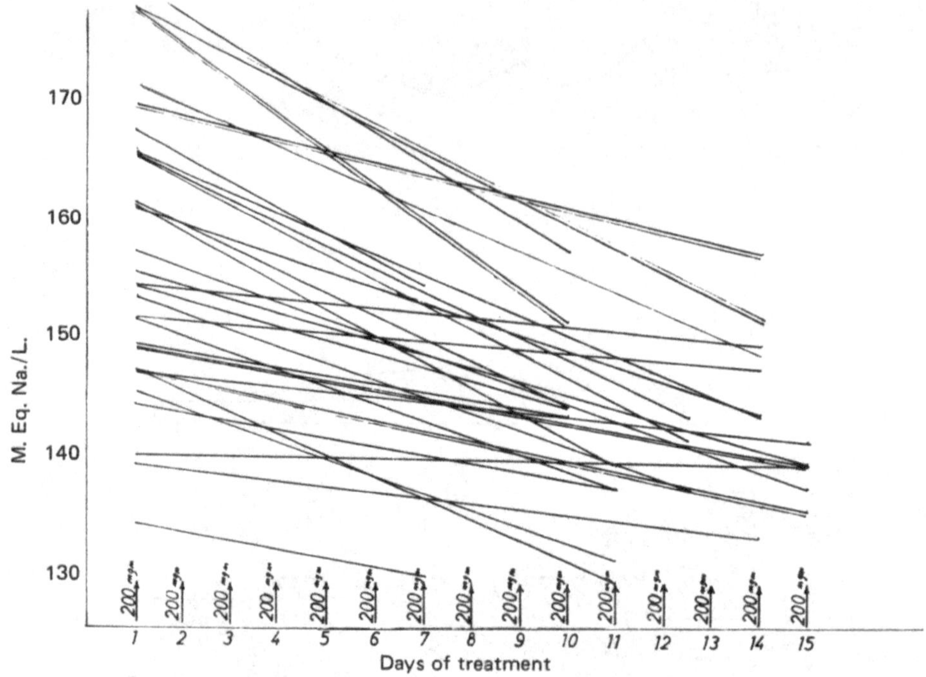

Scattergram for the serum sodium before and after the administration of natural progesterone for toxaemic patients

Fig. 4

Fig. 5 shows the very little variation in level of serum potassium in EPH-gestosis patients under progesterone therapy.

3. *Changes in serum uric acid:*

In 29 out of the 40 cases (72.5%) there was a definite drop in the serum uric acid starting from the 4th day of progesterone therapy. The drop varied between 1.5 and 2.5 mgm/100 ml after two weeks of treatment.

In 5 cases there was no such change inspite of the favourable clinical response, and in 3 others there was a rise of 0.2 to 0.5 mgm uric acid/100 ml of serum.

Fig. 6 demonstrates the reduction in the serum uric acid under natural progesterone therapy.

4. *Blood urea:*

In 11 out of the 40 cases (27.5%) of pre-eclamptic toxaemia was the blood urea reduced. In the rest of the cases the blood urea remained unchanged (23 cases) or even increased (6 cases).

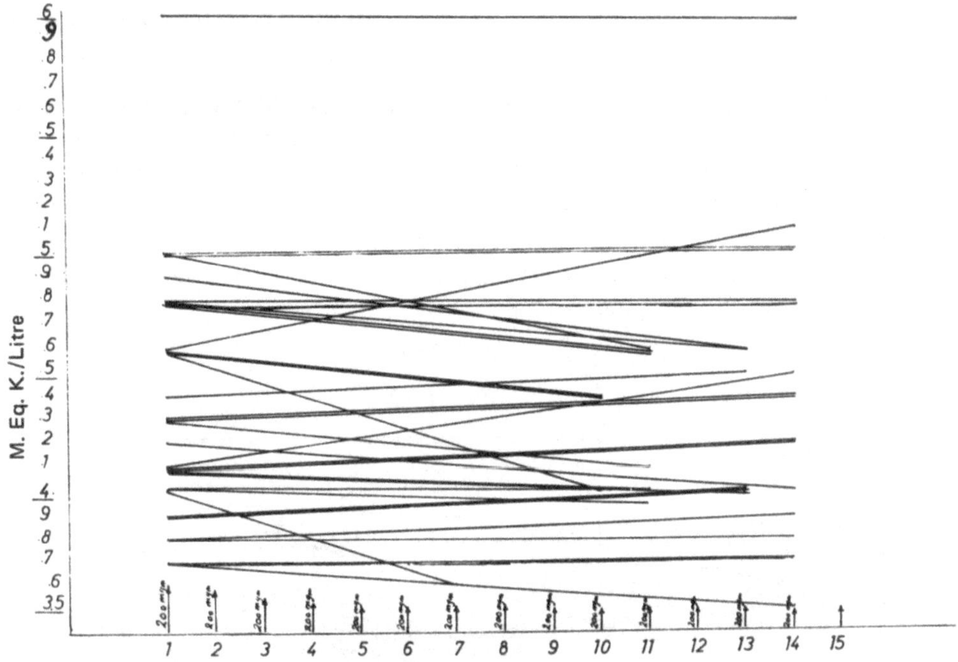

Scattergram of serum potassium before and after the administration of natural progesterone for toxaemic patients

Fig. 5

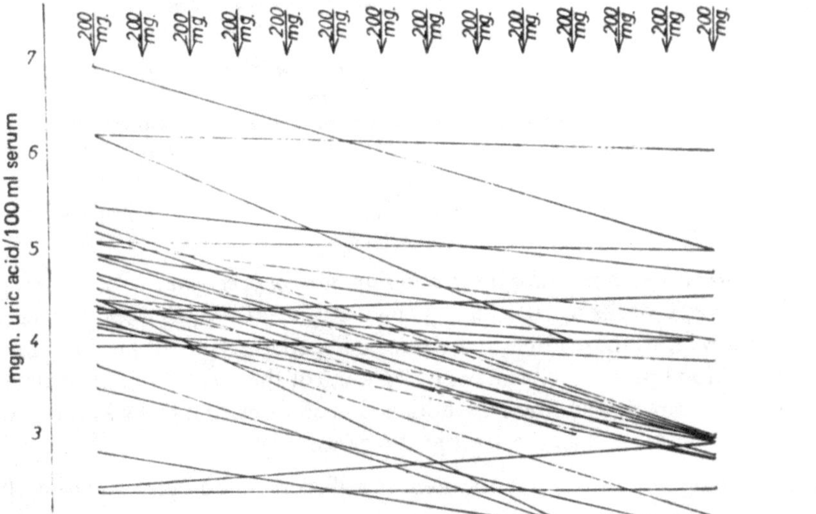

Scattergram of the serum uric acid before and after natural progesterone therapy

Fig. 6

5. *Urea clearance:*

The urea clearance before treatment varied between 55 and 100% of the normal levels. Two weeks after starting progesterone therapy improvement to above 75% of the normal values occurred in 22 cases (55%), no change appeared in 12 cases whose urea clearance before treatment was above 75%, and in 5 cases the clearance dropped below 55% of the normal.

Fig. 7 is a scattergram demonstrating the improvement in urea clearance in EPH-gestosis under the effect of progesterone.

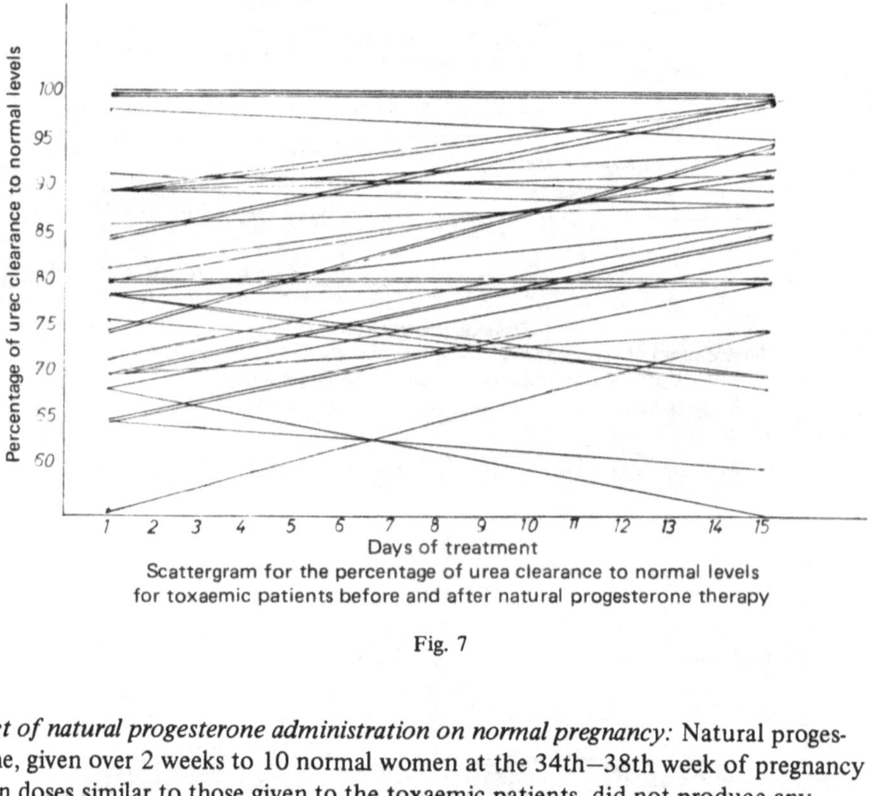

Scattergram for the percentage of urea clearance to normal levels for toxaemic patients before and after natural progesterone therapy

Fig. 7

Effect of natural progesterone administration on normal pregnancy: Natural progesterone, given over 2 weeks to 10 normal women at the 34th–38th week of pregnancy and in doses similar to those given to the toxaemic patients, did not produce any change in the blood pressure. A diuresis of 20–50% of the mean 24-hour volume of urine prior to treatment was, however, obtained in all cases, and this was accompanied with a gain in weight less than the average in 6 cases.

The serum sodium, potassium and uric acid, as well as the blood urea and urea clearance were not changed.

Obstetric management: Labour was induced in 15 cases (17.5%) at the 37th–38th week of pregnancy. Labour pains started spontaneously in 10 cases at the 40th week of gestation and in 14 cases 1–2 weeks before term. Cesarean section was resorted to in one case for a central placenta preaevia.

Delivery was unassisted in 23 cases, extraction by forceps was required in 8 cases and by the vacuum extractor in 3 cases, and labour was terminated by cesarean section in 5 cases, apart from the one case of ceasarean section done for placenta praevia.

Only two foetal deaths occurred. One of them was the outcome of a fulminating EPH-gestosis case, while the second case was not responding to progesterone therapy, intra-uterine foetal death was diagnosed 4 days before its spontaneous delivery.

Discussion

It has been widely assumed that progesterone is a salt retaining hormone. This assumption was favoured by the fact that progesterone administration could maintain the life of adrenalectomised aminals (*Gaunt* [5], *Pfieffer* and *Hooker* [18]). It also produced desoxycorticosterone-like reduction of the urinary sodium-potassium ratio in adrenalectomised rats when given in large doses (*Kagawa* [10]). These findings could be explained by the close structural similarity of progesterone to desoxycorticosterone which is a strong sodium retaining corticosteroid.

However, *Landau* [12 and 13] had clearly shown that progesterone had a natriuretic action which could not be elicited in adrenal deficient subjects unless aldosterone or desoxycorticosterone were administered. Therefore, they ascribed this natriuretic effect to inhibition of adrenal salt retaining hormones at a renal level. *Landau* and *Lugibihl* [14] assumed that the natriuretic influence of progesterone in normal subjects is due to competitive inhibition of endogenous aldosterone. Progesterone may be considered an aldosterone antagonist. They showed that discontinuance of progesterone treatment caused sodium retention which might be due to compensatory oversecretion of aldosterone.

Armstrong [1] first described the hypotensive action of progesterone in hypertensive rats, dogs and human beings suffering from essential hypertension. *Genest* [6] found that progesterone lowered the blood pressure of hypertensive patients. *Melby* [16] found that when progesterone was administered to patients suffering from the syndrome of idiopathic oedema characterised by generalised oedema, diminished urinary sodium excretion and hyperaldostenuria, they experienced a diuresis with a high excretion of sodium and water within 24 hours after a single injection of 500 mg of 17-hydroxyprogesterone capronate and remained oedema-free for 7 to 10 days.

Landau [12] and *Kyle* and *Hess* [11] showed that progesterone had a protein catabolic action. *Landau* and *Lugibihl* [14] found that progesterone lowered the total circulating amino acid nitrogen level whereas blood urea nitrogen did not decline. The increment in urinary nitrogen was urea. The urinary amino-acid nitrogen output did not rise. They concluded that the end product of the protein, catabolised as a result of the influence of progesterone, was urea. They suggested hat the progesterone enhanced the utilisation of amino acids of exogenous and endogenous origin by the liver.

The observations made in this work confirmed the hypotensive and diuretic effect of progesterone in EPH-gestosis. It improves the kidney function and it has no side effect on either the mother or the newborn. In 80% of the cases under study it controlled the process of toxaemia with a well maintained hypotensive action. None of our cases went into the convulsive state under progesterone medication. All the newborns did not manifest any abnormality in the genital organs. Our findings would support the previous observations made by *Dumitresco* [3] who demonstrated a diuretic and a hypotensive effect of progesterone on pregnancy toxaemia.

Abstract

Progesterone was used as the main line of therapy in 40 cases of EPH-Gestosis and it was also given to 10 normal pregnant women as a control group.

A significant fall in both the systolic and diastolic blood pressures was observed in 80% of the toxaemic patients. All cases showed marked increase in the 24 hour urinary output with an apparent loss of weight. Serum uric acid showed a significant drop and the urea clearance values have also improved. The serum sodium showed an apparent decline while the serum potassium did not show any marked variation.

The serum uric acid, urea clearance, blood urea, serum sodium and serum potassium remained unchanged in the control group.

References

[1] *Armstrong, J. G.:* Proc. Soc. Exp. Biol. Med. 102 (1959) p. 452–455.

[2] *Corbit, J. D.:* Amer. J. Med. Sci. 201 (1941) p. 876–884.

[3] *Dumitresco, P., E. Popsco* and *P. Medinisco:* Gynec. and Obstet. 65 (1966) p. 275.

[4] *Foa, P. P., N. L. Foa* and *M. M. Peet:* Amer. J. Med. Sci. 204 (1942) p. 350–356.

[5] *Gaunt, R., W. O. Nelson* and *E. Loomis:* Proc. Soc. Exp. Biol. Med. 39 (1938) p. 319–322.

[6] *Genest, J., W. Nowaczynski, E. Koiw, T. Sandor* and *P. Biron:* Ciba Intern. Symp. on Essential Hypertension, Bern (1960) p. 126–146.

[7] *Grollman, A.:* Amer. J. Physiol. 151 (1947) p. 373–379.

[8] *Gross, F., H. Brunner* and *M. Ziegler:* Recent progress in hormone research 21 (1965) p. 119–167.

[9] *Harrison, T. R., A. Grollman* and *J. R. Williams:* Amer. J. Physiol. 128 (1940) p. 716–724.

[10] *Kagawa, C. M.:* Soc. Exp. Biol. Med. 99 (1958) p. 705–707.

[11] *Kyle, L. H.* and *W. C. Hess:* J. Clin. Endocr. Met. 15 (1955) p. 879.

[12] *Landau, R. L., D. M. Bergenstal, K. Lugibihl* and *M. E. Kascht:* J. Clin. Endocr. Met. 15 (1955) p. 1194–1215.

[13] *Landau, R. I.* and *K. Lugibihl:* J. Clin. Endocr. 18 (1958) p. 1237–1245.

[14] *Landau, R. L.* and *K. Lugibihl:* Recent Progress in hormone research 17 (1961) p. 249–281.

[15] *Mc-Farlane, C. N.:* J. Obstet. and Gynaec. Brit. Commonwealth 70 (1963) p. 63.

[16] *Melby, J. C.:* Recent progress in hormone research 17 (1961) p. 249–281.

[17] *Page, E. W.* and *M. B. Glendening:* Proc. Soc., Exp. Biol. Med. 82 (1953) p. 466–468.

[18] *Pfeiffer, C. A., C. W. Hooker:* Amer. J. Physiol. 131 (1940) p. 441–448.

Reaction of the Fetus to Labour-Stress

Intérêt de l'épreuve de tolérance foetale à la contraction utérine dans le dépistage de la souffrance foetale au cours des gestoses

H. Hajeri, G. Winisdoerffer, G. Muller, P. Beauvais, E. Philippe, J. Dreyfus

Service de Gynécologie-Obstétrique, Hôpital Civil de Haguenau, France

Introduction

A l'unité obstétricale, de l'Hôpital Civil de Haguenau, (Médecin-Chef: Dr. *J. Dreyfus*), nous avons mis au point une méthode d'exploration de la fonction respiratoire du complexe foeto-placentaire, dénommée épreuve de tolérance foetale à la contraction utérine et dérivée du test à l'ocytocine décrit en 1964 par l'Ecole de Montevideo.

Cette méthode d'évaluation de la réserve foetale, que l'on sait diminuée au cours des gestoses, consiste à étudier la réaction cardiaque du foetus au stress physiologique que représente la contraction utérine (C.U.) artificiellement induite ou spontanément présente. Dans ce but, l'activité utérine et le rythme cardiaque foetal sont enregistrés simultanément et respectivement par tocographie externe et cardiotachygraphie stéthographique.

Matériel et méthode

Cette épreuve fonctionnelle dont la durée totale est d'environ 60 minutes connait trois modalités techniques:

le test à l'ocytocine proprement dit,
l'équivalent-test à l'ocytocine,
et le couplet Amnioscopie-Phonocardiotachygraphie.

Elle a été pratiquée dans l'immense majorité des cas au-delà de la 35è semaine, période au cours de laquelle, la thérapeutique de sauvetage foetal est possible. Elle n'a pas été exclusive: nous avons également eu recours à d'autres méthodes d'exploration bien connues à savoir le dosage de l'oestriolurie, l'analyse cyto-hormonale du frottis vaginal et l'amnioscopie.

Notre expérience personnelle porte sur 117 épreuves fonctionnelles concernant 46 cas de gestoses répertoriées selon la classification de *Goecke* et dont les placenta ont été examinés par le Professeur *Philippe* de l'Institut d'Anatomie-pathologique de Strasbourg.

Plusieurs critères ont été retenus pour apprécier la valeur de cette exploration fonctionnelle.

1. Comparaison avec:
   le dosage de l'oestriol urinaire,
   le colpocytogramme,
   l'amnioscopie.
2. Confrontation des résultats avec:
   les données de la tachymétrie per-partale,
   l'état néo-natal immédiat jugé selon le schéma établi par Apgar,
   le degré de maturité du nouveau-né apprécié d'après les courbes de *Lubchenko,*
   l'existence d'une souffrance néo-natale (S.N.N.) ou, au contraire, la bonne adaptation du nouveau-né à la vie extra-utérine.

Nous avons adopté le concept de S.N.N. défini par *J. M. Levy* et coll. dans leur rapport au XXIIè Congrès des Pédiâtres de langue française et classé les S.N.N. selon le schéma que, nous-mêmes, avions proposé dans une communication à ce même congrès.

Classification des S. N. N.

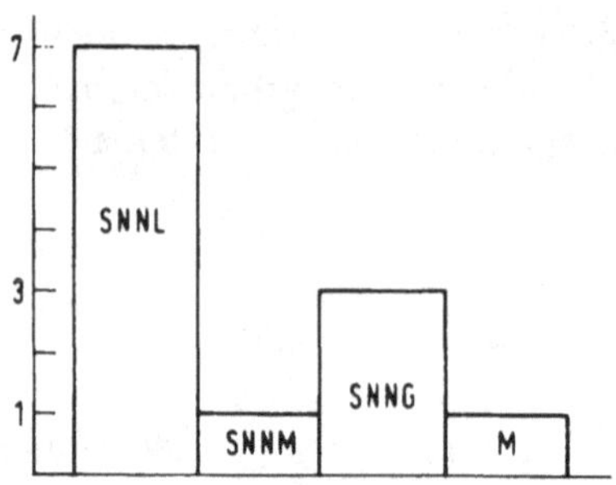

12 cas

Légères = 7
Moyennes = 1 Neuro
Graves = 3 Neuro
Malf. = 1

Résultats

L'interprétation des tracés tocophonocardiotachygraphiques selon les normes bien connues d'analyse de la courbe de fréquence cardiaque foetale nous a permis de définir trois modalités de réponse cardiaque foetale à l'épreuve de la contraction utérine:

I. *Epreuves positives:*
Elles représentent 34,78% des cas et ont été classées pathologiques sur la base de l'un et/ou l'autre des critères suivants.
tachycardie secondaire marquée,
rythme plat net,
ralentissements précoce, tardif ou variable, modérés ou sévères avec ou sans bradycardie résiduelle.

Tab. 1. Résultats des épreuves fonctionnelles et Index Gestosique.

Index	Nombre de cas	Epreuve positive	Limite	Epreuve negative
1	2	–	–	2
2	12	3	2	7
3	11	3	3	5
4	9	4	2	3
5	4	2	2	0
6	7	3	1	3
8	1	1	–	–
Total	46	16	10	20

II. *Epreuves à la limite de la normale:*
Elles constituent 21,73% des cas et sont définies par l'un et/ou l'autre phénomène(s) suivant(s):
variations prolongées modérées,
rythme plat intermittent ou fréquence cardiaque à ondulations serrées,
ralentissements précoce, tardif ou variable, simples et légers.

III. *Epreuves négatives:*
Elles représentent 43,47% des cas. Leur normalité est fondée sur l'absence de toute variation de la fréquence cardiaque foetale et leur pourcentage correspond à celui des rythmes stables observés lors de la période de dilatation dans les grossesses dites à „haut risque".

La mise en parallèle de ces résultats et des données de la clinique nous a permis de tirer trois conclusions qui, étant donné le nombre limité de cas, ne sont fournies qu'à titre provisoire:

1. *Existence d'une corrélation entre la gravité de la gestose et la perturbation de l'épreuve fonctionnelle.*
En d'autres termes, celle-ci est plus fréquemment pathologique lorsque l'Index Gestosique est élevé.

2. *Absence de réponse cardiaque foetale pathognomonique d'une gestose.*
Tout au plus peut-on souligner la prépondérance des ralentissements tardifs. Sur ce point, nous sommes en désaccord avec les conclusions émises par *Ionascu.*

3. Pas de parallélisme entre la gravité des variations de la courbe de fréquence cardiaque foetale et la valeur de l'Index Gestosique.

Appréciation de la valeur des résultats de l'épreuve fonctionnelle:

A. La confrontation des données de l'état néo-natal avec les modalités réactionnelles du coeur foetal à l'épreuve de la C.U., suggère les remarques suivantes:

I. *Tachymétrie per partum:*
Les anomalies du rythme cardiaque foetal observées pendant la grossesse se retrouvent lors du travail. Il s'agit donc bien de manifestations de souffrance foetale que l'on peut dépister précocement par le biais de l'E.T.F.C.U.

II. *Score d'Apgar:*

1. Une épreuve positive est en corrélation significative avec un état de dépression marquée du nouveau-né (Apgar ≤ 7) et témoigne donc d'une S.F.C. dans 65% des cas environ.

2. Une épreuve à la limite de la normale est assimilable en pratique à un test négatif.

3. Il y a discordance entre les données de l'épreuve et celles de l'état néo-natal immédiat, que l'on peut ainsi chiffrer:
12,5% de faux positifs,
10% de faux négatifs.

Tab. 2.

		Rythme plat isolé 2 cas	Ralentissement précoce simple 1 cas	Ralentissements tardifs 9 cas		Ralentissements variables 4 cas			
				Avec B. R.	Simples	Sévères			Modérés
						Avec B. R.	Simples isolés	Simples associés	
Tachymetrie		10-73 2 cas	80 1 cas	9-53-77 3 cas	2-5-13-17-81-87 6 cas	89 1 cas		18-22 2 cas	48 1 cas
Index Gestosique		2 6	5	6-4-4	2-4-5 4-6-2	8		3 3	3
Contexte neo-natal	Apgar deprimé	2	1	2	3	1		1	1
	Hypotrophie	1	1	1	1	1		1	–
	S. N. N.	1 (Décès) 1 enfant césarien	1	2 + 1 enfant césarien	1			0	0

Tab. 3. Score d'Apgar, Gestoses.

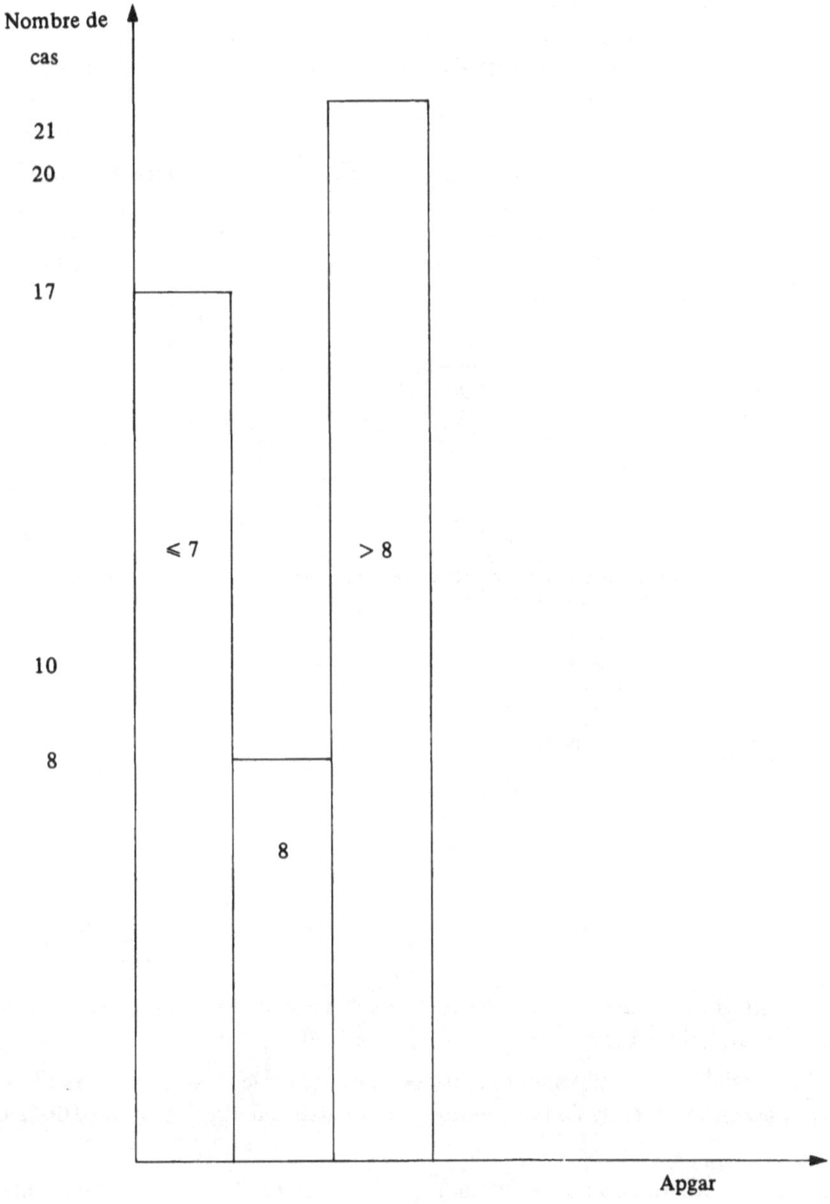

III. *Hypotrophie foetale:*
L'épreuve de tolérance foetale à la C.U. s'est révélée pathologique dans tous les cas de foetus hypotrophiques.

IV. *Souffrance néo-natale:*

1. 60% environ des nouveau-nés risquent de présenter une S.N.N. lorsque l'E.T.F.C.U. est pathologique.
2. Un tel risque est réduit à 26% lorsque l'épreuve est négative.
3. Le pourcentage de faux négatifs reste théoriquement fixé à 10% des cas environ.

Tab. 4. Score d'Apgar a la naissance et réponse cardiaque foetale pendant la grossesse.

Apgar	Epreuves positives	Epreuves à la limite de la normale	Epreuves négatives	Faux positifs	Faux négatifs
≤ 7 17 cas	11 64,70%	4	2	2/16 12,5%	2/20 10%
8 8 cas	3	2	3	–	–
> 8 21 cas	2 9,52%	4	15	–	–

Tab. 5. Comparaison de la valeur des deux explorations (Score d'Apgar)
Oestriolurie E. T. F. C. U.

Apgar	03 pathologique	Epreuve positive
≤ 7 11 cas	7 63,43%	7 63,43%
8 7 cas	2	3
> 8 15 cas	2 13,33%	0 0%

B. De la comparaison, dans 33 cas, des résultats de l'épreuve fonctionnelle et du dosage de l'oestriolurie, il ressort que:

1. Une corrélation sensiblement identique existe entre les résultats de ces deux explorations et l'état de l'enfant in utéro, à la naissance et pendant la période néo-natale.
2. Dans l'évaluation du risque foetal, les données de l'E.T.F.C.U. semblent plus précises.

3. Ces deux explorations peuvent paraître complémentaires et le sont en effet. Leur association permet de mieux cerner le problème du diagnostic de la S.F.C. sans garantir toutefois de façon absolue contre le risque d'une fausse sécurité.

Tab. 6. Réaction à la contraction utérine du coeur des hypotrophiques.

Foetus	Epreuves positives	Limite	Normale
Hypotrophiques 6 cas	6 100%	0	0
De poids normal pour l'age de la grossesse 40 cas	10 25%	10 25%	20 50%

Tab. 7. Score d'Apgar et oestriolurie.

Apgar	Oestriolurie patho.	03 Normale	Faux positif	Faux négatif
⩽ 7 11 cas	7 63,43%	4 36,36%	2/11 18,18%	4/22 18,18%
8 7 cas	2	5	–	–
> 8 15 cas	2 13,33%	13 86,66%	–	–

Tab. 8. Comparaison de la valeur des deux explorations hypotrophie foetale Oestriolurie E. T. F. C. U.

Foetus	03 Pathologique	Epreuve positive
Hypotrophiques 4	3 75%	4 100%
De poids normal pour l'âge de la grossesse 29	8 27,58%	6 20,68%

Tab. 9. Comparaison de la valeur des deux explorations
S. N. N.

Periode neonatale	03 Pathologique	Epreuve positive
S. N. N. 7	5 71,42%	4 57,14%
Normale 26	6 23,07%	6 23,07%

Tab. 10. Résultats des épreuves de tolérance foetale à la C. U. dans les cas de S. N. N.

Période néo-natale	Epreuves positives	Epreuves limite	Epreuves négatives	Présumés faux positifs	Présumés faux négatifs
S. N. N. 12 cas	7 58,33%	3 25%	2 16,66%	9/16 56,25%	2/20 10%
Normale 34	9 26,47%	7 20,58%	18 52,94%	–	–

Conduite thérapeutique et conclusions

L'E.T.F.C.U. dont nous venons d'apprécier la valeur diagnostique et pronostique présente un réel intérêt dans le dépistage de la S.F.C. au cours des gestoses. Sans être absolue, sa valeur n'en est pas moins réelle et se formule comme suit:

1. La stabilité du rythme cardiaque témoigne d'un bienêtre foetal dans l'immense majorité des cas. Ce n'est que dans 10% des cas que cette modalité de réponse ne concorde pas avec la condition réelle du foetus in utéro.

2. Les anomalies du rythme cardiaque foetal sont la manifestation d'un état de S.F.C. dans 65 à 87,5% des cas. Par contre dans 12,5% des cas, elles ne correspondent pas à la réalité des faits et constituent plutôt une fausse alarme.

3. Les erreurs de diagnostic inhérents à la pratique de l'E.T.F.C.U. nous paraissent tenir d'une part à des questions d'ordre technique et méthodologique et d'autre part aux difficultés que soulèvent l'analyse de la courbe de F.C.F. et l'interprétation physiopathologique de ses variations.

4. Le dosage de l'oestriolurie et l'épreuve de tolérance foetale à la C.U. apparaissent comme deux méthodes complémentaires permettant de mieux cerner le problème du diagnostic de la souffrance foetale chronique au cours des gestoses.
Sur la base de leurs résultats ci-dessus mentionnés et compte tenu des conclusions tirées d'un travail global portant sur 207 épreuves fonctionnelles concernant 91 grossesses „à haut risque", la ligne thérapeutique suivante peut être tracée:

a) L'extraction de l'enfant d'emblée par voie haute est indiquée lorsqu'on relève:
un rythme plat répété et/ou des ralentissements sévères tardifs ou variables avec bradycardie résiduelle,
un résultat pathologique du dosage de l'oestriol urinaire et des ralentissements tardifs sévères et répétés à l'E.T.F.C.U.

b) Dans tous les autres cas la conduite thérapeutique sera discutée en fonction du contexte clinique général et obstétrical.

Telle est la substance de notre expérience et telles sont les perspectives que l'on peut y discerner. Il va sans dire que bien des points restent à éclaircir et que les conclusions que nous venons de formuler n'ont aucun caractère définitif et demandent confirmation par un travail portant sur un nombre de cas nettement plus élevé. Un tel travail est en cours depuis un an dans notre service.

Short, Preliminary Reports of Study-Groups on Gestosis

Study group "Edema, Electrolytes, Metabolism" in EPH-Gestosis

N. A. M. Bergstein, P. J. Boodt, A. C. Drogendyk, G. Pardi, L. Tervilä, B. Vedra

Zevenaar, Holland, Kampsingel 72
Amsterdam, Holland, Academisch Ziekenhuis der Vrye Universiteit de Boelelaan 1117
Milano, Italy, Clinica "L. Mangiagalli", Via Commenda 12
Lahti, Finland, Kaupunginsairaala
Praha – Podolí, ČSSR, Institute for the care of mother and child

Purposes

The aim of the study group is to study
1. the pathogenesis of edema of pregnancy, both gestotic and non gestotic
2. the pathogenesis of salt and water retention in EPH-gestosis

Edema

Edema is defined – according to the definition of the O.G. – as gestotic if it is pretibial and can be observed after a night's rest.

This definition is an arbitrary one. Scientific proves are lacking that edema which disappears after night's rest is of different origin and has nothing to do with EPH-gestosis. Therefore we feel that more knowledge is needed of both gestotic and non gestotic edema. The following questions – and many others – are to be answered:
1. what is the difference of "gestotic" and "non gestotic" edema-fluid especially regarding proteins?
2. what is the difference of microproteinuria between the healthy controls, non gestotic edema and gestotic edema? – Cases with clinical proteinuria are to be excluded!
3. how does the gestotic edema develop? Is it preceeded by "orthostatic edema"? Is it accompanied by increasing microproteinuria? What is the participation of orthostasis in the development of "gestotic" edema?
4. what is the interrelationship between weight gain, development of edema and placental steroids? The interrelationship between weight gain, edema and weight of placenta?

Because it is difficult to answer the 1st question – which is basical – we can draw our attention to the permeability of glomerular capillaries for proteins. The working hypothesis can be accepted that the greater the permeability of glomerular capillaries for proteins the greater the permeability of the capillaries also in other tissues. Where the hydrostatic influences are cooperating, like in lower extremities, edema will develop. The greater the quantities of proteins in urine, the greater quantities of proteins can be expected also in other tissues.

These questions can be answered by means of a follow up study.

Follow up study

Material: 30–50 women beginning between the 8th and 12th week of pregnancy – calculated from the 1st day of the last regular bleeding –. Chronic renal or cardiovascular diseases are to be excluded.

To be followed:

1. weight gain – measured exactly with the precision of 50–100 g under strictly standard conditions –: up to the 28th week every 4 weeks, then every 2 weeks up to the 36th week, then weekly. Free diet.
2. development of edema: pitting of dorsum pedis, ankles, pretibial pitting, pitting of abdominal wall, of face is to be registered on every visit. Edema observed by the patient herself in the evening only should also be registered.
3. microproteinuria: presence of albumin, transferrin and imunoglobulin-G – ev. of other proteins – in urine should be examined on every visit. The last evening sample on the day before the visit and the first morning sample on day of the visit.
4. blood proteins: changes of albumin and immunoglobulin-G.
5. estriol/24 hours: after the 30th week estriol excretion should be followed in order to answer the question whether the weight gain is correlated to the estrogens.
6. other hormones – if possible –.

This follow-up study could answer the question whether clinical proteinuria develops suddenly or is preceeded by increasing microproteinuria, whether the appearance of edema could be correlated with some changes in microproteinuria – indicating changes in general capillary permeability –, whether there is a correlation between the weight gain and development of microproteinuria, of the quantity of some placental steroids.

Metabolism of electrolytes

The aim of this study: in nonpregnant individuals the homeostasis of the volume of extracellular fluid is well understood. There is a lack of understanding of how this system is operating during pregnancy.

Some of the following questions are to be answered:

1. There is a generally accepted opinion that in the EPH-gestosis salt and water is retained in abnormal quantity. What does it exactly mean? By which mechanism is salt retained? Under which conditions?
2. What is the role of the renin-angiotensin-aldosteron system in the retention of salt and water? What is the role of ADH? How is this system operating during pregnancy, normal and pathologic?
3. The interrelationship between aldosteron and progesteron: aldosteron excretion is closely depending on body posture: in upright posture it increases, at bed rest it decreases. Does pregnandiol excretion follow the changes of aldosteron?

Material

Three groups of patients should be studied: controls, edema, edema-hypertension-proteinuria. 8–10 individual in each group.

Method

The day of admission to the hospital is the day zero.

Day 1: strict bed rest for the next 24 hours. Normal diet. No therapy.

Day 2: activity out of bed for the 12 hours from 6 a.m. to 6 p.m. Bed rest for the next 12 hours at night.

The experiment begins by passing water at 6 a.m. This sample of urine is not collected. The samples of urine are collected in four 12-hour periods the quantity is measured exactly. The body weight is measured exactly twice a day: 6 a.m., 6 p.m., 6 a.m., 6 p.m. and 6 a.m. Blood samples are taken before breakfast.

Blood is examined for:
1. creatinine
2. Na, K, Cl
3. total plasma proteins
4. hemoglobine and hematocrit
5. urea
6. uric acid

Urine is examined for:
1. creatinine
2. Na, K, Cl
3. urea
4. if possible: aldosteron and pregnandiol

Comments

I have tried to propose these two studies according to our discussion in Fiesole. With both of the proposed studies I have certain experiences so that I am of the opinion that they are easy to perform. The only difficulty is the method of microproteinuria.

Regarding this method: as far as I am informed, Behring Werke, Marburg an der Lahn, Germany, is producing so called Partigen Platten, which is an equipment for assessing the spectrum of proteins. The principle of the method: immunoprecipitation in agar. The greater the concentration of the specific protein in urine, the greater is the precipitation circle in agar. The specific protein in urine represents the antigen, agar contains specific antiserum. For our study the most important proteins are those with the smallest molecule: albumin, transferrin and imunoglobulin-G. It is of course possible to examine the whole spectrum.

I am sure that every immunologist will be able to give further information.

Because it will need some time to coordinate the investigation of microproteinuria, I should recommend to start both studies. The samples of urine can be collected and kept frozen in a ice-box for many weeks. During the next months I shall try to supply you with further information.

I am prepared to answer every question regarding the methodology. Further, if somebody would have interrest to come and see our Institute in Prague for some time, he will be wellcomed. I can arrange a room free of charge in the Institute.

Short Report about the Research Program of the Study Group of Proteinuria/Organization Gestosis

This research program was the topic of the meeting of our study group at the 4th Meeting of Organization Gestosis in Florence. The following members of study group proteinuria were present:

A. Cretti, Bialystok, Poland
H. P. McEwan, Glasgow, Great Britain
J. W. W. Studd, Birmingham, Great Britain
M. D. Simanowitz, London, Great Britain
E. Tucci, Milano, Italy

The members of the group are of the opinion that the first aim is to make the definition of the signs of gestosis, as proposed by O.G., more widely accessible.

In the definition of proteinuria the level of proteinuria is given as estimated by the method of *Esbach* and the paper-sticks method. But there are countries where the method by *Esbach* is not used at all, and the paper-sticks method is not used in hospitals. In effort to make our definitions more widely accessible it seems justified to add also the cut-of-points for other methods, besides the method of *Esbach* and the paper-sticks method.

As far as we know the most widely used methods – besides *Esbach* and papersticks – are the procedure of heating the urine with acetic acid, the procedure with sulfosalycilic acid and the procedure with nitric acid. So one of our aims will be finding out the data of corresponding values of proteinuria, resulting from various method of estimation.

At present we have such data from the comparison between the paper-sticks method and the biuret method, this study was made by Dr. *Studd.* The following table contains these corresponding values, as related to classification of severity of proteinuria in points of Gestosis Index:

points of Gestosis Index	0	1	2	3
Biuret method	0	100 mg/%	101–250 mg/%	more than 250 mg/%
paper-sticks method	0	trace +	+ + to + + +	+ + + to + + + +

Such a study was also done on the comparison between the Biuret method and the method with sulfosalycilic acid. It remains to make the comparison of these three methods, basing on the data from the literature.

As far as we know there was probably no study done on the comparison between the results from the Biuret method – which remains the basic method for all comparisons – and the results from the method of heating the urine with acetic acid and the method with nitric acid. The members of the study group have divided between themselves the geographical regions for searching in the literature, how much and how far the studies were done on this problem. But as the number of publications grows immensely, all members of Organization Gestosis are kindly invited to take part in this searching.

Another important problem is the estimation of proteinuria in single specimens. In the definition of proteinuria and in the Gestosis Index, proposed by O.G., the cut-of-points are given as related to 24 h urine. Of course the estimation of proteinuria in 24 h collection of urine is the most reliable method and we think that it should remain in our definition. But it is obvious that the collection of 24 hours urine is not everywhere easily to perform, especially not in the out-patients practice. Our proposed criteria of diagnosis and classification should be easily accessible not only in hospitals but also for the general practitioner or for a midwife in small villages.

There is also another reason for giving in the definition of proteinuria also the value for single specimen. Let us consider a patient with severe gestosis who was just admitted to the hospital. Shall we wait full 24 hours for the result of proteinuria estimation? Certainly this would be not the best way. We should know immediately how far advanced are the renal lesions because it has important implications for the management. Therefore in such a case we estimate the proteinuria in single specimen, besides of determining the proteinuria in 24 h urine. This single portion should be any single specimen, not necessarily the first morning specimen, because of the decrease in urine output during the night and therefrom the increase of protein concentration, with the consequence of to high proteinuria estimation result.

But what is the value of proteinuria in single specimen corresponding to the given value of proteinuria in 24 h collection of urine? Corresponding at least to some extent? This is not known. The members of study group proteinuria feel that there should be some studies done on this problem. The hope is expressed that Organization Gestosis could support financially these studies.

Study Groups Endocrinology/Placental Insufficiency

Members

P. J. Keller, Zurich; *G. Zucconi,* Florence; *S. Severi,* Florence; *P. Curiel,* Florence; *H. Janisch,* Vienna; *J. Spona,* Vienna; *J. Andor,* Basle; *A. R. Genazzini,* Siena; *H. van der Crabben,* Düsseldorf; *C. Werner,* Düsseldorf; *K. H. Mosler,* Würzburg; *G. B. Massi,* Rome; *J. Stastny,* Geneva; *B. Salvadori,* Parma.

Collaboration not yet confirmed

C. Lauritzen, Ulm; *W. D. Lehmann,* Ulm; *J. W. Dudenhausen,* Berlin; *K. Hammacher,* Basle; *P. G. Crosigniani,* Milan.

Project: Studies on the endocrine and enzymatic activity of the human placenta in EPH-gestosis.
Comparison of various methods for monitoring placental and fetal distress in EPH-gestosis.

Patients: 100 cases of EPH-gestosis
(Edema, proteinuria > 0.5 g/d, blood pressure $> 140/90$ 24 hours after admission in the hospital; GI $\geqslant 4$)

Parameters: Oestriol (blood)
Progesterone (blood)
HPL (Human placental lactogen) (blood)
HCG (Human chorionic gonadotrophin) (blood)
HSAP (Heat-stable alcaline phosphatase) (blood)
17β-HO (17β-Hydroxysteroid-oxydoreductase) (blood)
Placental morphology
CTG (Cardiotocography)
pH-values in fetal blood
Apgar score

In addition in a limited number of cases according to facilities:
Oestriol (Amniotic fluid)
HCG (Amniotic fluid)
Placental blood flow
DHAS-test

Organization: All centers are contributing 10 or more suitable cases, which are followed until labour. All materials (serum, CTG-strips, placental pieces) are analyzed in the following reference laboratories:

Plasma oestriol, Florence
Plasma progesterone, Zurich
Plasma HCG, Vienna
Plasma HPL, Siena
HSAP, Düsseldorf
17β-HO, Düsseldorf
Amniotic fluid, Rome
CTG, Basle/Berlin
Placental histology, Düsseldorf
Computer program, Würzburg

DHAS-tests and placental blood flow are performed and analyzed in centers having own faculities for these methods.

Forms, mailing boxes and further instructions will be prepared and provided as soon as possible. After approvement by all members, a computer program will be established.

Preliminary results may be expected within one year, final correlation of all parameters should be worked out 1972/73.

Das Arbeitsprogramm der Studiengruppe Vaginale Zytologie

Dr. *Jan Židovský,* CSc., F.I.A.C.

Auf der Tagung der Organisation Gestose in Florenz (Fiesole) haben sich nur zwei zytologische Arbeiter zusammengetroffen: Dr. *Židovský* aus Prag und Dr. *Sammour* aus Cairo.

Die weitere zwei angemeldeten Teilnehmer Prof. *Watteville* und Dr. *Rosenblatt* aus Genf sind nicht gekommen.

Aus diesem Grunde war es deshalb nicht möglich, ein Arbeitsprogramm auf der breiteren internationalen Basis zu entfalten.

Aufgrund eines Austausches der beiderseitigen Erfahrungen (Dr. *Židovský*, Dr. *Sammour*) wird binnen eines Halbjahres ein schriftlicher ausführlicher Bericht mit dem definitiven Programm ausgearbeitet werden. Dieser Bericht wird Dr. *Rippmann,* dem Sekretär der Organisation Gestose übergeben werden.

Bis heute sind in der Weltliteratur nur wenige Erwähnungen über die Möglichkeiten bei der zytodiagnostischen Lösung der Problematik der EPH-Gestose.

Die neuesten zytologischen Arbeiten (*Wood* u. a., *Židovský* u. a.) geben schon genügende Möglichkeiten bei der Lösung der rechtzeitigen Diagnose der Beschädigung der Frucht bei EPH-Gestose. Es wäre darum sehr gelegen, diese zytodiagnostischen Möglichkeiten auf einer großen Zahl der Fälle auf den verschiedenen Arbeitsorten zu bestätigen.

Darum folgt auch das Arbeitsprogramm der cytologischen Studiengruppe für die nächste Zeit aus diesen zwei Aspekten:

1. Aus dem cytomorphologischen Aspekt (*Židovský*), d. h. auf einer großen Zahl der Fälle bisherige zytologischen Kriterien der rechtzeitigen Diagnose der Beschädigung des Kindes bei EPH-Gestose zu beweisen. Diese Kriterien beruhen auf der Pathognomonität des Befundes des ungünstigen „Terminzytotypen" III oder IV vor der 38. Woche der Schwangerschaft.

   Die Pathognomonität des „ungünstigen" Cytotype III, IV, ist je größer desto größer ist die zeitliche Entfernung dieser Cytotypen vor der 38. Schwangerschaftswoche. Wir wollen auch diesen zytomorphologischen Aspekt mit einer Korrelation der Oestriolbefunde ergänzen.

2. Aus dem *histochemischen Aspekt:* An der Arbeitsstelle Doktor Sammours aus Cairo werden die histochemischen Parameter des Scheidenabstriches analysiert: Lactodehydrogenase und alkalische Phosphatase in der Beziehung zur Therapie der EPH-Gestose und der Beschädigung des Kindes.
   In den endgültigen Schlußfolgerungen werden diese zwei Aspekte integriert in Beziehung zur komplexen Möglichkeit der rechtzeitigen Diagnose der Beschädigung des Foeten bei EPH-Gestose.
   Dieses vorläufige Arbeitsprogramm ist inzwischen bescheiden, aber es wird erwartet, daß auf dem Grunde verbreiteten Internationalen Kontaktes, werden diese zwei Arbeitsthemen um weitere Aspekte verbreitet.
   Man kann schon heute sagen, daß die Zytodiagnostik in der Beziehung zur EPH-Gestose eine vielversprechende Möglichkeit in der klinisch-praktischen Aplikation gibt.

Rapport der Psychosomatischen Arbeitsgruppe

Vorsitz: Prof. Dr. med. *Labhardt,* Basel
Teilnehmer: Dr. med. *Eicher,* Heidelberg, Dr. med. *Molinsky,* Düsseldorf,
Frau Dr. med. de *Senarclens,* Genf, Herr u. Frau Dr. med. *Siedentopf,* Frankfurt

Allgemeine Feststellungen

Das Problem psychosomatischer Zusammenhänge bei Gestosen ist komplex. Viele glauben an derartige Relationen können sie aber nur unklar umschreiben. Die Arbeitsgruppe wird im nächsten Jahre eine Präzision gewisser Fragen anstreben und versuchen, Hinweise für praktische Tätigkeit und wissenschaftliche Forschung zu geben. Besonders diskutiert wurde die Methodik des Vorgehens: Psychiatrisch-psychologische Exploration oder wissenschaftliche Testuntersuchungen?

Arbeitsplan

1. Eruierung von Meinungen über das Problem psychosomatischer Zusammenhänge bei Gestosen:
   a) von Ärzten, bzw. ärztlichen Publikationen,
   b) von den Patientinnen selbst,
   c) Meinung der Arbeitsgruppe.

2. Das Gestoseproblem im Lichte emotionalen Erlebens der gesamten Gravidität. Beziehungen zur Frühgravidität, klinische Untersuchung, evtl. mit testpsychologischen Untersuchungen (Frau Dr. med. *Siedentopf,* Herr Dr. med. *Eicher*).

3. Allgemein psychiatrische Untersuchung von Gestosepatientinnen. Heredität – Kindheit – frühere psychische Erkrankungen – Persönlichkeitsstruktur. Frage des Zeitpunktes der Untersuchung?

Die erwähnten Arbeiten sollen zunächst streng limitiert sein und können zunächst nur einige grundlegende Fragen beantworten. Größere Untersuchungen, evtl. testpsychologischer Art, erfordern für ihre statistische Stichhaltigkeit ein großes Krankengut und exakte Auswertung.

Grundlagen der Untersuchung betr. Patientengut

EPH-Patientinnen und PH-Patientinnen.
Patientinnen mit dem alleinigen Symptom „Ödem" sind möglicherweise psychosomatisch sehr interessant, sollen aber eine eigene Untersuchungsgruppe bilden (Zusammenhängende Emotionalität–Ödem sind bereits bekannt und können evtl. als Grundlage verwendet werden).
Gesunde Schwangere.

Die Arbeitsgruppe wird voraussichtlich im Mai 1972 zusammentreffen.

Representatives of the Organisation Gestosis
Vertreter der Organisation Gestose
Représentants de l'Organisation Gestose
Rappresentanti dell'Organizzazione Gestosi

Australia:	Prof. *H. M. Carey* – Royal Hospital for Women Paddington N.S.W./Australia
Austria:	Prof. *E. Leinzinger* – University Maternity Hospital Linz/Austria
Benelux: (Belgium, Holland, Luxemburg)	Dr. *Ch. Rippert,* at present: Maternity Hospital 5001 Aarau/Switzerland
Bulgaria:	P.D. Dr. *B. D. Boschkov* – "Christo Smirnenski" 1e Sofia 21/Bulgaria
Chile:	Dr. *Ronald Sievers* – Corporacion de Beneficensia Osorno, Casilla 163 Osorno/Chile
Costa Rica:	Dr. *Arturo Esquivel,* G. – P.O. Box 5689 San José/Costa Rica
Czechoslovakia:	Doz. *B. Vedra* – Research Institute Mother and Child, Podoli Prague 4/CSSR
Danmark:	Prof. *Dyre Trolle* – Kvindekliniken, Rigs Hospitalet 2100 Kopenhagen/Danmark
DDR:	Prof. *H. Kyank* – University Maternity Hospital Rostock/DDR
Ecuador:	Dr. *F. Gutiérrez* – Maternitad Enrique Sotomayor, P.O. Box 540 Guavaquil/Ecuador
Egypt:	Prof. Dr. *Maher Mahran* – Department of Obstetrics and Gynecology Ain Shams University Cairo/Egypt
Finland:	Prof. *P. Vàra* – 2nd University Maternity Hospital Helsinki/Finland
France:	Prof. *H. Henrion* – 16, rue Chardon – Lagache Paris 16e/France
Germany:	P.D. Dr. *C. Goecke* – University Maternity Hospital Würzburg/Germany
Greece:	P.D. Dr. *A. Gouscos* – 5, Skoufa Str. Athen (136)/Greece
Honduras:	Dr. *J. Radegundo Garcia G.* – Clinica Raudales Midence, 4a. avenida No. 426, Comayagüela, D.C. Honduras, C.A.

Hungary:	P.D. Dr. *B. Zsolnay* – Semmelweiss University, Maternity No 2 Ul. ut 78/a Budapest VIII/Hungary
Iceland:	Prof. *Petur H. J. Jakobsson* – President of the Icelandic Gynaecologic Society, The National Maternity Hospital, Post Box 1036 Reykjavik/Iceland
Italy:	Prof. *G. Massone* – Dept. Obstetr. Gynaec., Hospital Frosinone/Italy
Israel:	Prof. *A. M. Davies* – Hebrew University, Hadassah Medical School Jerusalem/Israel
Ivory Coast:	Dr. *J. Ritter* – Faculté de Médecine, B.P. 20.632 Abidjan/Ivory Coast
Japan:	Prof. *E. Nishida* – Dept. Obstetr. Gynaec., School of Medicine Kanazawa University 920 Kanazawa/Japan
Kenya:	Prof. *D. F. Horrobin* – University College Nairobi, Dept. of Medical Physiology, P.O. Box 30197 Nairobi/Kenya
Mexico:	Prof. *M. Lopez-Llera* – Hospital de Ginec-Obstetrica No 2 Mexico City/Mexico
Nigeria:	Dr. *S. B. Kuku,* M.B., M.R.C.O.G., Lagos University Teaching Hospital Private Mail Bag 12003 Lagos/Nigeria
Norway:	Dr. *Arne Strand* – Kvinneklinikken, Riks Hospitalet Oslo/Norway
Panama:	Prof. *R. Esquivel* – Ministerio de Salud, Chief Obstetric Service Hospital Santo Tomas, Apartado 957 Panama
Paraguay:	Dr. *Angel Morassi* – Hospital de Clinicas Sala III, Casilla Correo 1589 Asunción/Paraguay
Poland:	Doz. *A. Cretti* – 2nd Maternity Hospital, Ul. Warszawaky 15 Bialystok/Poland
Philippines:	Prof. *G. T. Aragon* – Dept. Obstetr. Gynaecol., Philippine General Hospital, College of Medicine U.P., 547 Herran Street, P.O. Box 593 Manila/Philippines
Rumania:	Prof. *N. Manescu* – III. Medizinische Klinik Timisoara/Rumania
Singapore:	Dr. *R. Sivasamboo* – Consultant Obstetrician and Gynaecologist Thomson Road General Hospital Singapore 11
South Africa:	Prof. *H. Geldenhuys* – Medical School, Dept. Obstetr. Gynaecol. Pretoria/South Africa
South Korea:	Dr. *Won Sup Oh,* M.D., D.G.O., D.C.P., Clinical Research Institute Catholic Medical Center, Myong Dong 2 KA 1 Seoul/South Korea

Spain:	P.D. Dr. *F. Bonilla-Musoles* – Cathedra di Obstetrica y Gynecologiy Universita Valencia/Spain
Sweden:	Dozent *H. Robbe* – Kvinnokliniken, Karolinska Sjukhuset 10401 Stockholm 60/Sweden
Switzerland:	Chairman: Prof. *H. Stamm* – Dept. Obstetr. Gynaecol. Hospital 5400 Baden/Switzerland
Switzerland:	Secretary: P.D. Dr. *E. T. Rippmann* – Maternity Hospital 5000 Aarau/Switzerland
Thailand:	P.D. Dr. *A. Uthaischand* – University Maternity Hospital Bangkok/Thailand
UdSSR:	Prof. *S. L. Persianinow* – Doz. H. Kirushenkow, Uliza Elanskow Moskwa/UdSSR
United Kingdom:	Prof. *G. W. Theobald* – 3 South Cliff Court, 11 South Cliff Eastbourne/Great Britain
United States:	Prof. *R. Vollman* – NIND/PRB, National Institutes of Health Bethesda, Maryland/USA
Uruguay:	Dr. *Luis F. Burjel* – Cerrito y Rincon Paysandu, Uruguay, South America
Zambia:	Prof. *Abu M. Hassim* – The University of Zambia, School of Medicine P.O. Box 2379 Lusaka/Zambia
AAMCH:	American Association for Maternal and Child Health Prof. *H. J. Fishbein* – 116 S Michigan Avenue Chicago, III. 60603/USA
BGG:	Büro für Geburtshilfe und Gynäkologie, Vereinigung deutsch sprechender Professoren und Privatdozenten für Geburtshilfe und Gynäkologie Prof. Dr. *Th. Koller* – Klingelbergstr. 3 4000 Basel/Switzerland
FIGO:	Fédération International des Gynécologies et Obstétriciens Prof. *H. de Watteville* – Dept. Obstetr. Gynaecol., University of Geneva 1200 Geneva/Switzerland
UPIGO:	Union Professionelle International des Obstétriciens et des Gynécologues Prof. *R. Wenner* – Dept. Obstetr. Gynaecol., Kantonsspital Liestal 4410 Liestal/Switzerland

Organisation Gestose

Es handelt sich um einen Zusammenschluß von Ärzten und Kliniken, die an der EPH-Gestose interessiert sind. Die O.G. (Organisation Gestose) hat sich folgende Aufgaben gestellt.

1. Bereinigung der Nomenklaturfrage, Internationalisierung einer einheitlichen Bezeichnung und Einteilung als Grundlage
   a) für Diagnose und Therapie
   b) für Vergleichsmöglichkeiten von Untersuchungsresultaten und Therapieerfolgen.

2. Standardisierung der Untersuchungsmethoden, so daß die *Art* der EPH-Gestose als einzige Variable übrig bleibt.

3. Errichtung einer Dokumentationszentrale mit
   a) Literatur über EPH-Gestose und Grenzgebiete
   b) Themenzentrum und Koordination von Arbeiten.

4. Konzentrierung von bestimmten Untersuchungsmethoden auf einzelne Kliniken, Forschergruppen oder Länder, je nach Interesse, Krankengut und Möglichkeiten.

5. Austausch von Forschern zwischen den einzelnen Untersuchungszentren, ev. auch Kliniken der Grenzgebiete einbeziehend.

6. Organisierung regelmäßiger Zusammenkünfte über das Thema EPH-Gestose. Forschungsresultate, Experimentelle Ergebnisse, Therapieerfolge, Nachkontrollen.

7. Therapiezentrale mit Ausarbeitung der neuesten und erfolgreichsten Vorschläge für Prophylaxe und Behandlung der EPH-Gestosen.

8. Anweisungen, Publikationen, Aufklärung, Fortbildungskurse, Kontakt zu den Massenkommunikationsmedien (Radio, Fernsehen, Presse).

Vorgeschlagene Bezeichnung: *EPH-Gestose*
EPH-Komplex

weil: E Ödeme
P Proteinurie
H Hypertonie

die 3 Kardinalsymptome und meistens die einzigen Symptome einer Gestose sind.

Definition:

E Ödeme:
Inadaequate Gewichtszunahme in der Schwangerschaft, meistens bedingt durch Wasseransammlung in den Geweben,
d. h. mehr als durchschnittlich 500 g/Woche
mehr als durchschnittlich 2000 g/Monat
mehr als durchschnittlich 13 kg/Schwangerschaft
Nachweisbare Beinödeme (prätibiale) sind dann ein Gestosesymptom, wenn sie nach Nachtruhe am Morgen nicht verschwunden sind (anamnestisch).
(Die übermäßige, alimentär bedingte Gewichtszunahme ist nicht abgetrennt, weil sie
1. schwierig zu erkennen ist,
2. weil Übergewicht an und für sich zur EPH-Gestose prädestiniert).

P Proteinurie:
Übersteigt die ausgeschiedene Eiweißmenge 0,5‰ Esbach im 24 h-Urin, so liegt eine Proteinurie vor.
(Die Methode nach Esbach wurde wegen ihrer Einfachheit beibehalten. Der Anteil der geformten Bestandteile des Sediments an der Proteinurie übersteigt nur selten die 0,5‰-Grenze bei fehlenden klinischen Zeichen eines Harnwegsinfektes).

H Hypertonie:
Letzter normaler Wert 135/85 mm/Hg,
erster pathologischer Wert 140/90 mm/Hg.
(Bei vorbestehender Hypertonie gilt ein BD-Anstieg von systolisch 30 mm/Hg und mehr und von diastolisch 15 mm/Hg und mehr als Hypertonie).

Einteilung:

I. Symptomatische Einteilung
Monosymptomatische EPH-Gestose
E = Ödeme
P = Proteinurie
H = Hypertonie
Polysymptomatische EPH-Gestose
Kombination von 2 oder allen 3 Symptomen
Imminente Eklampsie E I
Objektive und subjektive Symptome * vorhanden
Convulsive Eklampsie E C

II. Pathogenetische Einteilung
1. Propfgestose
a) vorbestehendes vaskuläres Leiden
b) vorbestehendes renales Leiden

2. Nicht aufgepropfte EPH-Gestose
   Transitorische EPH-Gestose
   Essentielle EPH-Gestose
3. Unklassifizierte Gestose

III. Konkomitierende Erkrankung
Vorbestehende Erkrankungen, die EPH-Symptome aufweisen, wobei sich die Symptome während der SS nicht verändern.
Konkomitierende Erkrankung + EPH-Gestose, chronische hypertensiv-vasculäre Erkrankung (ohne EPH-Gestose).

* Objektive und subjektive Symptome der Eclampsia Imminens EI (drohende Eklampsie):
objektive: Hyperreflexie
Motorische Unruhe
Bewußtseinsstörung
Plötzliche Verschlechterung (auch Cyanose)
subjektive: Kopfschmerzen
Sehstörungen
Akute Oberbauchsymptomatik

Gestose Index (G.I.):

Ähnlich wie beim Apgar-Score wird versucht, ein Beurteilungsschema in Form eines Punktesystems anzuwenden:
1. Es bezieht sich auf die 3 Cardinalsymptome E, P und H.

	0	1	2	3	Dat.	Dat.	Dat.	Dat.
Ödeme n. Bettruhe	keine	tibiale	generalisierte	–				
Proteinurie in ‰ n. Esbach	< 0,5	0,5– 2	2– 5	> 5				
Blutdruck systol.	< 140	140–160	160–180	> 180				
Blutdruck diastol.	< 90	90–100	100–110	> 110				
			Gestose Index					

Symptome der Eclampsie imminens EI ja ☐ nein ☐

Symptome der Eklampsie EC ja ☐ nein ☐

2. Die addierte Summe gibt den *momentanen* Zustand an. Der Zustand der Patientin kann deshalb nur durch fortlaufende und wiederholte Bestimmung des Gestose-Index beurteilt werden.
3. Da die imminente oder drohende Eklampsie E I und die Eklampsie E C dabei nicht zahlenmäßig erfaßt werden können, werden sie als Extragruppe aufgeführt. Die Zahl des Gestose-Index soll beigegeben werden.

Wir erbitten die Anwendung des G.I. auf Ihr Gestosematerial und Veröffentlichung Ihrer Resultate mit Orientierung der O.G.

Weitere Unterlagen und Informationen sind erhältlich durch

O.G.
Organisation Gestose

Sekretariat:
PD Dr. E. T. Rippmann
Frauenklinik
CH-5000 Aarau

Organisation Gestosis

This is an association of scientists and clinics, interested in the EPH-Gestosis. The O.G. (Organisation Gestosis) plans to work on the following subjects:

1st Internationalizing nomenclature and classification
 a) as basis for diagnosis and therapy
 b) to be able to compare results of investigations and therapy.

2nd Standardizing methods of investigation so that only the *type* of EPH-gestosis varies.

3rd Center of documentation, providing
 a) literature on the EPH-gestosis and special fields concerned
 b) pertinent subjects to be worked on and coordination of research program.

4th Concentrating special methods of research on different centers, according to interests, research teams, possibilities and material.

5th Exchange of scientists between the different centers, obstetrical services, laboratories as well as special clinics.

6th Organisation of regular meeting and congresses concerning the problem of the EPH-Gestosis to present results of clinical experimental research, of therapy and of long term follow-up.

7th Recommendation for the newest and most successful measures for prophylaxis and treatment of the EPH-gestosis.

8th Recommendations, publications, orientation and information, post graduate training and contact to the lay press, radio, television etc.

P.S.: Over the past several yeras the reprint most in demand in America has been on "Toxemias of Pregnancy" (new and better: *EPH-gestosis*).

Suggested Name: *EPH-gestosis*
EPH-Complex
EPH-Syndrome

because: E Edema
P Proteinuria
H Hypertension

are the 3 cardinal symptoms and usually the only symptoms of a gestosis.

Definition:

E Edema:
Excessive (inadequate) increase of body-weight during pregnancy, usually due to fluid retention.
i.e. more than 500 g/week
more than 2000 g/month } average
more than 13 kg/entire pregnancy
Demonstrable pretibial edema are of gestosis origine, if they are still present after a night's bedrest.

P Proteinuria:
Protein in the 24 h urine specimen, more than 0,5‰ Esbach (or similar quantitative test like paper sticks) is pathological.

H Hypertension:
Last normal reading 135/85 mm/Hg
first pathological reading 140/90 mm/Hg,
in primary hypotension rise of 30 mm/Hg or more systolic and/or rise of 15 mm/Hg or more diastolic.

Classification:

I. Symptomatic Classification: all cases
1. Monosymptomatic EPH-gestosis (EPH-Complex, EPH-Syndrome)
E = Edema
P = Proteinuria
H = Hypertension
2. Polysymptomatic EPH-gestosis (EPH-Complex, EPH-Syndrome)
Combination of 2 or all 3 symptoms.
3. Imminent (impending) eclampsia E I
Objective and subjective * symptoms.
4. Eclampsia E C
Convulsive eclampsia, seizures

II. Pathogenetic classification:
1. Superimposed gestosis
a) preexisting vascular disease
b) preexisting renal disease
2. Transient (essential) gestosis
no signs and symptoms after puerperium.
3. Unclassified gestosis

III. Concomitant disease:
1. Preexisting disease, presenting EPH-symptoms not changing during pregnancy.
2. Concomitant disease and EPH-gestosis, e.g. chronic hypertensive-vascular disease (without EPH-gestosis).
3. other cases

** Objective and subjective symptoms of imminent (impending) eclampsia E I:

Objective: Hyperreflexis
Motoric excitation
Impared consciousness
Sudden deterioration (also cyanosis)

Subjective: Headaches
Visual disturbances
Acute symptoms of the upper abdomen

Gestosis Index (G.I.):

Similar to the Apgar-Score, we have tried to classify the severity of the cases:
1. It concerns the 3 cardinal symptoms E, P and H.
2. The added sum indicates the *actual* condition of the patient. A prognosis can only be established if the figure of the G.I. is repeated frequently.
3. Since imminent (impending) eclampsia E I and eclampsia E C cannot be described in the type of scoring system, we have added these two extra groups with the letters E I and E C to the figure of the Gestosis Index.

	0	1	2	3	Date	Date	Date	Date
Edema after bedrest	none	tibiale	generalised	–				
Proteinuria in ‰ Esbach	< 0,5	0,5– 2	2– 5	> 5				
Bloodpressure systol.	< 140	140–160	160–180	> 180				
Bloodpressure diastol.	< 90	90–100	100–110	> 110				
			Gestosis Index					

Symptoms of imminent eclampsia EI yes ☐ no ☐
Symptoms of eclampsia EC yes ☐ no ☐

We suggest urgently to apply the Gestosis Index to your cases of EPH-gestosis. We ask for publication of your results and information of the Organisation Gestosis.

For further documentation and information please write to:

O.G.
Organisation Gestosis

Secretary:
PD Dr. E. T. Rippmann
Maternity Hospital
CH-5000 Aarau

Organisation Gestose

Il s'agit d'une association de chercheurs et cliniciens dont l'intérêt se porte sur la gestose-EPH. L'O.G. (Organisation Gestose) poursuit les buts suivants:

1e Internationalisation de nomenclature et classification
   a) comme base de diagnostic et de thérapeutique,
   b) en vue de comparer les résultats de recherches et de thérapie.

2e Standardisation des méthodes de recherche, de façon que seul varie le *type* de la gestose-EPH.

3e Centralisation de documentation, livrant
   a) la littérature sur la gestose-EPH et les domaines spéciaux annexes,
   b) les sujets adéquates de recherches, et la coordination des programmes d'investigation.

4e Concentration dans divers centres des méthodes spéciales de recherche, selon les inérêts, les groupes de chercheurs, les possibilités et le matériel.

5e Echange de chercheurs entre les différents centres, services obstétricaux, laboratoires, ainsi que cliniques spécialisées.

6e Organisation de meetings et de congrès, débattant des problèmes de la gestose-EPH, exposant les résultats des recherches cliniques expérimentales, des thérapeutiques et des observations à long terme.

7e Recommandation des plus récentes et efficaces mesures de prophylaxie et de traîtement de la gestose-EPH.

8e Recommandation, publication, orientation et information. Post-graduate training et contacts avec la presse laique, la radio, la télévision.

Terme proposé: Gestose-EPH
Complexe-EPH
Syndrome-EPH

car: E Edèmes
P Protéinurie
H Hypertension

sont les trois symptômes cadinaux et d'ordinaire les seuls symptômes d'une gestose.

Définitions:

E Edèmes:

Augmentation excessive (inadéquate) du poids pendant la grossesse, due d'ordinaire à une rétention de liquide,

p.ex. plus de 500 g/semaine
plus de 2000 g/mois } en moyenne
plus de 13 kg/en fin de grossesse

Les édèmes prétibiaux apparents sont d'origine gravidique quand ils sont encore présents après une nuit de repos.

P Protéinurie:

Plus de 0,5 g/‰ d'albumine à l'*Esbach* (ou déterminée d'après papiers colorimétriques ou autre méthode quantitative similaire) sont pathologiques.

H Hypertension:

Valeur-limite supérieure normale 135/85 mm/Hg,
première valeur pathologique 140/90 mm/Hg.
Dans les cas d'hypotension primaire augmentation systolique de 30 mm/Hg ou plus et/ou augmentation diastolique de 15 mm/Hg ou plus.

Classification:

I. Classification symptomatique: tous les cas
1. Gestose-EPH monosymptomatique (Complexe-EPH, Syndrome-EPH)
E = Edèmes
P = Protéinurie
H = Hypertension
2. Gestose-EPH polysymptomatique (Complexe-EPH, Syndrome-EPH)
Association de 2 ou des 3 symptômes.
3. Eclampsie imminente (menace d'eclampsie) E I
Symptômes objectifs et subjectifs *.
4. Eclampsie E C
éclampsie convulsive, attaques.

II. Classification pathogénétique:
1. Gestose superposée
a) maladie vasculaire préexistante
b) maladie rénale préexistante
2. Gestose transitoire (essentielle)
aucun signe ou somptôme après les couches
3. Gestose non-classifiée.

III. Maladies concomitantes:
1. Maladies préexistantes, présentant des symptômes EPH, ne changeant pas en cours de grossesse.

2. Maladie concomitante et gestose-EPH
   p.ex. maladie hypertensive-vasculaire chronique (sans gestose-EPH).
3. Autres cas.

* Symptômes objectifs et subjectifs de l'éclampsie imminente (menaçante) E I:

Objectifs: Hyperréflexie
excitation motrice
concience altérée
déterioration soudaine (cyanose aussi)

Subjectifs: Céphalées
troubles visuels
symptômes de l'abdomen aigu supérieur

Index-Gestose (G.I.):

Semblable au Score-Apgar: essai de graduation de la sévérité des cas.
1. Concerne les 3 symptômes cardinaux E, P et H.
2. La sommation des chiffres indique l'état *actuel* de la malade. Un pronostic ne peut être établi que si le chiffre de G.I. est répété fréquement.
3. Etant donné que l'éclampsie imminente E I et l'éclampsie E C ne peuvent être décrites par un tel système d'évaluation numérique, nous avons ajouté ces deux groupes spéciaux à l'aide des lettres E I et E C au schéma de l'Index-Gestose.

	0	1	2	3	Date	Date	Date	Date
Edèmes après repos	inexistant	prétibiaux	généralisés	–				
Protéinurie en ‰ Esbach	< 0,5	0,5– 2	2– 5	> 5				
Tension artérielle systolique	< 140	140–160	160–180	> 180				
Tension artérielle diastolique	< 90	90–100	100–110	> 110				
			Index-Gestose					

Symptomes d'éclampsie imminente EI oui ☐ non ☐
Symptomes d'éclampsie EC oui ☐ non ☐

Nous suggérons instamment d'appliquer l'index-Gestose à vos cas de gestose-EPH. Nous vous prions de publier vos résultats, en informant l'Organisation Gestose.

Documentation et information aditionnelle peut être obtenue par

O.G.
Organisation Gestose

Secrétariat:
PD Dr. E. T. Rippmann
Maternité
CH-5000 Aarau

Walter de Gruyter
Berlin · New York

E. T. Rippmann

EPH-Gestose

Oktav. XII, 238 S. 35 Strichzeichnungen u. 42 Autotypien. 1972.
Geb. DM 78,– ISBN 3 11 004009 3

Gitsch – Palmrich

Gynäkologisch-operative Anatomie

Einfache und erweiterte Hysterektomie

Ein Atlas

Anhang: Die Radioisotopen-Radikaloperation. Mit Geleitworten von H. Husslein u. I. Amreich. Bildteil: Hans Lang. Quart. VI, 162 S. Mit 200, z. T. mehrfarb. Abb. 1972. Geb. DM 160,–
ISBN 3 11 993480 8

H. W. Boschann

Gynäkologische Zytodiagnostik für Klinik und Praxis

2., völlig überarb. Aufl. der „Praktischen Zytologie". Groß-Oktav. Etwa 180 S. Mit 28 Abb., davon 18 farb., 110 Strichzeichn. 1972.
Geb. etwa DM 50,– ISBN 11 003981 8

Gerhard Martius

Geburtshilfe in Stichworten

Unter Mitarbeit von Ulrich Magnus
Klein-Oktav. 447 S. 1972. Kart. DM 14,80 ISBN 3 11 004270 3
(Sammlung Göschen Bd. 7003)

K. H. Mosler

Fetale Herzaktion und Tokographie

Ultrasonographie

Atlas für die Geburtshilfe

Unter Mitarbeit von Edgar Kitz
Quart. XII, 105 S. Mit 78 Abb. 1972. Kart. DM 56,–
ISBN 3 11 004225 8

FSC
www.fsc.org
MIX
Papier | Fördert
gute Waldnutzung
FSC® C083411

Kolibri 360 GmbH
Ferdinand-Jühlke-Straße 7
99095 Erfurt, Deutschland
produktsicherheit@kolibri360.de